ANTIPHOSPHOLIPID SYNDROME

Edited by **Alena Bulikova**

Antiphospholipid Syndrome
Edited by Alena Bulikova

Published by InTech

Janeza Trdine 9, 51000 Rijeka, Croatia

Publishing Process Manager Dragana Manestar

Technical Editor Teodora Smiljanic

Cover Designer InTech Design Team

Additional hard copies can be obtained from orders@intechopen.com

Antiphospholipid Syndrome, Edited by Alena Bulikova
p. cm.
ISBN 978-953-51-0526-8

For EU product safety concerns:
IN TECH d.o.o., Prolaz Marije Krucifikse Kozulić 3, 51000 Rijeka, Croatia,
info@intechopen.com or visit our website at intechopen.com.

Meet the editor

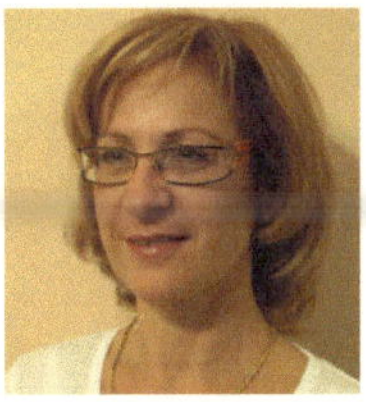

Dr Alena Buliková, M.D., Ph.D., is the Deputy Chief at Department of Clinical Haematology, University Hospital Brno, Czech Republic. She graduated in 1985 cum laude from Faculty of Medicine at Masaryk University Brno where she also obtained her M.D. degree. She trained at Internal Medicine and Teaching Clinic in Zlín, and at Medical Department Haemato-Oncology University Hospital Brno. She has been working with the Department of Clinical Haematology at the same hospital since 1990. She received a degree as Internist in 1990, the second degree in Haematology in 1994. She obtained her Ph.D. degree from Masaryk University in Brno in 2006 for her thesis on antiphospholipid antibodies. She is a co-author on thirteen books and the first author of 23 articles between, among other publications.

Contents

Preface

Immunity seems to be a fascinating system in the human body, whose role has never been understood in detail, despite the great progress in our knowledge about its role, regulation and its disorders. The same goes for autoimmunity diseases as well as antiphospholipid antibodies presence and antiphospholipid syndrome.

Due to humoral nature of these autoantibodies they can impact every tissue and due to their heterogeneity and complex actions they can be connected with wide spectrum of clinical manifestations. This leads to the fact that almost every medical doctor, regardless of his or her specialty, can come across a patient affected by some of these manifestations. This is why it is necessary to share the knowledge possessed by experts in this subject with the aim to help patients with antiphospholipid antibodies presence. Finally, this is why this book is presented to a wide range of readers. Forty seven contributors from nine countries bring together their knowledge and also their own experience from different fields of their professional work with the aim of providing a valuable resource for improving some of the points of view, decisions and treatment success in the antiphospholipid antibodies positive patients' management.

May the authors' hopeful expectations fulfil.
May the readers find the answers for their questions.
May the patients with antiphospholipid syndrome meet the doctor who has read this book that had changed his/her knowledge.

Best regards.

Alena Buliková, M.D., Ph.D.
University Hospital Brno
Czech Republic

Section 1

Introduction

Introductory Chapter

Antiphospholipid Syndrome: Changing Knowledge During the Time – The "Four P" Pattern

Alena Buliková
Department of Clinical Haematology, University Hospital Brno
Medical Faulty of Masaryk's University Brno
Czech Republic

1. Past

When searching the history of antiphospholipid antibodies one must meet cornerstone in Graham Hughes's descriptions of antiphospholipid syndrome in his "Prosser-White Oration" to the British Society of Dermatology in 1983 (Hughes GRV; 1984). The main points of his lecture can be found in different publications (Hughes GRV; 1984, Hughes GRV; 1999, Khamastha MA; 2000) and they are still truthful although they have been expressed almost thirty years ago. He finished his own work (Hughes GRV 1980; Hughes GRV; 1983) and crowned also another authors' important publication and observations. Some of these should be mentioned like the presence of false positive Wasserman reactions and also presence of circulating coagulants in patients with systemic lupus erythematosus (Laurel BB, Nilsson IM; 1957), the association of such circulating anticoagulants with thromboses (Bowie EJW et al 1983) and term "lupus anticoagulant" designation (Feinstein DI, Rapaport SI; 1972). The publication concerning association of these autoantibodies with foetal losses (Boey ML, et al; 1983) or the article which was directed to laboratory diagnostics (Harris EN, et al; 1983) arose almost at the same time as the Hughes's syndrome description.

The next important milestone emerged in 1990 when three independent working groups described the role of β_2-glycoprotein I as a target antigen in antiphospholipid antibodies' action (Galli M, et al; 1990, Matsura E, et al; 1990, McNeil HP, et al; 1990). This discovery substantially changed point of view of many of the researchers and also clinical practisers in the topic and it led to research of β_2-glycoprotein I structure, function and confirmation of significance of its antibodies presence during the next years.

As the important fact in our knowledge in antiphospholipid antibodies presence has to be stressed that laboratory investigation of lupus anticoagulants bodies has been under a control almost from the earliest time of their "standard" guidelines formulation (Exner T, et al; 1991, Barna LK, Triplett DA; 1991). The same situation is true in other antiphospholipid antibodies' detection and the experts have been searching continuously the solution to this problem until nowadays. Descriptions of the clinical manifestation of antiphospholipid antibodies' presence accompanied by antiphospholipid syndrome's definition were created in patients with systemic lupus erythematosus in the late eightieths and early ninetieths

(Alacrón-Segóvia D, et al; 1989a, Alacrón-Segóvia D, et al. 1992) and the definition and description of primary and also catastrophic antiphospholipid syndrome (Asherson RA, et al. 1989, Alacrón-Segóvia D, et al; 1989b) arose at the almost same time. This effort had led to so call Sapporo criteria of antiphospholipid syndrome which were generally accepted and widely used for many years (Wilson WA, et al; 1998).

2. Presence

Let's start "presence" twenty years after the antiphospholipid syndrome's description with two really important publications by Monica Galli (Galli M, et al; 2003a, Galli M, et al; 2003b) which summarised association of different type of antiphospholipid antibodies and their clinical significance in patients based on meta-analyses. The international consensus statement for definition of catastrophic antiphospolipid was published at the same year (Asherson RA, et al; 2003) and it was based on agreement by international workshop (during the international congress on antiphospholipid antibodies at Taormina, Italy 2002). The information from these articles has retained its importance until now.

The antiphopholipid syndrome's definition changed after discussion which started in international congress on antiphospholipid antibodies at Syndey 2004 (Miyakis S, at al. 2006). This consensus statement also determined non-criteria manifestations of antiphospholipid antibodies like thrombocytopenia, nephropathy and cardiac valve disease or livedo reticularis.

The important debate concerning serological criteria occurred at the pages of Journal of Thrombosis and Haemostasis in years 2007-2009 (Swadzba J, et al; 2007, Ruffatti A, et al; 2008, Galli M, et al; 2008, Pengo V; 2008, Tripodi A; 2008, Swadzba J et at; 2009, Ruffatti A, et al; 2009). The main finding from this debate seemed to be recommendation that the "cut off" in anticardiolipin antibodies' testing should be defined separately for thrombotic risk assessment and for pregnancy complication (Rufatti A, et al. 2008) and confirmation of the fact that the highest risk of clinical manifestation of antiphospholipid syndrome depends on the "triple positivity" of antiphospholipid antibodies, which means presence of lupus anticoagulant, significant positivity of anticardiolipin antibodies IgG and anti- β_2-glycoprotein I antibodies. Recommendation for lupus anticoagulant detection was also updated recently (Pengo V, et al; 2009, Tripodi A; 2009). The whole laboratory diagnostic process has been summarised in important publications (Gianacopulous B, et al; 2009, Pengo V, et al. 2010, Roubey RAS; 2010) including clinical meaning and critical analysis of different results.

An attempt to summarise briefly current knowledge in pathophysiology of antiphospholipid antibodies' action is a real "mission impossible". The same is true for the attempt to only list important researchers on the field. The compact overview bring Giannakopoulos (Giannakopoulos B, et al; 2007) or Meroni (Meroni PL; 2008). The role of prothrombotic and proinflammatory phenotype of endothelial cells, monocytes and platelets via direct action of antiphosholipid antibodies has been summarised by Pierangelli (Pierangelli SS, et al;2006). The connection between antiphospholipid antibodies, complement and foetal losses has been described for the first time by Holers (Holers VM, et al; 2002) and this research led to next association with tissue factor's role (Redecha P, et al; 2007). The most recent knowledge in pathophysiology of antiphospholipid antibodies was widely discussed at the 13th international congress on anthiphospholipid antibodies, which was held in April 2010 at Galveston, Texas, USA. The role of innate immunity was described by Rauch (Rauch J, et al; 2010). The role of tissue factor was summarised by Boles and Mackman (Boles J, Mackman N; 2010). The pathophysiology of β_2-glycoprotein I was discussed by Matsuura (Matsuura E, et al. 2010), the role of the receptor LRP8 by de Groot (de Groot PG, et al. 2010) and involvement of protein C pathway by Urbanus (Urbanus RT, de Last B; 2010). The annexin A5-mediated mechanism in pregnancy losses and thrombosis was clarified by Rand (Rand JH, et al. 2010). These are the most important but definitely not all publications concerning antiphospholipid antibodies pathophysiology at this congress.

3. Perspectives

The great progression of our knowledge in antiphospholipid antibodies, their action and clinical manifestation is attended by arising of new questions and problems to be solved. Some of these have been opened by Lockshin many years ago (Lockshin MD; 2000) and not all of them have been answered until now. Many different experts of various specialisations like investigators, animal models experts, laboratory diagnosis specialists, clinicians and epidemiologists assign a lot of important tasks. Some of them should be mentioned.

3.1 Other autoantibodies

Evidence is increasing that a lot of other autoantibodies could be found in patients with antiphospholipid syndrome and/or with another clinical manifestation of antiphospholipid antibodies (Shoenfeld Y, et al; 2008). What is their role and how they could be involved in antiphospholipd syndrome diagnose?

3.2 Other diagnostic tools

Some new diagnostic procedures, which seem to bring new information for antiphospholipid antibodies' positive patients, have been described recently. The first of all is evaluation of circulating antibodies against domain I of β_2-glycoprotein I (de Laat B, et al 2005, de Laat B, et al. 2009). The positive finding correlates with thrombotic and obstetric history in IgG type of these autoantibodies. Next example is ELISA detection of IgG phosphatidylserine-dependent antiprothrobmin antibodies which seem to be associated with antiphospholipid syndrome manifestation and also with lupus anticoagulant presence (Atsumi T, Koike T; 2010). The open question is also the meaning of finding of the presence of autoantibodies directed to phospholipid itself (Tebo AE, et al. 2008). These examples belong to the most important discoveries which should be verified in daily clinical practice.

3.3 Therapy of antiphospholipid syndrome and antiphospholipid antibodies presence

The standard approach of the management of the antiphospholipid syndrome's manifestation has been described and accepted widely (Derksen RHWM, de Groot PG; 2010, Cervera R, et al; 2010). Other thing is primary prophylaxis of thromboembolic event in patient with asymptomatic course. Some recommendation but also controversy information in this field exist (Erkan D, et al; 2007, Metjian A, Lim W; 2009), but these patients' management has been considered as the open question until now. The new approaches with new directions which need to prove their action are under investigation. Some of new antithrombotic drugs have proved their effectiveness in patient with thromboembolic disease when they were compared with vitamin K antagonists. The direct oral thrombin inhibitor dabigatran has a predictable anticoagulant effect and its safety profile is similar to that of warfarin (Schulman S, et al; 2009). Also rivaroxaban, an oral factor Xa inhibitor offers a simple, single-drug approach to the treatment of venous thrombosis that may improve the benefit-to-risk profile of anticoagulation (Bauersachs R, et al as the Einstein Investigators; 2010). These drugs are fixed-dose oral agents which do not appear to require routine laboratory monitoring and they may have a potential role in the management of patients in certain clinical manifestation of antiphospholipid syndrome. Among patients with acute venous thromboembolism approximately 10% have antiphospholipid antibodies and therefore it is likely that those patients were included in the study population in the dabigatran and rivaroxaban trials (Cohen H, Machin SJ; 2010). The potential advantages of these drugs in antiphospholipid antibodies positive patients have to be mentioned. The first of all is well known complicated laboratory monitoring in vitamin K dependent oral anticoagulant in the cases of lupus anticoagulants presence (Tripody A, et al; 2001). The second reasons which could favourite the new antithrombotic drugs is the fact that warfarin failures more frequently in secondary prevention in venous thromboembolisms in antiphospholipid antibodies than in other indications (Ames PRJ, et al; 2005, Wittkowsky AK, et al; 2006, Kearon C, et al; 2008).

Another approaches which could be involved in antiphospholipid antibodies positive persons management in future is potential immunomodulatory effect of some drugs. There are involved for example tissue factor up-regulation's inhibition, nuclear factor κB up-regulation's inhibition, p38 mitogen activated protein kinase up-regulation's inhibition, role of hydroxychloroquine, statins, anti-C5 monoclonal antibodies action or those against the lymphocytes bearing CD 20 receptor (rituximab) and other therapeutic modalities which role is supported only by animal models or only by episodic experiences in human (Pierangeli SS, Erkan D; 2010).

Vitamin D inhibits proinflamatory processes by suppressing the enhanced activity of immune cells that take part in autoimmune reactions. Shoenfeld Y, et al. intend to determine basal levels of vitamin D in patient with antiphospholipid syndrome and to identify those who require vitamin D supplementation, and to establish the therapeutic dose (Arnson Y, et al; 2007, Rotar Z, et al; 2009).

3.4 Other point of interest for the future

Future direction for antiphospholid syndrome research should concern some more opened questions. In aetiology of antiphospholipid antibodies the problems of infections, tumours, drugs and genetic predisposition could be involved. The meaning and managing of clinical manifestations associated with antiphopsholipid antibodies presence in which thromboembolic events are not suppose to be involved in clinical course also remains to be established (Shoenfeld Y, et al; 2008).

The next directions of the investigation at the field should be directed in paediatric patients. It includes newborns born to antiphospholipid antibodies positive mothers and their long-term clinical and immunological follow-up, paediatric antiphospholipid syndrome registry and clinical and laboratory differences between paediatric and adult patient with antipphospholipid syndrome (Rotar Z, et al; 2009, Avcin T, Silverman ED; 2007).

The really open field for next investigation seems to be mechanisms of antiphospholipid antibodies generation and action. The questions concerning why they occur or not, which pathways could be involved in their generation and next action, what are predisposing risk factors for their formation and clinical manifestation and many other still waiting for their solution.

4. Persons

It has been mentioned before and it will be mentioned once again later in this book that the problem of antiphospholipid antibodies and their effect really need interdisciplinary approaches. The leading persons in discovery of current knowledge of antiphospholipid antibodies and their action, clinical manifestation, detection and management are listed at the references of this chapter bellow, they belong to contributors of the next chapters of this book or they are mentioned in the references in these chapters. But, it should be stressed out, that persons themselves, theirs' contributions and publications, imagine and experiences and their willingness to share their knowledge are necessary requirements which could lead to important progress at the topic.

5. References

Alacrón-Segóvia D, Deléz M, Oria CV, et al. Antiphospholipid antibodies and the antiphospholipid syndrome in systemic lupus erythematosus. A perspective analysis of 500 consecutive patients. Medicine 1989a; 68: 353-365

Alacrón-Segóvia D, Sánches_Guerrero J. Primary antiphospholid syndrome. J Rheumatol 1989b; 16: 768-772

Alacrón-Segóvia D, Peréz-Vézquez ME, Villa AR, et al. Preliminary classification criteria for the antiphospholipid syndrome within systemic lupus erythematosus. Sem Arthr Rheumat 1992; 21: 275-285

Ames PRJ, Ciampa A, Margaglione M et al. Bleeding and re-thrombosis in primary antiphospholipid syndrome on oral anticoagulation. Thromb Haemost 2005; 93: 694-699.

Arnson Y, Amital H, Shoenfeld Y. Vitamin D and autoimmunity: new aetiological and therapeutic consideration. Ann Rheumat Dis 2007; 66: 1137-1142

Asherson RA, Khamashta M, Ordi-Ros J. The "primary" antiphospholipid syndrome. Major clinical and serological features. Medicine 1989; 68: 366-375

Asherson RA. The catastrophic antiphospholipid syndrome. J Rheumatol 1992; 19: 508-512

Asherson RA. Catastrophic antiphospholipid syndrome. International consensus statement on classification criteria and treatment guidelines. Lupus 2003; 12: 530-534

Atsumi T, Koike T. Antiprothrombin antibody: why do we need more assays. Lupus 2010; 19: 436-439

Avcin T, Silverman ED. Antiphospholipid antibodies in pediatric systemic lupus erythematosus and the antiphospholipid syndrome. Lupus 2007; 16: 627-633

Barna LK, Triplett DA. A report of the first international workshop for lupus anticoagulant identification. Clin Exp Rheumatol 1991; 9: 557-567

Bauersachs R, Berkowitz SD, Brenner B, et al as "The Einstein investigators". Oral rivaroxaban for symptomatic venous thromboembolism. N Engl J Med 2010; 363: 2499-2510

Boey ML, Colaco CB, Gharavi AL, et al. Thrombosis in SLE: striking association with the presence of circulation lupus anticoagulant. BMJ 1983; 287: 1023

Boles J, Mackman N. Role of tissue factor in thrombosis in antiphospholipid antibody syndrome. Lupus 2010; 19: 370-378

Bowie EJW, Thompson JH jr, Pascuzzi CA, Owen CA jr. Thrombosis in systemic lupus erythematosus despite circulation anticoagulants. J lab Clin Med 1963; 62: 416-430

Cervera R, on behalf of the "CAPS registry project group". Catastrophic antiphospholipid syndrome (CAPS): update from the "CAPS Registry". Lupus 2010; 19: 412-418

Derksen RHWM, de Groot PG. Towards evidence-based treatment of thrombotic antiphospholipid syndrome. Lupus 2010; 19: 470-474

Cohen H, Machin SJ. Antithrombotic treatment failures in antiphospholipid syndrome: the new anticoagulants? Lupus 2010; 19: 486-491

Erkan D, Harrison MJ, Levy R et al. Aspirin for primary thrombosis prevention in the antiphospholipid syndrome. Arthrit Rheumat 2007; 56: 2382-2391

Exner T, Triplett DA, Taberner D, Machin SJ. Guidelines for testing and revised criteria for lupus anticoagulants. SSC subcommittee for the standardization of lupus anticoagulants. Thromb and Haemost 1994; 65: 320-322

Feinstein DI, Rapapport SI. Acquired inhibitors of blood coagulation. Prog Hemost Thromb 1972; 1: 75-95

Galli M, Comfurius P, Maassen C, et al. Anticardiolipin antibodies (ACA) directed not to cardiolipin but to a plasma protein cofactor. Lancet 1990; 335: 1544-1547

Galli M, Luciani D, Bertolini G, Barbui T. Lupus anticoagulants are stronger risk factors for thrombosis than anticardiolipin antibodies in the antiphospholipid syndrome: a systematic review of the literature. Blood 2003a; 101: 1827-1832

Galli M, Luciani D, Bertolini G, Barbui T. Anti- β_2-glycoprotein I, antiprothrombin antibodies, and the risk of thrombosis in the antiphospholipid syndrome. Blood 2003; 102: 2717-2722

Galli M, Reber G, de Moerloose P, deGroot PG. Invitation to a debate on the serological criteria that define the antiphopsholipid syndrome. J Thromb Haemost 2008; 6: 399-401.

Giannakopoulos B, Passam F, Rahgozar S, Krilis SA. Current concepts on the pathogenesis of the antiphospholipd syndrome. Blood 2007, 109; 422-430

Giannakopoulos B, Passam F, Ioannou Y, Krilis SA. How we diagnose the antiphospholipid syndrome. Blood 2009; 113: 985-994

De Groot PG, Derksen RHWM, Urbanus RT. The role of LRP8 (ApoER2') in the pathophysiology of antiphospholipid syndrome. Lupus 2010; 19: 389-393

Harris EN, Gharave AE, Boey ML, et al. Anticardiolipin antibodies: detection by radioimmunoassay and association with thrombosis in SLE: Lancet 1983; 2: 1211-1214

Holers VM, Girardi G, Mo L, et al. C3 activation is required for anti-phospholipid antibody-induced fetal loss. J Ex Med 2002; 195: 211-220

Hughes GRV. Central nervous system lupus-diagnosis and treatment. J Rheumatol 1980; 7: 405-411

Hughes GRV. Thrombosis, abortion, cerebral disease, and the lupus anticoagulant. BMJ 1983; 287: 1088-1089

Hughes GRV. Connective tissue disease and the skin: the 1983 Prosser-White oration. Clin Exp Dermatol 1984; 9: 535-544

Hughes GRV. Hughes' syndrome: The antiphospholipid syndrome. A historical view. Lupus 1998, Suppl. 2: S1-S4

Kearon C, Julian JA, Kovacs MJ et al. Influence of thrombophilia on risk of recurrent venous thromboembolism while on warfarin: results from a randomized trial. Blood 2008; 112: 4432-4436

Khamastha MA. Hughes Syndrome: History. In Khamastha MA (Ed): Hughes Syndrome: Antiphospholipid syndrome. Springer-Verlag London Berlin Heidelberg 2000; 3-7

Lockshin MD. Prognosis and future directions. In HKhamashta MA (Ed). Hughes syndrome. Antiphospholipid syndrome. Springer-Verlag London 2000: 459-462

de Laat B, Derksen RHWM, Urbanus RT, de Groot PG. IgG antibodies that recognize epitope Gly40-Arg43 in domain I of β_2-glycoprotein I cause LAC and their presence correlates strongly with thrombosis. Blood 2005; 105: 1540-1545.

de Laat B, Pengo V, Pabinger I, et al. The association between circulating antibodies against domain I of beta2-glycoprotein I and thrombosis.an international multicenter study. J Thromb Haemost 2009; 7: 1767-1773

Laurel BB, Nilsson IM. Hypergamaglobulinaemia, circulating anticoagulant and biologic false positive Wassermann reactions. J Lab Clin Med 1957; 49: 694-707

Matsuura E, Igarashi Y, Fujimoto M, at al. Anticardiolipin cofactor(s) and differential diagnosis of autoimmune disease. Lancet 1990; 336: 177-178

Matsuura E, Shen L, Matsunami Y, et al. Pathophysiology of β_2-glycoprotein I in antiphospholipid syndrome. Lupus 2010; 379-384

McNeil HP, Simpson RJ, Chesterman CN, Krilis SA. Anti-phospholipid antibodies are directed a complex antigen that includes a lipid-binding inhibitor of coagulation. Proc Natl Acad Sci 1990; 87: 4120-4124

Meroni PL. Pathogenesis of the antiphospholipid syndrome. An additional example of the mosaic of autoimmunity. J Autoimmunity 2008; 30: 99-103

Miyakis S, Lockshin MD, Atsumi T, et al. International consensus statement on update of an update of the classification criteria for definite antiphospholipid syndrome (APS). J Thromb Haemost 2006; 4: 295-306

Pengo V. A contribution to the debate on the laboratory criteria that define the antiphospholipid syndrome. J Thromb Haemost 2008; 6: 1048-1049

Pengo V, Tripodi A, Reber G, et al. Update of the guidelines for lupus anticoagulant detection. J Thromb Haemost 2009; 7: 1737-1740

Pengo V, Banzato A, Bison E, et al. Antiphosholipid syndrome: critical analysis of the diagnostic path. Lupus 2010; 19: 428-431

Pierangeli SS, Chen PP, Gonzalez EB. Antiphospholipid antibodies and the antiphospholipid syndrome: an update on treatment and pathogenic mechanisms. Curr Opin in Hematology 2006; 13: 366-375

Pierangeli SS, Erkan D. Antiphospholipid syndrome treatment beyond anticoagulation: are we there yet. Lupus 2010; 19: 475-485

Rand JH, Wu X-X, Quinn AS, Taatjes DJ. The annexin A5-mediated pathogenetic mechanism in antiphospholipid syndrome: role in pregnancy losses and thrombosis. Lupus 2010; 19: 460-469

Rauch J, Dieudé M, Subang R, Levine JS. The dual role of innate immunity in the antiphospholipid syndrome. Lupus 2010; 19: 347-353

Redecha P, Tilley R, Tencati M, et al. Tissue factor: a link between C5a and neutrophil activation in antiphospholipid antibodiy induced fetal injury. Blood 2007; 110: 2423-2431

Roubey RAS: Risky business: the interpretation, use, and abuse of antiphospholipid antibodies tests in clinical practice. Lupus 2010; 19: 440-445

Rotar Z, Rozman B, de Groot PG, et al. Sixth meeting of the European Forum on antiphospholipid antibosies. How to improve the understanding of the antiphospholipid syndrome. Lupus 2009; 18: 53-60

Ruffatti A, Olivieri S, Tonello M, et al. Influence of different IgG anticardiolipin antibody cut-off values on antiphospholipid syndrome classification. J Thromb Haemost 2008; 6: 1693-1696.

Ruffatti A, Pengo V. Antipospholipid syndrome classification criteria: comments to the Letter of Jakub Swadzba and Jacek Musial. J Thromb Haemost; 7: 503-504

Schulman S, Kearon C, Kakkar AK, et al. Dabigatran versus warfarin in the treatment of acute venous thromboembolism. N Engl J Med 2009; 361: 2342-2352

Shoendfeld Y, Twig G, Katz U, Sherer Y. Autoantibody explosion in antiphospholipid syndrome. J Autoimmunity 2008a; 30: 74-83

Shoenfeld Y, Meroni PL, Cervera R. Antiphospholipid syndrome dilemmas still to be solved: 2008 status. Ann Rheumat Dis 2008b; 67: 438-442

Swadzba J, Iwaniec T, Szczeklik A, Musial J. Revised classification criteria for antiphospholipid syndrome and the thrombotic risk in patients with autoimmune disease. J Thromb Haemost 2007; 5: 1883-1889.

Swadzba J, Musial J. Letters to the Editor. More on: The debate on antiphospholipid syndrome classification criteria. J Thromb Haemost 2009; 7: 501-502.

Tebo AE, Jaskowski TD, Phansalkar AR, et al. Diagnostic performance of phospholipid-specific assays for the evaluation of antiphospholipid syndrome. Am J Clin Pathol 2008; 129: 870-875.

Tripodi A, Chantaraggkul V, Clerici M, et al. Laboratory control of oral anticoagulant treatment by INR system in patient with antiphospholipid syndrome and lupus anticoagulant. Result of a collaborative study involving nine commercials thromboplastins. Br J Haematol 2001; 115: 672-678

Tripodi A. More on: criteria to define the antiphospholipid syndrome. J Thromb Haemost 2008; 6: 1049-1050.

Tripodi A. Testing for lupus anticoagulants: all that a clinician should know. Lupus 2009; 18: 291-298

Urbanus RT, de Laat B. Antiphospholipid antibodies and the protein C pathway. Lupus 2010; 394-399

Wilson WA, Gharavi AE, Koike T, et al. International consensus statement on preliminary classification for definite antiphospholipid syndrome. Arthritis Rheumatol 1999; 42: 1309-1311

Wittkowsky AK, Downing J, Blackburn J, Nutescu E. Warfarin-related outcomes in patients with antiphospholipid antibody syndrome managed in an anticoagulation clinic. Thromb Haemost 2006; 96: 137-141

Section 2

Pathophysiologic Mechanisms Involved in Antiphospholipid Antibodies Action

1

β_2-Glycoprotein I – A Protein in Search of Function

Anthony Prakasam and Perumal Thiagarajan
Department of Pathology, Michael E. DeBakey Veterans Affairs Medical Center, Houston, Texas
Departments of Pathology and Medicine, Baylor College of Medicine, Houston, Texas
USA

1. Introduction

β2-glycoprotein I is a lipid-binding 50-kDa glycoprotein that circulates in plasma at a concentration of approximately 4 μM (200 μg/ml). The amino acid sequence of human β2-glycoprotein I was completely determined (1), the cDNAs have been isolated (2, 3) and the crystal structure has been solved (4). β2-glycoprotein I is a member of the so-called "complement control protein" (CCP) superfamily, whose members are identified by the presence of one or more of a motif containing a characteristic disulfide bond pattern (5). These motifs are called CCP or sushi domains. CCP repeats are units of approximately 60 amino acids with a relatively invariant arrangement of 2 disulfide bonds and a number of other highly conserved residues. Other members of the CCP superfamily include at least 12 complement proteins, the B subunit of blood clotting factor XIII, haptoglobin, the interleukin 2 receptor and selectins. β2-glycoprotein I is made up entirely of five CCP repeats. CCP5 diverges from the norm for CCPs, including CCPs 1-4 in that it has a relatively unique pattern of 3 disulfide bridges (6), and contains a positively-charged sequence, CKNKEKKC (residues 281-288), that mediates its binding site for anionic phospholipid (7). The crystal structure of β2-glycoprotein I showed the four CCP domains 1-4 are arranged like a beads on a sting and CCP5 folds back giving fishhook-like conformation. The CCP5 contains a central spiral structure with positively charged motif CKNKEKKC close to a hydrophobic patch (LAFW). B2-glycoprotein I anchors to the anionic phospholipid membrane surface via CCP5 with its hydrophobic loop adjacent to the positively charged lysine rich region in CCP5. Subsequently, β2-glycoprotein I penetrates the membrane interfacial headgroup region. This binding restricts the mobility of the lipid side chains and aggregates the vesicles without inducing fusion (8-10). In addition to anionic phospholipids, β2-glycoprotein I binds to sulfatide (11), heparin (12), complement C3 (13), annexin A2 (14), platelet glycoprotein Ib (15), megalin (16), apolipoprotein receptor 2' (17) von Willebrand factor (18, 19) and possibly many others ligands. The solution structure of β2-glycoprotein I was studied by small angle X-ray scattering (20), the experimentally derived curves fitted poorly to the simulated scattering curves calculated from the crystallographic coordinates of human b2GPI, suggesting different conformation in solution. Recent studies with negative staining electron microscopic studies showed β2-glycoprotein I can exist in two different conformations - a circular conformation due to the interaction of CCP1 with CCP5 and an open elongated conformation consistent with the fishhook-like structure seen in the crystallographic studies (21). In closed conformation β2-glycoprotein I bind less well to anionic phospholipids or to complement C3 (13). Binding to anionic phospholipids, and possibly other ligands stabilizes the elongated conformation (22). Circulating plasma β2-glycoprotein I contains free thiols and these moieties are proposed to interaction with platelets and endothelium, protecting these cells from oxidative stress (18). Oxidized form β2-glycoprotein I is increased in patients with thrombosis (23). Oxidized β2-glycoprotein I induces human dentritic cell maturation and promotes a T helper type I response (24). These studies imply the antibody response to β2-glycoprotein I are due post translational modifications due to oxidative stress.

β2-glycoprotein I was designated as apolipoprotein H initially as it could be isolated from very low density lipoprotein fractions and had high affinity for triglyceride-rich particles (25). However, recent studies do not suggest an interaction between β2-glycoprotein I with either high or low density lipoproteins (26).

Despite the extensive physicochemical characterization, the physiological role of β2-glycoprotein I remains uncertain. Based on several *in vitro* studies, a wide range of functions have been attributed such as regulation of coagulation (27), modulation of complement activity and clearance of apoptotic cells from the circulation (28). In this review, we will summarize newer data on the possible physiological role of β2-glycoprotein I.

2. Modulation of hemostasis

Since β2-glycoprotein I is the target of the majority of antiphospholipid antibodies associated with thrombosis, an anticoagulant function for β2-glycoprotein I was anticipated. Anionic phospholipid surfaces play an essential role in normal hemostasis by providing a site for the assembly of enzyme-cofactor complexes involved in virtually every step of the enzymatic cascade that results in the generation of fibrin, which polymerizes to form an insoluble fibrin clot. In normal cells, anionic phospholipids such as phosphatidylserine are present only in the inner leaflet of the membrane bilayer. Platelets externalize anionic phospholipid when stimulated by agonists. Binding of β2-glycoprotein I to anionic phospholipid vesicles (29) and platelets (30, 31) is accompanied by inhibition of phospholipid-dependent coagulation tests (27, 32), suggesting a likely physiological role of β2-glycoprotein I in the regulation of coagulation, particularly on activated platelets and possibly on other cell surfaces. In addition, β2-glycoprotein I inhibits the contact activation of the intrinsic coagulation pathway (15, 33). β2-glycoprotein I binds to factor XI with an affinity equivalent to that of high molecular weight kininogen. The binding inhibits the activation to factor XI by thrombin and FXIIa. This was suggested to be a mechanism, by which β2-glycoprotein I may modulate thrombin generation. β2-glycoprotein I also binds to heparin - a fact used in its isolation (12, 29). Heparin binding site had been localized to the positively charged CCP5 (12). Heparin also promotes plasmin cleavage of β2-glycoprotein I at Lys317-Thr318 bond (34). Plasmin-cleaved β2-glycoprotein I has markedly decreased affinity for anionic phospholipid. This form of cleaved β2-glycoprotein I is seen in patients treated with streptokinase and in patients with disseminated intravascular coagulation (35), showing this cleavage reaction can occur in vivo during accelerated fibrinolysis.

Several procoagulant effect of β2-glycoprotein I have also been described. β2-glycoprotein I binds to thrombin and protects it from inactivation by heparin cofactor II/heparin complex (36). Furthermore, Mori et al (37) showed β2-glycoprotein inhibited activated protein C inactivation of factor Va - an effect diminished by the addition of phospholipids. At similar concentration, β2-glycoprotein I inhibited weakly factor Va- and phospholipid-dependent prothrombinase activity. The depletion of beta β2-glycoprotein I from plasma led to only a slight shortening of the diluted Russell's viper venom-dependent clotting time, but to a strong and significant potentiation of the anticoagulant activity of APC. These results suggest that under certain physiological conditions β2-glycoprotein I may have procoagulant function.

In contrast to these hemostatic activities demonstrated in vivo, neither the β2-glycoprotein I-deficient mice (generated by homologous recombination) nor β2-glycoprotein I-deficient individuals exhibit any bleeding manifestations (38-40). On the contrary, β2-glycoprotein I-deficient mice have diminished rate of thrombin generation compared with normal or even with heterozygous mice. No significant differences in clotting time were observed in plasma from these three genotypes when measured by dRVVT, dKCT, aPTT, and protein C pathway assays (41). Hereditary deficiency of β2-glycoprotein I was reported since 1968 (42), and its potential association with risk of thrombosis had been examined. Bansci *et al.* (43) have described two brothers with total deficiency of β2-glycoprotein I, one of whom had experienced recurrent unexplained thrombosis by age 36. However, six other heterozygous individuals (ages 9-73) from this family and the proband's brother with homozygous deficiency were free of thrombosis. Takeuchi et al (39) described two asymptomatic individuals with complete deficiency of β2-glycoprotein I. The routine coagulation assays were normal. A slight shortening of the DRVVT was observed in these individuals, which interestingly were not corrected by exogenous addition of β2-glycoprotein I.

Thrombosis is a complex multigene phenotype (44). Because of the large number of genes that influence this phenotype teasing out the role of β2-glycoprotein I in in this prothrombotic phenotype will be difficult. It is also possible that the thrombosis seen with antiphospholipid antibodies is not related to any of interaction identified above.

3. β2-glycoprotein I as an opsonin

The term opsonins is used to refer molecules that target a cell for phagocytosis. A number of observations suggest β2-glycoprotein I can be an opsonin for clearance of anionic phospholipid vesicles containing surfaces from the circulation. In normal cells, anionic phospholipids such as phosphatidylserine are present only in the inner leaflet of membrane bilayer. There is transbilayer movement of phosphatidylserine during apoptosis and phosphatidylserine exposed can be a tag for their clearance by macrophages (45-47). In artificial membranes, the phosphatidylserine content has to be at least 5-10% before a significant binding of β2-glycoprotein I could be observed (48). Nevertheless, the binding of β2-glycoprotein I to phosphatidylserine containing surfaces such as apoptotic cells and platelet microvesicles have been shown (49, 50). In addition to the anionic phospholipids, β2-glycoprotein I is also shown to bind the Ro/SSA, a 60 kDa a nuclear antigen and target of autoantibodies in primary Sjogren syndrome (19). Ro/SSA translocates to cell surface during apoptosis and can serve as additional binding site. The complex of anionic phospholipid and ß2-glycoprotein I are taken into a receptor-mediated pathway by macrophages and possibly endothelial cells also. The phagocytic receptors mediating the uptake have been shown to be toll-like receptor 4 in macrophages (51) and lipoprotein receptor related family members (49). In endothelial cells toll-like receptor 2 and 4 (52, 53), annexin A2 (14), and apolipoprotein E receptor 2 (54) have been implicated. Deficiencies of factors, implicated in the removal of apoptotic cells such as lactadherin and Gas6 receptors, are associated with systemic lupus erythematosus and autoimmunity (55). However, no immunological dysfunction is reported in β2-glycoprotein I deficiency.

β2-glycoprotein I may also have a role in the clearance of exogenous liposomes. Liposomes have been used extensively as vehicles for drug delivery and following in vivo infusions, liposomes are preferentially taken up by the mononuclear phagocytic cells of the reticuloendothelial system (56). In 1982, Wurm et al (57) showed that infusion of ß2-glycoprotein I in rats results in an accelerated clearance of triglyceride-rich vesicles from the circulation. The clearance of liposomes by the phagocytic cells, is markedly affected lipid composition of the liposomes and anionic phospholipid containing are cleared very rapidly from blood (56). By analyzing the proteins that associate with the liposomes in blood, Chonn et al. have identified β2-glycoprotein I as a major protein associated with rapidly cleared liposomes and noted that pretreating the mice with anti-β2-glycoprotein I antibodies markedly increased the circulating half-life of the liposomes (58). It is interesting to note that in 1982, Wurm et al (57) showed that infusion of ß2-glycoprotein I in rats results in an accelerated clearance of triglyceride-rich vesicles from the circulation.

The complement system is involved in the clearance of dead cells and debris from the circulation and recently a role for β2-glycoprotein I its regulation has been identified (13). The elongated and open conformation of β2-glycoprotein I binds to C3 and induces a conformational changes so that the regulator factor H binds. As factor H promotes factor I-induced the cleavage of C3, β2-glycoprotein I acts as special cofactor for factor H and factor I. The enhanced the degradation of C3 limits further complement amplification. Deficiencies of complement factor H and I are associated atypical hemolytic uremic syndrome and no such association has been described for β2-glycoprotein I.

4. A role in gestation

Because of the association with fetal loss and anti-β2-glycoprotein I antibodies, a role in gestation has been proposed. Infusion of cyanine labeled β2-glycoprotein I in mice show preferential localization on the endothelium of uterine vessels and at the implantation sites in pregnant mice (59), suggesting a role in early gestation. However, the β2-glycoprotein I null mice were fertile and carried viable fetuses to term and there were no thrombosis in placental vessels (60). Nevertheless, there was an 18% reduction in the number of viable implantation sites and reduced fetal weight and fetal:placental weight ratio in late gestation in β2-glycoprotein I null mice.

5. β2-glycoprotein I and angiogenesis

β2-glycoprotein I is enzymatically cleaved by plasmin at the peptide bond between Lys317-Thr318 to form a cleaved form β2-glycoprotein I (61, 62). This form is seen in the circulation in patients with increased fibrinolysis. The cleaved form of β2-glycoprotein I binds to plasminogen and inhibits plasmin generation. In addition to modulating fibrinolysis, a role in angiogenesis had been proposed for the cleaved form of β2-glycoprotein I. The cleaved form of β2-glycoprotein I inhibits endothelial cell proliferation in vitro, inhibits neovascularization into subcutaneously implanted angiogenic matrices and the growth of orthotopic prostate cancer in C57BL/6 mice (63, 64). The cleaved β2-glycoprotein I strongly reduced HUVEC growth and proliferation as evidenced by the MTT and BrdU assay and delayed cell cycle progression arresting endothelial cells in the S-and G2/M-phase (65). However, the cleaved form of β2-glycoprotein I can also be promote angiogenes is as it binds angiostatin 4.5 (plasminogen kringle 1-5) and attenuates its antiangiogenic property (66). The murine β in vivo apparently displayed only mild anti-angiogenic properties. β2-glycoprotein I deficient mice developed larger tumors with more vessels than β2-glycoprotein I replete mice but no survival benefit is conferred to tumor bearing animals regardless of β2GPI status raising questions about the its pathophysiological role in tumorigenesis(66).

6. Conclusion

Since its discovery in the sixties and following the recognition that it is the antigenic target for antiphospholipid antibodies in nineties, several structural and functional studies have been described. However, there is no convincing pathogenetic mechanism or theoretical framework for the hypercoagulable state associated with antibodies to this protein. Many hypotheses have been proposed based on in vitro findings and most of them revolve on the anionic phospholipid binding properties of β2-glycoprotein I. At least two patients are described with antiphospholipid syndrome who had mutations in β2-glycoprotein I rendering it in capable of binding phospholipids (67, 68), questioning its phospholipid binding in pathogenesis. These findings underscore the importance finding its physiological function to elucidate the mechanism of thrombosis seen with antibody to this molecule.

7. Acknowledgment

Supported by a Merit Review Grant from the Veterans Affairs Research Service.

8. References

[1] Lozier, J., Takahashi, N., and Putnam, F.W. 1984. Complete amino acid sequence of human plasma beta 2-glycoprotein I. *Proc Natl Acad Sci U S A* 81:3640-3644.

[2] Steinkasserer, A., Estaller, C., Weiss, E.H., Sim, R.B., and Day, A.J. 1991. Complete nucleotide and deduced amino acid sequence of human beta 2-glycoprotein I. *Biochem J* 277 (Pt 2):387-391.

[3] Day, J.R., O'Hara, P.J., Grant, F.J., Lofton-Day, C., Berkaw, M.N., Werner, P., and Arnaud, P. 1992. Molecular cloning and sequence analysis of the cDNA encoding human apolipoprotein H (beta 2-glycoprotein I). *Int J Clin Lab Res* 21:256-263.

[4] Schwarzenbacher, R., Zeth, K., Diederichs, K., Gries, A., Kostner, G.M., Laggner, P., and Prassl, R. 1999. Crystal structure of human beta2-glycoprotein I: implications for phospholipid binding and the antiphospholipid syndrome. *EMBO J* 18:6228-6239.

[5] Reid, K.B., and Day, A.J. 1989. Structure-function relationships of the complement components. *Immunol Today* 10:177-180.

[6] Kato, H., and Enjyoji, K. 1991. Amino acid sequence and location of the disulfide bonds in bovine beta 2 glycoprotein I: the presence of five Sushi domains. *Biochemistry* 30:11687-11694.

[7] Hunt, J., and Krilis, S. 1994. The fifth domain of beta 2-glycoprotein I contains a phospholipid binding site (Cys281-Cys288) and a region recognized by anticardiolipin antibodies. *J Immunol* 152:653-659.

[8] Willems, G.M., Janssen, M.P., Pelsers, M.M., Comfurius, P., Galli, M., Zwaal, R.F., and Bevers, E.M. 1996. Role of divalency in the high-affinity binding of anticardiolipin antibody-beta 2-glycoprotein I complexes to lipid membranes. *Biochemistry* 35:13833-13842.

[9] Hammel, M., Schwarzenbacher, R., Gries, A., Kostner, G.M., Laggner, P., and Prassl, R. 2001. Mechanism of the interaction of beta(2)-glycoprotein I with negatively charged phospholipid membranes. *Biochemistry* 40:14173-14181.

[10] Gushiken, F.C., Le, A., Arnett, F.C., and Thiagarajan, P. 2002. Polymorphisms beta2-glycoprotein I: phospholipid binding and multimeric structure. *Thromb Res* 108:175-180.

[11] Merten, M., Motamedy, S., Ramamurthy, S., Arnett, F.C., and Thiagarajan, P. 2003. Sulfatides: targets for anti-phospholipid antibodies. *Circulation* 108:2082-2087.

[12] Guerin, J., Sheng, Y., Reddel, S., Iverson, G.M., Chapman, M.G., and Krilis, S.A. 2002. Heparin inhibits the binding of beta 2-glycoprotein I to phospholipids and promotes the plasmin-mediated inactivation of this blood protein. Elucidation of the consequences of the two biological events in patients with the anti-phospholipid syndrome. *J Biol Chem* 277:2644-2649.

[13] Gropp, K., Weber, N., Reuter, M., Micklisch, S., Kopka, I., Hallstrom, T., and Skerka, C. {beta}2 glycoprotein 1 ({beta}2GPI), the major target in anti phospholipid syndrome (APS), is a special human complement regulator. *Blood.*

[14] Ma, K., Simantov, R., Zhang, J.C., Silverstein, R., Hajjar, K.A., and McCrae, K.R. 2000. High affinity binding of beta 2-glycoprotein I to human endothelial cells is mediated by annexin II. *J Biol Chem* 275:15541-15548.

[15] Shi, T., Iverson, G.M., Qi, J.C., Cockerill, K.A., Linnik, M.D., Konecny, P., and Krilis, S.A. 2004. Beta 2-Glycoprotein I binds factor XI and inhibits its activation by thrombin and factor XIIa: loss of inhibition by clipped beta 2-glycoprotein I. *Proc Natl Acad Sci U S A* 101:3939-3944.

[16] Moestrup, S.K., Schousboe, I., Jacobsen, C., Leheste, J.R., Christensen, E.I., and Willnow, T.E. 1998. beta2-glycoprotein-I (apolipoprotein H) and beta2-glycoprotein-I-phospholipid complex harbor a recognition site for the endocytic receptor megalin. *J Clin Invest* 102:902-909.

[17] van Lummel, M., Pennings, M.T., Derksen, R.H., Urbanus, R.T., Lutters, B.C., Kaldenhoven, N., and de Groot, P.G. 2005. The binding site in {beta}2-glycoprotein I for ApoER2' on platelets is located in domain V. *J Biol Chem* 280:36729-36736.

[18] Passam, F.H., Rahgozar, S., Qi, M., Raftery, M.J., Wong, J.W., Tanaka, K., Ioannou, Y., Zhang, J.Y., Gemmell, R., Qi, J.C., et al. Redox control of beta2-glycoprotein I-von Willebrand factor interaction by thioredoxin-1. *J Thromb Haemost* 8:1754-1762.

[19] Reed, J.H., Giannakopoulos, B., Jackson, M.W., Krilis, S.A., and Gordon, T.P. 2009. Ro 60 functions as a receptor for beta(2)-glycoprotein I on apoptotic cells. *Arthritis Rheum* 60:860-869.

[20] Hammel, M., Kriechbaum, M., Gries, A., Kostner, G.M., Laggner, P., and Prassl, R. 2002. Solution structure of human and bovine beta(2)-glycoprotein I revealed by small-angle X-ray scattering. *J Mol Biol* 321:85-97.

[21] Agar, C., van Os, G.M., Morgelin, M., Sprenger, R.R., Marquart, J.A., Urbanus, R.T., Derksen, R.H., Meijers, J.C., and de Groot, P.G. Beta2-glycoprotein I can exist in 2 conformations: implications for our understanding of the antiphospholipid syndrome. *Blood* 116:1336-1343.

[22] Pengo, V., Biasiolo, A., and Fior, M.G. 1995. Autoimmune antiphospholipid antibodies are directed against a cryptic epitope expressed when beta 2-glycoprotein I is bound to a suitable surface. *Thromb Haemost* 73:29-34.

[23] Ioannou, Y., Zhang, J.Y., Qi, M., Gao, L., Qi, J.C., Yu, D.M., Lau, H., Sturgess, A.D., Vlachoyiannopoulos, P.G., Moutsopoulos, H.M., et al. Novel assays of thrombogenic pathogenicity for the antiphospholipid syndrome based on the detection of molecular oxidative modification of the major autoantigen ss2-glycoprotein I. *Arthritis Rheum.*

[24] Buttari, B., Profumo, E., Mattei, V., Siracusano, A., Ortona, E., Margutti, P., Salvati, B., Sorice, M., and Rigano, R. 2005. Oxidized beta2-glycoprotein I induces human dendritic cell maturation and promotes a T helper type 1 response. *Blood* 106:3880-3887.

[25] Lee, N.S., Brewer, H.B., Jr., and Osborne, J.C., Jr. 1983. beta 2-Glycoprotein I. Molecular properties of an unusual apolipoprotein, apolipoprotein H. *J Biol Chem* 258:4765-4770.

[26] Agar, C., de Groot, P.G., Levels, J.H., Marquart, J.A., and Meijers, J.C. 2009. Beta2-glycoprotein I is incorrectly named apolipoprotein H. *J Thromb Haemost* 7:235-236.

[27] Nimpf, J., Bevers, E.M., Bomans, P.H., Till, U., Wurm, H., Kostner, G.M., and Zwaal, R.F. 1986. Prothrombinase activity of human platelets is inhibited by beta 2-glycoprotein-I. *Biochim Biophys Acta* 884:142-149.

[28] Balasubramanian, K., Chandra, J., and Schroit, A.J. 1997. Immune clearance of phosphatidylserine-expressing cells by phagocytes. The role of beta2-glycoprotein I in macrophage recognition. *J Biol Chem* 272:31113-31117.

[29] Wurm, H. 1984. beta 2-Glycoprotein-I (apolipoprotein H) interactions with phospholipid vesicles. *Int J Biochem* 16:511-515.

[30] Schousboe, I. 1980. Binding of beta 2-glycoprotein I to platelets: effect of adenylate cyclase activity. *Thromb Res* 19:225-237.

[31] Nimpf, J., Wurm, H., and Kostner, G.M. 1985. Interaction of beta 2-glycoprotein-I with human blood platelets: influence upon the ADP-induced aggregation. *Thromb Haemost* 54:397-401.

[32] Bevers, E.M., Janssen, M.P., Comfurius, P., Balasubramanian, K., Schroit, A.J., Zwaal, R.F., and Willems, G.M. 2005. Quantitative determination of the binding of beta2-glycoprotein I and prothrombin to phosphatidylserine-exposing blood platelets. *Biochem J* 386:271-279.

[33] Schousboe, I., and Rasmussen, M.S. 1995. Synchronized inhibition of the phospholipid mediated autoactivation of factor XII in plasma by beta 2-glycoprotein I and anti-beta 2-glycoprotein I. *Thromb Haemost* 73:798-804.

[34] Ohkura, N., Hagihara, Y., Yoshimura, T., Goto, Y., and Kato, H. 1998. Plasmin can reduce the function of human beta2 glycoprotein I by cleaving domain V into a nicked form. *Blood* 91:4173-4179.

[35] Horbach, D.A., van Oort, E., Lisman, T., Meijers, J.C., Derksen, R.H., and de Groot, P.G. 1999. Beta2-glycoprotein I is proteolytically cleaved in vivo upon activation of fibrinolysis. *Thromb Haemost* 81:87-95.

[36] Rahgozar, S., Giannakopoulos, B., Yan, X., Wei, J., Cheng Qi, J., Gemmell, R., and Krilis, S.A. 2008. Beta2-glycoprotein I protects thrombin from inhibition by heparin cofactor II: potentiation of this effect in the presence of anti-beta2-glycoprotein I autoantibodies. *Arthritis Rheum* 58:1146-1155.

[37] Mori, T., Takeya, H., Nishioka, J., Gabazza, E.C., and Suzuki, K. 1996. beta 2-Glycoprotein I modulates the anticoagulant activity of activated protein C on the phospholipid surface. *Thromb Haemost* 75:49-55.

[38] Sheng, Y., Reddel, S.W., Herzog, H., Wang, Y.X., Brighton, T., France, M.P., Robertson, S.A., and Krilis, S.A. 2001. Impaired thrombin generation in beta 2-glycoprotein I null mice. *J Biol Chem* 276:13817-13821.

[39] Takeuchi, R., Atsumi, T., Ieko, M., Takeya, H., Yasuda, S., Ichikawa, K., Tsutsumi, A., Suzuki, K., and Koike, T. 2000. Coagulation and fibrinolytic activities in 2 siblings with beta(2)-glycoprotein I deficiency. *Blood* 96:1594-1595.

[40] Yasuda, S., Tsutsumi, A., Chiba, H., Yanai, H., Miyoshi, Y., Takeuchi, R., Horita, T., Atsumi, T., Ichikawa, K., Matsuura, E., et al. 2000. beta(2)-glycoprotein I deficiency: prevalence, genetic background and effects on plasma lipoprotein metabolism and hemostasis. *Atherosclerosis* 152:337-346.

[41] Miyakis, S., Robertson, S.A., and Krilis, S.A. 2004. Beta-2 glycoprotein I and its role in antiphospholipid syndrome-lessons from knockout mice. *Clin Immunol* 112:136-143.

[42] Cleve, H. 1968. [Genetic studies on the deficiency of beta 2-glycoprotein I of human serum]. *Humangenetik* 5:294-304.

[43] Bancsi, L.F., van der Linden, I.K., and Bertina, R.M. 1992. Beta 2-glycoprotein I deficiency and the risk of thrombosis. *Thromb Haemost* 67:649-653.

[44] Zoller, B., Garcia de Frutos, P., Hillarp, A., and Dahlback, B. 1999. Thrombophilia as a multigenic disease. *Haematologica* 84:59-70.

[45] Navratil, J.S., and Ahearn, J.M. 2001. Apoptosis, clearance mechanisms, and the development of systemic lupus erythematosus. *Curr Rheumatol Rep* 3:191-198.

[46] Ravichandran, K.S., and Lorenz, U. 2007. Engulfment of apoptotic cells: signals for a good meal. *Nat Rev Immunol* 7:964-974.

[47] Casciola-Rosen, L., Rosen, A., Petri, M., and Schlissel, M. 1996. Surface blebs on apoptotic cells are sites of enhanced procoagulant activity: implications for coagulation events and antigenic spread in systemic lupus erythematosus. *Proc Natl Acad Sci U S A* 93:1624-1629.

[48] Thiagarajan, P., Le, A., and Benedict, C.R. 1999. Beta(2)-glycoprotein I promotes the binding of anionic phospholipid vesicles by macrophages. *Arterioscler Thromb Vasc Biol* 19:2807-2811.

[49] Maiti, S.N., Balasubramanian, K., Ramoth, J.A., and Schroit, A.J. 2008. Beta-2-glycoprotein 1-dependent macrophage uptake of apoptotic cells. Binding to lipoprotein receptor-related protein receptor family members. *J Biol Chem* 283:3761-3766.

[50] Nomura, S., Komiyama, Y., Matsuura, E., Kokawa, T., Takahashi, H., and Koike, T. 1993. Binding of beta 2-glycoprotein I to platelet-derived microparticles. *Br J Haematol* 85:639-640.

[51] Lambrianides, A., Carroll, C.J., Pierangeli, S.S., Pericleous, C., Branch, W., Rice, J., Latchman, D.S., Townsend, P., Isenberg, D.A., Rahman, A., et al. Effects of polyclonal IgG derived from patients with different clinical types of the antiphospholipid syndrome on monocyte signaling pathways. *J Immunol* 184:6622-6628.

[52] Alard, J.E., Gaillard, F., Daridon, C., Shoenfeld, Y., Jamin, C., and Youinou, P. TLR2 is one of the endothelial receptors for beta 2-glycoprotein I. *J Immunol* 185:1550-1557.

[53] Pierangeli, S.S., Vega-Ostertag, M.E., Raschi, E., Liu, X., Romay-Penabad, Z., De Micheli, V., Galli, M., Moia, M., Tincani, A., Borghi, M.O., et al. 2007. Toll-like receptor and antiphospholipid mediated thrombosis: in vivo studies. *Ann Rheum Dis* 66:1327-1333.

[54] Romay-Penabad, Z., Aguilar-Valenzuela, R., Urbanus, R.T., Derksen, R.H., Pennings, M.T., Papalardo, E., Shilagard, T., Vargas, G., Hwang, Y., de Groot, P.G., et al. Apolipoprotein E receptor 2 is involved in the thrombotic complications in a murine model of the antiphospholipid syndrome. *Blood* 117:1408-1414.

[55] Nagata, S., Hanayama, R., and Kawane, K. Autoimmunity and the clearance of dead cells. *Cell* 140:619-630.

[56] Senior, J.H. 1987. Fate and behavior of liposomes in vivo: a review of controlling factors. *Crit Rev Ther Drug Carrier Syst* 3:123-193.

[57] Wurm, H., Beubler, E., Polz, E., Holasek, A., and Kostner, G. 1982. Studies on the possible function of beta 2-glycoprotein-I: influence in the triglyceride metabolism in the rat. *Metabolism* 31:484-486.

[58] Chonn, A., Semple, S.C., and Cullis, P.R. 1995. Beta 2 glycoprotein I is a major protein associated with very rapidly cleared liposomes in vivo, suggesting a significant role in the immune clearance of "non-self" particles. *J Biol Chem* 270:25845-25849.

[59] Agostinis, C., Biffi, S., Garrovo, C., Durigutto, P., Lorenzon, A., Bek, A., Bulla, R., Grossi, C., Borghi, M.O., Meroni, P., et al. In vivo distribution of {beta}2 glycoprotein I under various pathophysiological conditions. *Blood.*

[60] Robertson, S.A., Roberts, C.T., van Beijering, E., Pensa, K., Sheng, Y., Shi, T., and Krilis, S.A. 2004. Effect of beta2-glycoprotein I null mutation on reproductive outcome and antiphospholipid antibody-mediated pregnancy pathology in mice. *Mol Hum Reprod* 10:409-416.

[61] Hunt, J.E., Simpson, R.J., and Krilis, S.A. 1993. Identification of a region of beta 2-glycoprotein I critical for lipid binding and anti-cardiolipin antibody cofactor activity. *Proc Natl Acad Sci U S A* 90:2141-2145.

[62] Yasuda, S., Atsumi, T., Ieko, M., Matsuura, E., Kobayashi, K., Inagaki, J., Kato, H., Tanaka, H., Yamakado, M., Akino, M., et al. 2004. Nicked beta2-glycoprotein I: a marker of cerebral infarct and a novel role in the negative feedback pathway of extrinsic fibrinolysis. *Blood* 103:3766-3772.

[63] Beecken, W.D., Engl, T., Ringel, E.M., Camphausen, K., Michaelis, M., Jonas, D., Folkman, J., Shing, Y., and Blaheta, R.A. 2006. An endogenous inhibitor of angiogenesis derived from a transitional cell carcinoma: clipped beta2-glycoprotein-I. *Ann Surg Oncol* 13:1241-1251.

[64] Sakai, T., Balasubramanian, K., Maiti, S., Halder, J.B., and Schroit, A.J. 2007. Plasmin-cleaved beta-2-glycoprotein 1 is an inhibitor of angiogenesis. *Am J Pathol* 171:1659-1669.

[65] Beecken, W.D., Ringel, E.M., Babica, J., Oppermann, E., Jonas, D., and Blaheta, R.A. Plasmin-clipped beta(2)-glycoprotein-I inhibits endothelial cell growth by down-regulating cyclin A, B and D1 and up-regulating p21 and p27. *Cancer Lett* 296:160-167.

[66] Nakagawa, H., Yasuda, S., Matsuura, E., Kobayashi, K., Ieko, M., Kataoka, H., Horita,T., Atsumi, T., Koike, T. 2009. Nicked β2-glycoprotein I binds angiostatin 4.5 (plasminogen kringle 1-5) and attenuates its antiangiogenic property. *Blood* 114:2553-2559.

[67] Passam, F.H., Qi, J.C., Tanaka, K., Matthaei, K.I., and Krilis, S.A. In vivo modulation of angiogenesis by beta 2 glycoprotein I. *J Autoimmun* 35:232-240.

[68] Nash, M.J., Camilleri, R.S., Liesner, R., Mackie, I.J., Machin, S.J., and Cohen, H. 2003. Paradoxical association between the 316 Trp to Ser beta 2-glycoprotein I (Beta2GPI) polymorphism and anti-Beta2GPI antibodies. *Br J Haematol* 120:529-531.

[69] Gushiken, F.C., Arnett, F.C., and Thiagarajan, P. 2000. Primary antiphospholipid antibody syndrome with mutations in the phospholipid binding domain of beta(2)-glycoprotein I. *Am J Hematol* 65:160-165.

2

Structural Changes in β_2-Glycoprotein I and the Antiphospholipid Syndrome

Çetin Ağar[1,2], Philip G. De Groot[2] and Joost C.M. Meijers[1]
[1]*University of Amsterdam*
[2]*University of Utrecht*
The Netherlands

1. Introduction

1.1 History of β_2-glycoprotein I

β_2-Glycoprotein I (β_2GPI) was described in literature for the first time in 1961 (Schultze et al., 1961) and seven years later the first β_2GPI deficient, seemingly healthy individual was identified (Haupt et al., 1968). β_2GPI's alternative name, apolipoprotein H, suggests a function in lipid metabolism, but this was based on a single publication that dates from 1979 in which it was shown that β_2GPI was distributed over different human lipoproteins (Polz & Kostner, 1979). Since 1983, the names β_2GPI and apolipoprotein H were used side by side for the same protein (Lee et al., 1983), and the official designation for the β_2GPI gene has become APOH. From 1990 on, the interest in this protein has increased significantly when β_2GPI was identified as the most important antigen in the antiphospholipid syndrome, which is amongst others characterized by the presence of antibodies directed to β_2GPI (McNeil et al., 1990; Galli et al., 1990). In 2010, a second three-dimensional conformation of β_2GPI was identified (Ağar et al., 2010) besides the known fishhook-like conformation that was suggested by the crystal structure of the protein (Bouma et al., 1999; Schwarzenbacher et al., 1999). In this chapter we will focus on this novel conformation of β_2GPI and discuss the consequences of the transition between the two conformations for β_2GPI on past but also on present findings.

1.2 Biochemistry of β_2-glycoprotein I

β_2GPI is a 43 kDa protein and consists of 326 amino acid residues (Lozier et al., 1984). β_2GPI is synthesized in the liver and it circulates in blood at variable levels (Rioche et al., 1974). β_2GPI is an anionic phospholipid binding glycoprotein composed of five homologous complement control protein repeats, CCP-I to CCP-V (Bouma et al., 1990; Schwarzenbacher et al., 1990). These CCPs are generally found in proteins from the complement system and mediate binding of complement factors to viruses and bacteria (Breier et al., 1970; Pangburn & Rawal, 2002). The first four domains contain approx. 60 amino acids each, whereas the fifth domain has a 6 residue insertion and an additional 19 amino acid C-terminal extension. The extra amino acids are responsible for the formation of a large positive charged patch within the fifth domain of β_2GPI (Hunt et al., 1993) that forms the binding site for anionic phospholipids (Figure 1).The crystal structure of β_2GPI has been solved in 1999 by two groups (Bouma et al., 1990; Schwarzenbacher et al., 1990), and revealed a structure that resembles a J-shaped fishhook. The phospholipid binding site is located at the bottom side of CCP-V and consists of two major parts, a large positive patch of 14 charged amino acid residues and a flexible hydrophobic loop. This flexible loop has the potential to insert into membranes (Planque et al., 1999).

1.3 β_2-Glycoprotein I and the antiphospholipid syndrome

The antiphospholipid syndrome (APS) is an auto-immune disease defined by the presence of antiphospholipid antibodies in blood of patients in combination with thrombotic complications in arteries or veins as well as pregnancy-related complications (Miyakis et al., 2006). In APS patients, the most common venous event is deep vein thrombosis and the most common arterial event is stroke. In pregnant women with APS early and late miscarriages can occur (Eswaran & Rosen, 1985). Next to miscarriages also placental infarctions, early deliveries and stillbirth have been reported (Lockshin et al., 1985; Branch et al., 1989; Birdsall et al., 1992). Antiphospholipid antibodies often occur transiently after infectious diseases, but there is a general consensus that these transient auto-antibodies are not related to an increased thrombotic risk (Miyakis et al., 2006). The syndrome occurs more in women than in men, and is most common in young to middle-aged adults but can also occur in children and the elderly. Among patients with systemic lupus erythematodes or lupus, the prevalence of antiphospholipid antibodies ranges from 12 to 30% for anticardiolipin antibodies, and 20 to 35% for lupus anticoagulant antibodies (Gezer et al., 2003). It is now generally accepted that the relevant auto-antibodies are not directed against phospholipids, but towards proteins bound to these phospholipids (Galli et al., 1990; McNeil et al., 1990; Bevers & Galli, 1990). β_2GPI has a relative low affinity towards these negatively charged phospholipids but its affinity increased more than 100-fold in the presence of auto-antibodies. Anti-β_2GPI antibodies were found to be the most prominent auto-antibodies in APS (de Groot & Meijers, 2011). Recently, three independent groups have shown the importance of antibodies against β_2GPI (Pierangelli et al., 1999; Jankowski et al., 2003; Arad et al., 2011) Mice that were challenged by injection of antiphospholipid antibodies had increased thrombus formation and foetal resorption (García et al., 1997; Ikematsu et al., 1998). Despite the wealth of data on the role of β_2GPI in the pathophysiology of APS, there were no convincing indications that help our understanding of the function of β_2GPI in normal physiology.

2. Conformations of β_2-glycoprotein I

2.1 β_2GPI exists in two conformations

There is overwhelming evidence that antibodies against β_2GPI can induce thrombosis in animal models (Blank et al., 1991; Pierangelli et al., 1999; Jankowski et al., 2003, Arad et al. 2011), but it was unclear which metabolic pathway was disturbed by the auto-antibodies. Nevertheless, the β_2GPI protein itself must hold an important functional clue that could lead us to both its function and its role in the antiphospholipid syndrome. Since patients with antiphospholipid antibodies do not have circulating antibody-antigen complexes despite the presence of large amounts of β_2GPI and antibodies in the circulation, the epitope for the auto-antibodies on β_2GPI must be cryptic. As a consequence, the conformation of β_2GPI in plasma must be different from the one coated on an ELISA tray in tests for the detection of antibodies. The crystal structure of β_2GPI revealed a fishhook-like shape of the molecule (Bouma et al., 1990; Schwarzenbacher et al., 1990) (Figure 1). Part of the epitope that is recognized by auto-antibodies is located in the first domain of β_2GPI (Iverson et al., 1998; de Laat et al., 2006). The crystal structure indicated that these amino acids are expressed on the surface of domain I of β_2GPI and should thus be accessible for auto-antibodies. But the lack of binding of antibodies to β_2GPI in solution fits better with a circular structure of β_2GPI, a structure that was originally suggested by Koike et al. (1998). Electron microscopy (EM) studies showed that when antibodies were bound to β_2GPI, the protein indeed showed a fishhook-like shape, but native β_2GPI in the absence of antibodies showed a closed 'circular' shape (Figure 2) in which domains I and V interact with each other (Agar et al., 2010).

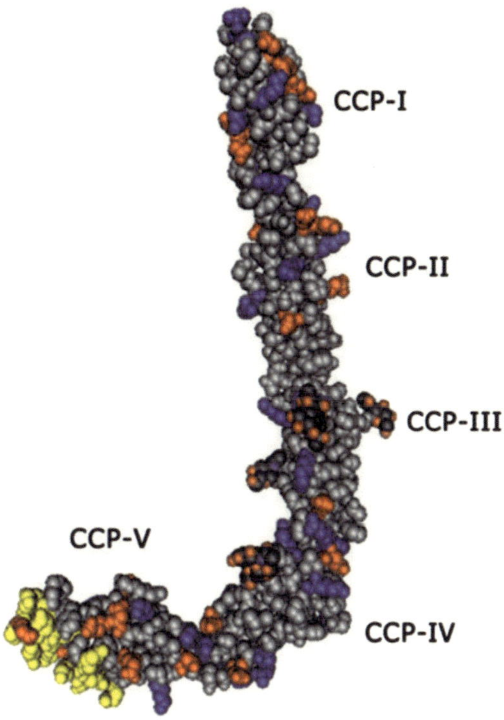

In blue the negatively charged amino acids are depicted and in red the positively charged amino acids. In yellow the large positive charged patch is shown within the fifth domain of β_2GP that forms the binding site for anionic phospholipids. Picture was made using Cn3D version 4.1, produced by the National Center for Biotechnology Information (http://www.ncbi.nlm.nih.gov).

Fig. 1. Crystal structure of β_2GPI with the five CCP domains (CCP-I to CCP-V).

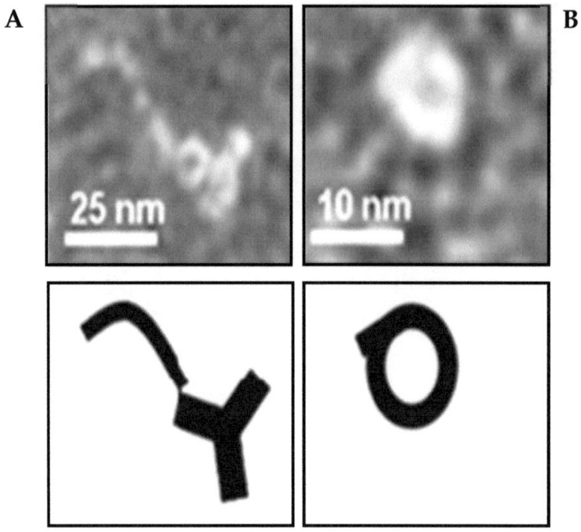

(A) Purified plasma β_2GPI in the presence of antibodies directed against domain I of β_2GPI shows on magnification an open fishhook-like shape of β_2GPI. (B) Magnification of purified plasma β_2GPI shows a circular conformation of the protein. This figure was modified from work originally published in *Blood.* C. Agar, G.M.A. van Os, M. Mörgelin, R.R. Sprenger, J.A. Marquart, R.T. Urbanus, R.H.W.M. Derksen, J.C.M. Meijers, P.G. de Groot. β_2-Glycoprotein I can exist in 2 conformations: implications for our understanding of the antiphospholipid syndrome. *Blood* 2010;116(8):1336-1343. © the American Society of Hematology.

Fig. 2. Electron microscopy analysis of β_2GPI.

By changing pH and salt concentrations, it was possible to convert β_2GPI from the native closed conformation into the open conformation and back (Agar et al., 2010). Analysis of EM pictures showed that more than 99% of plasma β_2GPI was in a closed conformation. These observations suggested that plasma β_2GPI circulates in a circular (closed) conformation, whereas after interaction with antibodies β_2GPI undergoes a major conformational change into a fishhook-like (open) structure.

2.1.1 Effect of the conformation of β_2GPI on coagulation

β_2GPI is present in high concentrations in plasma, and depletion of β_2GPI from normal plasma does not influence the results of coagulation assays (Oosting et al., 1992; Willems et al., 1996). When antibodies toward β_2GPI were added to plasma, clotting times prolonged in a β_2GPI-dependent way. This effect of anti-β_2GPI antibodies is known as lupus anticoagulant (LA) activity. A LA could also be seen with open β_2GPI (Agar et al., 2010). When closed native β_2GPI was added to normal plasma or β_2GPI-depleted plasma, no effect on an activated partial thromboplastin time (aPTT)-based clotting assay was observed.

When open β_2GPI was added to plasma or β_2GPI-depleted plasma, the aPTT prolonged. Addition of antibody and open β_2GPI together to normal plasma gave an additional anticoagulant effect on top of the effect of open β_2GPI alone (Agar et al., 2010). The presence of β_2GPI in a certain conformation is dependent on the presence of anionic surfaces but also on the method of purification of β_2GPI. As was described by Agar et al (2010), the conformation of β_2GPI is dependent on the pH and salt concentration used during the purification of native β_2GPI. The structure of β_2GPI needs confirmation before doing experiments with purified β_2GPI.

Schousboe (1985) was the first who described β_2GPI as a plasma inhibitor of the contact activation of the intrinsic blood coagulation pathway. With the current knowledge of the two conformations (Agar et al., 2010), these studies were most likely performed with the open conformation of β_2GPI, the only conformation that gives a prolongation in an aPTT. Furthermore, it was suggested that β_2GPI inhibited coagulation by inhibition of activation of coagulation factor XII (Henry et al., 1988) and coagulation factor XI (Shi et al., 2004). It is likely, that also these observations were obtained with the open 'activated' conformation of β_2GPI. The purification method that all these groups used included the use of perchloric acid, and these harsh conditions may have induced a conformational change of closed native β_2GPI into the open activated conformation of β_2GPI. It is highly recommended that the conformation of β_2GPI is confirmed in coagulation tests or by electron microscopy. It is expected that in the near future specific immunological assays will become available to determine the specific conformational state of β_2GPI.

2.2 Functional consequence of the conformations of β_2GPI

Lipopolysaccharide (LPS), a major constituent of the outer membrane of Gram-negative bacteria, plays a role in activating the hosts' immune response by binding to white blood cells (van der Poll & Opal, 2008). Analysis of electron microscopy pictures of β_2GPI incubated with LPS, showed that LPS was bound to domain V of β_2GPI and thereby induced a conformational change to the open conformation of β_2GPI (Figure 3) and showed the same fishhook-like shape when β_2GPI was bound to anionic surfaces or antibodies (Agar et al., 2011a).

A functional consequence of β_2GPI binding to LPS was investigated in an *in vitro* cellular model of LPS-induced tissue factor (TF) expression. Native plasma-purified β_2GPI dose-dependently inhibited LPS induced TF expression both in monocytes and endothelial cells (Agar et al., 2011a). Furthermore, in an *ex vivo* whole blood assay β_2GPI inhibited LPS induced interleukin-6 expression, an inflammatory marker in innate immunity. Furthermore, an *in vivo* relevance was found of the interaction between β_2GPI and LPS in plasma samples of 23 healthy volunteers intravenously challenged with LPS (de Kruif et al., 2007). A reduction of 25% of baseline values was observed of β_2GPI immediately after LPS injection, suggesting an *in vivo* interaction between β_2GPI and LPS.

Also, a highly significant, negative association was found between plasma levels of β_2GPI and plasma levels of inflammatory markers TNFα, IL-6 and-IL-8 after the LPS challenge. In agreement to this, there was a highly significant inverse relation between the baseline β_2GPI levels and the observed temperature rise upon LPS challenge (Agar et al., 2011a). Subsequently, a significant difference in β_2GPI levels was observed between non-sepsis

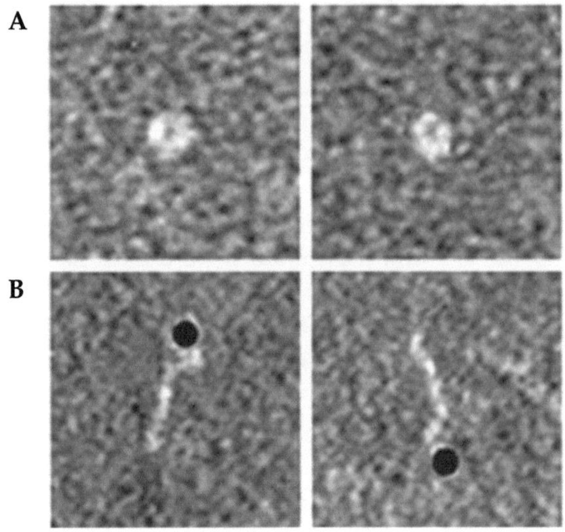

(A) Magnifications of purified plasma β_2GPI show a circular conformation. (B) Purified plasma β_2GPI in the presence of gold-labeled (black dots) LPS shows on magnification an open fishhook-like shape of β_2GPI. This figure was modified from work originally published in *Blood.* C. Agar, P.G. de Groot, M. Mörgelin, S.D.D.C. Monk, G. van Os, J.H.M. Levels, B. de Laat, R.T. Urbanus, H. Herwald, T. van der Poll, J.C.M. Meijers. β_2-Glycoprotein I: a novel component of innate immunity. *Blood* 2011;117(25):6939-6947. © the American Society of Hematology

Fig. 3. Electron microscopy analysis of β_2GPI and LPS.

and sepsis patients in the intensive care unit. β_2GPI levels returned to normal after recovery, again suggesting an *in vivo* interaction between β_2GPI and LPS. The reduction in β_2GPI levels after LPS challenge coincided with an uptake of β_2GPI by monocytes. When β_2GPI binds to LPS, it changes conformation after which the LPS-β_2GPI complex is taken up by monocytes. Interestingly, the binding of this complex could be dose-dependently inhibited by receptor associated protein, indicating that binding of β_2GPI is mediated via a receptor of the LRP-family (Lutters et al., 2003; Pennings et al., 2006; Urbanus et al., 2008).

The ability of native β_2GPI to inactivate LPS *in vivo* might offer opportunities to use β_2GPI for the treatment of sepsis. β_2GPI binds to LPS via domain V of β_2GPI. It seems logical to use domain V of β_2GPI, and not the whole molecule for sepsis treatment. The use of the whole protein could induce the formation of auto-antibodies against the cryptic epitope located in domain I, which could lead to the development of APS (McNeil et al., 1990). The use of only domain V could potentially avoid the development of the pathological auto-antibodies against β_2GPI.

2.2.1 Evolutionary conservation of the LPS binding site in β_2GPI

A survey of the genome sequences of 40 vertebrates and of the fruit fly and roundworm, revealed a 14% amino acid homology with β_2GPI from the fruit fly *Drosophila melanogaster* and a 17% homology with the roundworm *Caenorhabditis elegans*, the most primitive organisms in which β_2GPI could be identified (Agar et al., 2011b). It was found that the majority of mammals showed 75% or higher homology for the complete human β_2GPI amino acid sequence. Remarkably, all mammals except the platypus, showed 100% homology for all 22 cysteine residues present in β_2GPI, which serve an important structural role in protein folding and stability.

Surface plasmon resonance experiments revealed that the peptide AFWKTDA comprising a hydrophobic loop within a large positively charged patch in CCP-V of β_2GPI, was able to compete for binding of β_2GPI to the LPS. This amino acid sequence within domain V was completely conserved in all mammals (Agar et al., 2011b). The same amino acid sequences also attenuated the inhibition by β_2GPI in a cellular model of LPS-induced tissue factor expression. This indicated that the AFWKTDA amino acid sequence found in the genome of all mammals is the LPS binding region within CCP-V of β_2GPI. From this it can be concluded that the LPS scavenging function is not only present in humans but evolutionary conserved throughout all mammals. This certainly emphasizes an important role for β_2GPI in biology, explains its high concentration in blood, its conformational change and suggests a general role in scavenging of unwanted toxic substances and cells.

2.3 β_2GPI as an overall scavenger

Analysis of the structure and function of β_2-GPI has induced a turn into our understanding of the antiphospholipid syndrome. For the last two decades the protein β_2GPI has been linked mainly to the regulation of coagulation, but recent developments (Agar et al., 2011a,b; Gropp et al., 2011) has broadened the focus on β_2GPI from coagulation to innate immunity. For many years the characterization of the antibodies was the line of approach to understand the pathophysiology of the syndrome, unfortunately with little success.

During the last years, more and more evidence has become available that β_2GPI is a more general scavenger in our circulation. Maiti et al (2008) showed a β_2GPI-dependent phosphatidylserine (PS) expressing apoptotic cell uptake by macrophages. Binding of β_2GPI to these cells caused recognition and uptake of the β_2GPI-apoptotic cell complex by the LRP receptor on macrophages. The receptor for binding to apoptotic cells was determined to be the Ro 60 receptor (Reed et al., 2008, 2009). Furthermore, another study suggested that the binding of β_2GPI to PS-expressing procoagulant platelet microparticles might promote their clearance by phagocytosis (Abdel-Monem et al., 2010).

Blood contains microparticles (MPs) derived from a variety of cell types, including platelets, monocytes, and endothelial cells. MPs are formed from membrane blebs that are released from the cell surface by proteolytic cleavage of the cytoskeleton (Owens & Mackman, 2011). MPs may be procoagulant because they provide a membrane surface for the assembly of components of the coagulation protease cascade. Importantly, procoagulant activity is increased by the presence of anionic phospholipids, particularly phosphatidylserine (PS), and the procoagulant protein tissue factor (TF), which is the major cellular activator of the clotting cascade (Owens & Mackman, 2011). Since microparticles are considered to be important in coagulation, the efficient recognition and removal of these particles is critical for the maintenance of homeostasis and resolution of inflammation.

It has been shown that autoantibodies to β_2GPI inhibit this uptake of microparticles and bound TF to induce a procoagulant state (Abdel-Monem et al., 2010). The role of TF was studied in a renal injury mouse model that shared many features with thrombotic microvascular disease (Seshan et al,. 2009). Both complement-dependent and complement-independent mechanisms were found to be responsible for endothelial activation and microvascular disease induced by antiphospholipid antibodies obtained from APS patients. The presence of antibodies against β_2GPI showed a disturbed uptake of microparticles leading to increased TF in the circulation, which on its turn caused renal injury. It was also shown that mice expressing low levels of TF were protected against this injury induced by the presence of the antiphospholipid antibodies (Seshan et al., 2009).

3. Conclusions and future perspective

In conclusion, over the last few years a wealth of interesting data has become available that increased our knowledge on β_2GPI. The discovery of the native state of β_2GPI as a circular protein explained the important paradox that antibodies and protein could circulate separately in blood. Also, other previously ascribed functions were probably functions of the protein induced by the harsh method of purification after which only the open, activated, conformation of the protein was obtained. Furthermore, the potential of antibodies, anionic phospholipids, LPS and probably even more agents to switch the conformation of β_2GPI from a circular to an open activated conformation has given a clue to its role as scavenger, since the open conformation can bind to and subsequently be taken up by cells such as monocytes and macrophages. A role of β_2GPI as overall scavenger in coagulation and innate immunity, two complex processes that are highly intertwined, may provide clues to one of the remaining questions in APS research, namely how binding of antiphospholipid antibodies to β_2GPI result in thrombosis. An interesting option is that β_2GPI disturbs the uptake of microparticles resulting in a procoagulant state due to increased levels of TF and anionic phospholipids in the circulation. If the formation and presence of antibodies against β_2GPI also disturbs the scavenging function of β_2GPI still needs to be proven.

By identifying agents that can switch the conformation of β_2GPI, other areas of biology can be identified where β_2GPI might play a role. With the evolutionary conservation that was observed for the protein, its role in biology must be significant. It goes beyond saying that the appreciation of the different conformations and the ability to switch conformation has provided an important basis for research in this area.

4. Acknowledgments

This research was supported in part by a grant from the Netherlands Organization for Scientific Research (ZonMW 91207002; JCM Meijers and PG de Groot) and an Academic Medical Center stimulation grant (JCM Meijers).

5. References

Abdel-Monem H, Dasgupta SK, Le A, Prakasam A & Thiagarajan P. (2010) Phagocytosis of platelet microvesicles and beta2- glycoprotein I. *Thromb Haemost.* 104(2), 335-341.

Agar C, van Os GM, Mörgelin M, Sprenger RR, Marquart JA, Urbanus RT, Derksen RH, Meijers JC & de Groot PG. (2010) Beta2-glycoprotein I can exist in 2 conformations: implications for our understanding of the antiphospholipid syndrome. *Blood.* 116(8), 1336-1343.

Agar C, de Groot PG, Mörgelin M, Monk SD, van Os G, Levels JH, de Laat B, Urbanus RT, Herwald H, van der Poll T & Meijers JC. (2011a) {beta}2-Glycoprotein I: a novel component of innate immunity. *Blood.* 117(25), 6939-6947.

Agar C, de Groot PG, Marquart JA & Meijers JCM. (2011b) Evolutionary conservation of the LPS binding site of beta2-glycoprotein I. *Thromb Haemost.* In press.

Arad A, Proulle V, Furie RA, Furie BC & Furie B. (2011) β_2-Glycoprotein-1 autoantibodies from patients with antiphospholipid syndrome are sufficient to potentiate arterial thrombus formation in a mouse model. *Blood.* 117(12), 3453-3459.

Bevers EM & Galli M. (1990) Beta 2-glycoprotein I for binding of anticardiolipin antibodies to cardiolipin. *Lancet.* 336(8720), 952-953.

Birdsall MA, Pattison NS & Chamley LW. (1992) Antiphospholipid antibodies in pregnancy. *J Obstet Gynaecol.* 32, 328-330.

Blank M, Cohen J, Toder V & Shoenfeld Y. (1991) Induction of anti-phospholipid syndrome in naive mice with mouse lupus monoclonal and human polyclonal anti-cardiolipin antibodies. *Proc Natl Acad Sci U S A.* 88(8), 3069-3073.

Bouma B, de Groot PG, van den Elsen JM, Ravelli RB, Schouten A, Simmelink MJ, Derksen RH, Kroon J & Gros P. (1999) Adhesion mechanism of human beta(2)-glycoprotein I to phospholipids based on its crystal structure. EMBO J. 18(19), 5166-5174.

Branch DW, Andrew R & Digre KB. (1988) The association of antiphospholipid antibodies with severe preeclampsia. *Obstet Gynaecol.* 73, 541-545.

Brier AM, Snyderman R, Mergenhagen SE & Notkins AL. (1970) Inflammation and herpes simplex virus: release of a chemotaxis-generating factor from infected cells. *Science.* 170(962), 1104-1106.

de Groot PG & Meijers JC. (2011) β(2)-Glycoprotein I: evolution, structure and function. J *Thromb Haemost.* 9(7), 1275-1284.

de Kruif MD, Lemaire LC, Giebelen IA, van Zoelen MA, Pater JM, van den Pangaart PS, Groot AP, de Vos AF, Elliott PJ, Meijers JC, Levi M & van der Poll T. (2007) Prednisolone dose-dependently influences inflammation and coagulation during human endotoxemia. *J Immunol.* 178(3), 1845-1851.

de Laat B, Derksen RH, van Lummel M, Pennings MT & de Groot PG. (2006) Pathogenic anti-beta2-glycoprotein I antibodies recognize domain I of beta2-glycoprotein I only after a conformational change. *Blood.* 107(5), 1916-1924.

Eswaran K & Rosen SW. (1985) Recurrent abortions, thromboses, and a circulating anticoagulant. *Am J Obst Gynecol.* 151(6), 751-752.

Galli M, Comfurius P, Maassen C, Hemker HC, de Baets MH, van Breda-Vriesman PJ, Barbui T, Zwaal RF & Bevers EM. (1990) Anticardiolipin antibodies (ACA) directed not to cardiolipin but to a plasma protein cofactor. *Lancet.* 335(8705), 1544-1547.

García CO, Kanbour-Shakir A, Tang H, Molina JF, Espinoza LR & Gharavi AE. (1997) Induction of experimental antiphospholipid antibody syndrome in PL/J mice following immunization with beta 2 GPI. *Am J Reprod Immunol.* 37(1), 118-124.

Giannakopoulos B, Passam F, Ioannou Y & Krilis SA. (2009) How we diagnose the antiphospholipid syndrome. *Blood.* 113(5), 985-994.

Gropp K, Weber N, Reuter M, Micklisch S, Kopka I, Hallström T & Skerka C. (2011) {beta}2 glycoprotein 1 ({beta}2GPI), the major target in anti phospholipid syndrome (APS), is a special human complement regulator. *Blood.* 118(10), 2774-2783.

Haupt H, Schwick HG & Störiko K. (1968) On a hereditary beta-2-glycoprotein I deficiency. *Humangenetik.* 5(4), 291-293.

Henry ML, Everson B & Ratnoff OD. (1988) Inhibition of the activation of Hageman factor (factor XII) by beta 2-glycoprotein I. *J Lab Clin Med.* 111(5), 519-523.

Hunt JE, Simpson RJ & Krilis SA. (1993) Identification of a region of beta 2-glycoprotein I critical for lipid binding and anti-cardiolipin antibody cofactor activity. *Proc Natl Acad Sci U S A.* 90(6), 2141-2145.

Ikematsu W, Luan FL, La Rosa L, Beltrami B, Nicoletti F, Buyon JP, Meroni PL, Balestrieri G & Casali P. (1998) Human anticardiolipin monoclonal autoantibodies cause placental necrosis and fetal loss in BALB/c mice. *Arthritis Rheum.* 41(6), 1026-1039.

Iverson GM, Victoria EJ & Marquis DM. (1998) Anti-beta2 glycoprotein I (beta2GPI) autoantibodies recognize an epitope on the first domain of beta2GPI. *Proc Natl Acad Sci U S A.* 95(26), 15542-15546.

Jankowski M, Vreys I, Wittevrongel C, Boon D, Vermylen J, Hoylaerts MF & Arnout J. (2003) Thrombogenicity of beta 2-glycoprotein I-dependent antiphospholipid antibodies in a photochemically induced thrombosis model in the hamster. *Blood.* 101(1), 157-162.

Koike T, Ichikawa K, Kasahara H, Atsumi T, Tsutsumi A & Matsuura E. (1998) Epitopes on beta2-GPI recognized by anticardiolipin antibodies. *Lupus.* 7 Suppl 2, S14-7.

Lee NS, Brewer HB Jr & Osborne JC Jr. (1983) beta 2-Glycoprotein I. Molecular properties of an unusual apolipoprotein, apolipoprotein H. *J Biol Chem.* 258(8), 4765-4770.

Lockshin MD, Harpel PC, Druzin ML,Qamar T, Magid MS, Jovanovic L & Ferenc M. (1985) Antibody to cardiolipin as a predictor of fetal distress or death in pregnancy patients with systemic lupus erythematosis. *N Eng J Med.* 313, 152-153.

Lozier J, Takahashi N & Putnam FW. (1984) Complete amino acid sequence of human plasma beta 2-glycoprotein I. *Proc Natl Acad Sci U S A.* 81(12), 3640-3644.

Lutters BC, Derksen RH, Tekelenburg WL, Lenting PJ, Arnout J & de Groot PG. (2003) Dimers of beta 2-glycoprotein I increase platelet deposition to collagen via interaction with phospholipids and the apolipoprotein E receptor 2'. *J Biol Chem.* 278(36), 33831-33838.

Maiti SN, Balasubramanian K, Ramoth JA & Schroit AJ. (2008) Beta-2-glycoprotein 1-dependent macrophage uptake of apoptotic cells.Binding to lipoprotein receptor-related protein receptor family members. *J Biol Chem.* 283(7), 3761-3766.

McNeil HP, Simpson RJ, Chesterman CN & Krilis SA. (1990) Anti-phospholipid antibodies are directed against a complex antigen that includes a lipid-binding inhibitor of coagulation: beta 2-glycoprotein I (apolipoprotein H). *Proc Natl Acad Sci U S A.* 87(11), 4120-4124.

Oosting JD, Derksen RH, Entjes HT, Bouma BN & de Groot PG. (1992) Lupus anticoagulant activity is frequently dependent on the presence of beta 2-glycoprotein I. *Thromb Haemost.* 67(5), 499-502.

Owens AP 3rd & Mackman N. (2011) Microparticles in hemostasis and thrombosis. *Circ Res.* 108(10), 1284-1297.

Pangburn MK & Rawal N. (2002) Structure and function of complement C5 convertase enzymes. *Biochem Soc Trans.* 30(Pt 6), 1006-1010.

Pennings MT, van Lummel M, Derksen RH, Urbanus RT, Romijn RA, Lenting PJ & de Groot PG. (2006) Interaction of beta2-glycoprotein I with members of the low density lipoprotein receptor family. *J Thromb Haemost.* 4(8), 1680-1690.

Pierangeli SS, Colden-Stanfield M, Liu X, Barker JH, Anderson GL & Harris EN. (1999) Antiphospholipid antibodies from antiphospholipid syndrome patients activate endothelial cells in vitro and in vivo. *Circulation.* 99(15), 1997-2002.

Polz E & Kostner GM. (1979) The binding of beta 2-glycoprotein-I to human serum lipoproteins: distribution among density fractions. *FEBS Lett.* 102(1), 183-186.

Rioche M & Masseyeff R. (1974) Synthesis of plasma beta 2 glycoprotein I by human hepatoma cells in tissue culture. *Biomedicine.* 21(10), 420-423.

Shi T, Iverson GM, Qi JC, Cockcrill KA, Linnik MD, Konecny P & Krilis SA. (2004) Beta 2-Glycoprotein I binds factor XI and inhibits its activation by thrombin and factor XIIa: loss of inhibition by clipped beta 2-glycoprotein I. *Proc Natl Acad Sci U S A.* 101(11), 3939-3944.

Schousboe I. (1985) beta 2-Glycoprotein I: a plasma inhibitor of the contact activation of the intrinsic blood coagulation pathway. *Blood.* 66(5), 1086-1091.

Schultze HE, Heide K & Haupt H. (1961) Uber ein bisher unbekanntes niedermolekulares beta2-globulin des Humanserums. *Naturwissenschaften.* 48, 719-721.

Schwarzenbacher R, Zeth K, Diederichs K, Gries A, Kostner GM, Laggner P & Prassl R. (1999) Crystal structure of human beta2-glycoprotein I: implications for phospholipid binding and the antiphospholipid syndrome. *EMBO J.* 18(22), 6228-6239.

Seshan SV, Franzke CW, Redecha P, Monestier M, Mackman N & Girardi G. (2009) Role of tissue factor in a mouse model of thrombotic microangiopathy induced by antiphospholipid antibodies. *Blood.* 114(8), 1675-1683.

Urbanus RT, Pennings MT, Derksen RH & de Groot PG. (2008) Platelet activation by dimeric beta2-glycoprotein I requires signaling via both glycoprotein Ibalpha and apolipoprotein E receptor 2'. *J Thromb Haemost.* 6(8), 1405-12.

van der Poll T & Opal SM. (2008) Host-pathogen interactions in sepsis. *Lancet Infect Dis.* 8(1), 32-43.

Willems GM, Janssen MP, Pelsers MM, Comfurius P, Galli M, Zwaal RF & Bevers EM. (1996) Role of divalency in the high-affinity binding of anticardiolipin antibody-beta 2-glycoprotein I complexes to lipid membranes. *Biochemistry*. 35(43), 13833-13842.

3

Genetics of Antiphospholipid Syndrome

Jesús Castro-Marrero, Eva Balada,
Josep Ordi-Ros and Miquel Vilardell-Tarrés
Systemic Autoimmune Diseases Research Unit,
Vall d'Hebron University Hospital Research Institute
Universitat Autónoma de Barcelona, Barcelona
Spain

1. Introduction

Antiphospholipid Syndrome (APS), also known as Hughes Syndrome in honor of the doctor who first described it, is an autoimmune disease characterized by clinical manifestations such as vascular thrombosis (both arterial and venous), and/or recurrent pregnancy loss along with the presence of persistently elevated antiphospholipid antibodies (aPL) titers in serum (Bertolaccini et al., 2006). The etiology of APS, however, is still unknown. Incidence of disease remains unknown; however, the reported prevalence of aPL in the general population is low (1-4.5%) and increases with age (http://www.orpha.net/data/patho/GB/uk-APS.pdf in Orphanet, INSERM MIM n° 107320). APS can involve almost any organ system, including a wide range of clinical manifestations. The clinical involvement of different organs and systems poses the question of whether the syndrome should be considered a true systemic autoimmune disease, rather than an acquired autoimmune coagulopathy (Shoenfeld et al., 2008). Patients with this syndrome often have systemic lupus erythematosus (SLE) or related autoimmune diseases. In this case, we refer to the disease as secondary APS. The syndrome may also occur in the absence of such diseases and it is then known as primary APS.

Most autoimmunes diseases (AID) have a genetic background, but this hereditary component is not as obvious as diseases which are transferred from a parent to his children in half of quarter of cases. On the other hand, it is relatively common that members of the same family will have different AID. The conclusions of the genetic research in the field of primary APS are that this syndrome is significantly different in its genetic aspects from Systemic Lupus Erythematosus (SLE) (even though secondary APS might occur during lupus). Like other autoimmune diseases, APS is a complex multifactorial and polygenic disorder caused by interactions between multiple genes of small to modest effect in combination with environmental factors. Although complex disorders often cluster in families, they do not have a clear-cut pattern of inheritance. This makes it difficult to determine a person's risk of inheriting or passing on these disorders (Horita et al., 2004).

There is little doubt as to the pathogenic role of aPL in determining the clinical manifestations of APS, even if their mechanism of action has not been fully clarified. Although the pathogenic role of aPL is widely accepted, the fact that aPL induces thrombotic events only occasionally suggests the need for a "seconf hit" to display the thrombogenic effect. The question of whether other environmental triggers or a genetic individual susceptibility can behave as a second hit is still open. Despite much research effort over the last 25 years, we do not know how aPL increases the risk of thrombosis and recurrent fetal loss in patients with APS. Many theories have been proposed to explain the increased thrombotic tendency in patients with aPL, but unfortunately none of them has been proven by convincing evidence.

2. Antiphospholipid antibody syndrome: Phenotype assessment

In the decades following the recognition of APS as a distinct entity, there came increasing calls for a consensus on the criteria required for accurate diagnosis of these patients. In response, an International workshop was held in Sapporo, Japan (Wilson et al., 1999) with the sole aim of producing classification criteria that would allow further investigation and study of the syndrome. This expert workshop's result was a group of criteria divided into clinical and laboratory findings. The stated requirements were that patients must meet at least one clinical and one laboratory criteria in order to be classified as having APS. The clinical manifestations focused on vascular thrombosis and obstetric complications whilst the laboratory criteria required the presence of either Lupus Anticoagulant (LAC) or Anticardiolipin antibodies (aCL). These antibodies had to be present on two separate testings at least six weeks apart. The Sapporo criteria were afterwards revised and updated in 2006. These updates resulted in two important amendments. Firstly, the addition of a new laboratory criteria, anti-beta 2 glycoprotein-I antibody. This antibody is now recognised as being crucial to APS pathogenesis and is in fact an independent risk factor for thromboses. Secondly, it was advised that the time delay between serological testing should be extended to twelve weeks instead of the original six so as to avoid positive results caused by transient rises in autoantibody titres. It should be noted that these criteria were not developed with clinical situations in mind but were specifically aimed at encouraging clinical trials in the area. Despite this, there remains no alternative for clinicians who simply need accurate guidance in providing valid diagnoses for their patients. As previously mentioned, the potential APS clinical manifestations are numerous and widespread. This can be illustrated by listing a myriad of clinical specialities that can be involved in a patient's management-rheumatology, neurology, cardiology, nephrology, endocrinology, gastroenterology, dermatology, surgery, haematology, intensive care, and obstetrics. The hallmarks of APS, as defined by the Sapporo criteria, are however limited to thromboses and obstetric complications.

Defining the phenotype correctly is an important issue in genetic studies of complex diseases as autoimmune diseases. In APS it appears quite difficult, since several clinical entities coexist. Many epidemiological and genetic studies assess the APS phenotype based on clinical criteria of thromboembolism or pregnancy morbidity, and laboratory findings of medium or high titers of antiphospholipid antibodies that are present on two or more occasions at least 12 weeks apart (Miyakis et al., 2006). These international consensus criteria were designed to facilitate clinical studies of treatment and causation in APS and were not intended to be diagnostic criteria for clinical practice. Nonetheless, these criteria can be useful to assess the applicability of the results of clinical trials to an individual patient or even for genetic studies in other populations. It is notable that patients with APS may have other clinical characteristics, including thrombocytopenia; livedo reticularis, valvular heart lesions and nephropathy, but these features are not formally part of the consensus diagnostic criteria. Similarly, these patients may have antiphospholipid antibodies other than LA, aCL and anti-β2-GPI, including antibodies against prothrombin and other phospholipids and proteins that are not included in the current consensus criteria. Another problem in defining the APS phenotype is that the clinical expression of disease may vary over time even within an individual, especially at older age. Thus, lack of a gold standard to diagnose APS, (variable clinical expression, variable age at onset, and variable progression of disease activity during lifetime) are providing some difficulties in the studies on the genetics of APS.

3. HLA and genetic susceptibility to antiphospholipid syndrome

The genetic predisposition for APS is partially explained in part by markers called Human Leukocyte Antigens (HLA). Some of these HLA molecules are associated to the presence of aPL (Horita et al., 2004): HLA-DR4, -DR7, -DRw53, and DQB1*0302 are associated with the presence of aCL that has been demonstrated in primary APS and can also be found in SLE, a disease with a completely different pattern of HLA allele association (HLA-DR2, -DR3, -DRw52). Therefore, it can be argued that both DR4 and DR7 are independently associated with aCL. According to published results, it seems that DRB1*0402 and DRB1*0403 are slightly more important than DR7 and that the association with DRw53 is only apparent because patients typing positive for DRw53 possess haplotypes that also contain either DR4 or DR7. Furthermore, it is hard to discriminate whether aCL and anti-beta-2GPI antibodies are more strongly associated with DR alleles or DQ alleles, because they are often in strong linkage disequilibrium. Alternatively, these alleles may be apparent only because of their linkage disequilibrium with an as yet unidentified primarily involved HLA locus, or they could act in cooperation with other genes, possibly even outside the MHC. For instance, some reports indicate that aCL are associated with C4A or C4B null alleles (Galeazzi et al., 2000). In addition, the different aPL (anticardiolipin antibodies, lupus anticoagulant, anti-β_2GPI antibodies, antiphosphatidylserine/prothrombin antibodies) show similar HLA association, again independent of the clinical context (primary APS or SLE), and across various ethnic groups.

The genetic findings in the research of APS can explain only partially the development of APS, and like in other AID, disease occurrence depends both on hereditary factors and environmental factors. There is increased prevalence of APS among family members, even though the genetic background of the syndrome is not completely understood. Yet, the chances of a family member of an APS patient also to develop APS are low. Furthermore, aPL are a heterogenous family of autoantibodies. Their presence is not always associated with the clinical manifestations of APS and even in experimental animal models not all aPL are of pathogenetic significance (Sebastiani et al., 2003). Many authors favour the hypothesis that the association of APS with HLA alleles is a consequence of the association of aPL with HLA alleles; therefore, it is reasonable to think that, like in SLE, HLA alleles account only in part for the genetic susceptibility to develop APS. In fact, it appears that some HLA alleles only determine the risk of susceptibility to producce aPL, and this is independent of the clinical context. Other genes, even outside the MHC, give their contribution to the development of this syndrome. For example, it has been shown that a polymorphism in domain 5 of beta-2 GPI, (a valine instead of a leucine at position 247), is correlated with anti-beta2-GPI antibodies production in patients with primary APS (Hirose et al., 1999); (Atsumi et al., 1999). This replacement of one aminoacid in the structure of beta2-GPI could turn this molecule immunogenic and may induce the production of anti-beta-2GPI autoantibodies.

As we will see, additional genetic risk factors for thrombosis have been described in patients with APS (Factor V Leiden, Methylenetetrahydrofolate-reductase (MTHFR), Homocysteine, Protein C or Protein S deficiency, Adquired Activated Protein C Resistence). The role of these genetically determined factors in APS is not completely clarified, but it appears that they can act as additional (to aPL) thrombogenic risk factors. In conclusion, immunogenetic studies suggest that APS is an independent entity from SLE, even if it can appear in the course of this latter disease. A genetic predisposition to APS can be at least in part explained with an influence of certain HLA alleles. However, these alleles could only be apparent because of their linkage disequilibrium with an as yet unidentified primarily involved HLA-locus, or they could act in cooperation with other genes, even residing outside the MHC. A recent advance in the field of molecular genetics has led to a better understanding of the genes predisposing to APS in both humans and laboratory animal models. The search for a more strongly associated polymorphim is actively pursued whenever new loci are identified in the HLA region. Identification of many more susceptibility genes provides key insights into the pathogenesis of APS, making new prophylactic and therapeutic approaches feasible.

3.1 HLA alleles, antiphospholipid antibodies and genetic susceptibility to the antiphospholipid syndrome

Like many other autoimmune diseases, this syndrome arises in a predisposed subject after antigenic stimuli from various sources. Proof of the genetic predisposition of APS lies in the observation of familial clustering of cases, greater prevalence of aPL in the serum of subjects sharing the same descent of patients, animal models (mice), and associations with HLA alleles. Many autoimmune diseases are associated with genes in the HLA region. In some autoimmune disorders, such as SLE, HLA antigens seem to be associated with specific autoantibodies, including anticardiolipin (aCL) and anti-beta-2 glycoprotein I (anti-beta2 GPI), rather than with the disease itself (Smolen et al., 1987); (Lulli et al., 1991). Thus, it appears that HLA genes may influence not only the expression of autoimmune diseases, but also the production of autoantibodies that can be found in these diseases. Many researchers in the field of immunogenetics have investigated possible associations between APS or the various antibodies directed against negatively charged phospholipids and HLA genes or their products. However, there is increasing evidence that aPL represent a heterogeneous group of antibodies, which includes lupus anticoagulant (LAC), aCL, anti-b2-GPI, antibodies to prothrombin, annexin V, phosphatidylethanolamine, phosphatidylserine and other oxidized phospholipids. Thus, it appears evident that the spectrum of associations with HLA alleles in APS might become clearer if more specific autoantibody subgroups are studied. As stated before, APS may exist both as a primary condition as well as in the setting of another autoimmune disease (mainly SLE), and this implies possible differences in the association with HLA alleles. The presence of aPL is not always associated with the clinical manifestations of APS, and even in experimental animal models not all aPLs are of pathogenetic significance. Some aPL bind preferentially to anionic phospholipids, whereas as others react with zwitterionic phospholipids, and their binding can be either enhanced or depressed by beta2-

GPI, depending on the source of aPL. Therefore, what we call "antiphospholipid antibodies" may comprise a group of antibodies whose unique common feature is their reactivity against phospholipids, but with different specificities and different HLA associations.

The question of whether a genetic predisposition to develop APS and to produce aPL exists can be examined both in animal models and in humans (Ahmed et al., 1993). It thus appears that the genetic background of mice can influence the production of aPL, and this production can be modulated by hormones. Nevertheless, it has not been clarified whether aPL are constitutively expressed by mice or induced by antigenic stimulation (Hashimoto et al., 1992). In humans, the contribution of immunogenetics to the development of aPL and APS has been addressed mainly by family-based studies and by population-based studies looking at the association with the HLA region.

3.1.1 Family-based studies

Familial occurrence of aPL with or without clinical evidence of APS has been documented since 1980. A genetic basis for aPL was suggested for the first time when a familial clustering of chronic false-positive syphilis test individuals were detected (McGhee-Harvey, 1966); in this case, aPL were observed many years before overt autoimmune disease developed. Familial occurrence of lupus anticoagulant (LA) was first described in three sets of siblings, two of which had more than one clinically affected member (Exner et al., 1980). Subsequent studies have reported that first-degree relatives of patients with SLE or primary APS have a higher incidence of aCL antibodies, suggesting a genetic predisposition to the development of these antibodies (Mackworth-Young et al., 1987); (Goldberg et al., 1995). Identification of several pedigrees with an increased frequency of aPL antibodies and the associated clinical manifestations further support the familial form of APS. In one of these studies, a large kindred in which nine individuals had aPL antibodies was described. Associated clinical manifestations included stroke, deep venous thrombosis, and recurrent abortions (Ford et al., 1990). A study also have described a family, including identical twins and their mother, in which all members had SLE and presented with different manifestations of APS. The mother and the twins shared the HLA haplotype that included DR4, DRw53 and DQw7, whereas C4A or C4B deficiencies could not be implicated in the autoimmune process (May et al., 1993). In another study, pedigrees with more than one affected member were examined for possible modes of inheritance and linkage to potential candidate genes (Goel et al., 1999). Thirty out of 101 family members from 7 families met diagnostic criteria for the syndrome. Segregation studies rejected environment and autosomal recessive models, and the data were fitted best by a dominant or codominant model. However, linkage analysis showed independent segregation of APS and several candidate genes.

In conclusion, family studies suggest a genetic predisposition to APS, either when it presents as a primary condition or when it is seen in the context of SLE. It appears that this genetic predisposition is in part accounted for the HLA system, the most consistent associations being those with DR4 and DRw53. Furthermore, it appears that LA and aCL are both associated with the same HLA antigens.

3.1.2 Population-based studies

In a study of primary APS and HLA associations, HLA-DQw7 (DQB1*0301 allele) was significantly associated with disease. All patients with DQw7 were HLA-DR4 or -DR5-positive

(Arnett et al., 1991). Asherson et al., reported on 13 English patients with primary APS, in which both HLA class I and HLA class II genes were examined by molecular methods (Asherson et al., 1992). They found that significant differences were limited to the HLA class II region. In fact, DR4 and DRw53 were found with increased frequency in patients compared with controls, whereas DR3 was absent in all patients. No significant associations between any DQB alleles or C4 or 21-hydroxylase gene polymorphisms and primary APS were found, and the prevalence of DQw7 was not significantly increased in patients.

More recently, Caliz et al., found that the haplotypes DQB1*0301/4-DQA1*0301/2-DRB1*04 and DQB1*0604/5/6/7/9-DQA1*0102-DRB1*1302 were more frequent in 53 white British patients with primary APS than in controls (Caliz et al., 2001). The most striking association was found between DQB1*0604/5/6/7/9-DQA1*0102-DRB1*1302 and the presence of anti-b2GPI antibodies in primary APS.

The DQB1*0301/DQA1*0301/DRB1*04 haplotype was also associated with antiphosphatidylserine/prothrombin autoantibodies (Bertolaccini et al., 2000). In another study on the same patients, Bertolaccini et al., evaluated the role of tumor necrosis factor-alpha (TNF-α), an immunomodulatory cytokine with prothrombotic action, encoded at the TNFA locus in the HLA class III region (Bertolaccini et al., 2001). They found significantly higher plasma TNF-alpha levels in patients with APS when compared with controls. In addition, they found a strong association between TNFA-238A polymorphism and APS, and a possible association of the TNFA-238A-DQB1*0303-DRB1*0701 haplotype with APS. However, they failed to demonstrate correlation between TNFA-238A and plasma TNF-alpha levels, suggesting that this polymorphism is not implicated in the elevation of TNF-alpha levels found in APS. It is possible that TNFA-238A polymorphisms associated with APS because of its linkage with the DRB1*0701-DQB1*0303 haplotype.

Another study reports the association of HLA-DR5 with primary APS in Mexican patients (Vargas-Alarcon et al., 1995). To assess whether the HLA profile of patients presenting with primary APS is different from that of patients with secondary APS, Freitas et al., studied 123 patients, 34 of whom presented primary APS and 35 secondary APS due to SLE, 54 SLE patients without APS, and 166 controls. Compared with controls, primary APS patients exhibited a non-significantly increased frequency of DRw53-associated alleles, and secondary APS patients presented an increased frequency of HLA-DRB1*03 alleles. In addition, HLA-DRB1*03 alleles were over-represented in secondary APS patients presenting aCL, in SLE patients as a whole, and in SLE patients without APS. Taken together, their results suggest that the HLA class II profile of primary APS is different from that of secondary APS (Freitas et al., 2004). Sánchez et al., examined the susceptibility of the polymorphisms at the HLA-DM locus (whose products are involved in the antigen processing pathway of HLA class II restricted antigen presentation) to aPL production in a white British population, and observed the skewed distribution of DMA alleles, including the increase of DMA*0102 in patients with aPL. However, this association could simply reflect the strong linkage disequilibrium between HLA-DM alleles and HLA-class II alleles (Sanchez et al., 2004).

Thus, population studies suggest that HLA genes have a role in conferring susceptibility to develop primary APS. DRB1*04, DR7, DRw53, DQB1*0301/4, DQB1*0604/5/6/7/9, DQA1*0102, and DQA1*0301/2, seem to be the relevant loci. HLA-DR4 seems to be more important in Anglo-Saxon populations, whereas DR7 emerges in populations of Latin origin. Results of those studies in which HLA polymorphisms have been investigated by molecular methods overlap those obtained by serological typing. It is difficult to discriminate whether DR loci contribute to this genetic susceptibility more than DQ loci, because they are in strong linkage disequilibrium.

4. Prothrombotic risk factors in antiphospholipid syndrome

Antiphospholipid antibodies (aPL) are related to thrombosis in APS and thromboses are, together with obstetric complications, the main clinical manifestations of APS. Numerous pathophysiological mechanisms have been suggested to explain thrombotic events in APS, in both arterial and venous territories, involving cellular mechanisms, plasma coagulation regulatory proteins, and fibrinolysis. However, although there is a clear epidemiological association, not all aPL-positive individuals experience such complications. The heterogeneity of thrombotic manifestations in APS suggests that other additional factors may contribute to determine the "prothrombotic profile" in these patients: First, several characteristics of aPL, such as the concentration, class/subclass, affinity, or charge, and several characteristics of the antigens, such as the concentration, size, location, or charge, may influence whether aPL will act as prothrombotic "in vivo" (Roubey, 1996); second, oral contraception, pregnancy, surgery, trauma, smoking, immobilization, and other environmental causes can modify the thrombotic risk; and third, individual patient variability due to a predetermined genetic profile can modulate the effect of aPL on hemostasis.

Thrombophilia can be (inherited) congenital, which is supposed to result from the interaction of multiple genetic backgrounds with environmental or acquired factors, such as aPLs or hyperhomocysteinemia, causing together the thrombus growth. There are two levels of prothombotic genetic characteristics potentially related to the clinical expression of APS, the major alterations consisting of deficiencies or polymorphisms clearly related to thrombosis (mainly related to venous thromboembolism), which are for this reason included in the usual thrombophilia test profiles, and a series of polymorphisms that have a little prothrombotic role on their own, but can significantly modify the effect of aPL on hemostasis.

The main genetic thrombophilic conditions in APS include: Major and minor thrombophilic defects.

5. Major thrombophilia alterations in antiphospholipid syndrome

Results of early genetic studies have established that two types of genetic thrombophilic defects cause venous thrombosis: loss-of-function mutations (Antithrombin [SERPINC1], Protein C [PROC] and Protein S [PROS1] deficiencies) and gain-of-function mutations (Factor V Leiden [F5] G1691A and Prothrombin [F2] G20210A mutation) (Reitsma et al., 2007). Combined, these loss and gain-of-function mutations account for about half of the genetic thrombosis risk. Therefore, there is every reason to believe that additional genetic causes of thrombosis remain to be discovered, and many attempts have been made and are still being made to identify them.

Congenital deficiencies of antithrombin and protein C are very uncommon and for this reason, the number of patients with these deficiencies is too small to allow an accurate assessment of the associated risk of thrombosis in APS (Brouwer et al., 2004). By contrast, low levels of free protein S are seen in a high number of APS patients, suggesting an acquired origin like high level of C4-binding protein. Although it is likely that these genetic defects may increase the risk of venous thromboembolism in patients with APS, only little is known about its possible interactions (Brouwer et al., 2004).

Anecdotically, a single patient suffering from recurrent thrombosis with type II plasminogen deficiency (a controversial thrombophilia factor deficiency) associated with APS and SLE has been described (Iguchi et al., 2002). This case may be coincidental or it may be that the plasminogen deficiency increased the thrombotic tendency of APS in this patient.

5.1 Antithrombin deficiency

Family studies in kindreds with antithrombin deficiency have revealed that antithrombin deficiency probably confers a higher risk of thrombosis than protein C or protein S deficiencies (Lane et al., 1996). The reported incidence of antithrombin deficiency in the general population varies from 0.17-0.20 % as revised by De Stefano *et al.* (De Stefano et al., 1996) which amounts to one-tenth of that for protein C deficiency. Despite this, it has 1-2% prevalence in patients with thrombosis (as against 2.5% for Protein C deficient patients). Thus, Antithrombin III deficiency appears to confer a higher thrombotic risk than Protein C and S deficiencies (Van Cott et al., 1998).

5.1.1 Antithrombin deficiency and risk of thrombosis

Affected patients have antithrombin levels between 40%-60% of normal and 70% of those affected experience thromboembolic events before the age of 50. Thrombotic episodes are rare before puberty in AT-deficient individuals. They start to occur with some frequency after puberty, with the risk increasing substantially with advancing age (Khan et al., 2006). In 1994, Tait et al. studied 9,669 blood donors in Scotland by taking blood samples and monitoring the donors for two years. Of the study participants, 107 were found to have an initial level of AT< 83 IU/dl. They were retested, and eventually, 16 donors where found to have congenital AT deficiency. The study suggested a prevalence of 1/600 or 1.65 per 1000 (95% CI of 0.95-2.27 per 1000). Two of the affected individuals had Type I deficiency while the other 14 had Type II. The study showed an overall prevalence of 1/4,400 for Type I AT deficiency and 1/630 for type II with an overall prevalence of AT deficiency at 1/630 in the population studied. It all brins up the important issue of whether AT deficiency itself, or in combination with other factors, would make a thromboembolic event likely in these individuals (Tait et al., 1994). Another challenge when testing for AT without other clinical information is that levels of antithrombin can be reduced in protein-losing states. Marked reductions in antithrombin levels occur in patients with liver disease as well as severe malnutrition and these may cause skewed results (Hoffman, 2000).

Using only an immunoassay for measuring plasma levels of AT, initial estimates of the prevalence of AT deficiency in the general Scottish population was 1 in 2,000 to 5,000. However, studies employing functional assays that measure AT-heparin cofactor activity have found that the prevalence of AT deficiency in the Scottish population is 1 in 250 to 500 (Tait et al., 1994). The majority of AT-deficient patients identified in these studies did not have a personal or familial history of thrombosis and had a type II defect with mutations at the heparin binding site. Among patients with a first thrombotic event, the prevalence of hereditary AT deficiency is approximately 0.5 to 1 %, being less common than factor V Leiden, the prothrombin gene mutation, or protein S/protein C deficiencies. A recent study showed that homozygous children of consanguineous parents who were asymptomatic carriers developed severe venous or arterial thrombosis in association with plasma AT-heparin cofactor levels below 10 percent of normal (Picard et al., 2003).

The thrombotic risk associated with AT deficiency, as with other inherited thrombophilias, has been assessed in two ways: evaluation of patients with deep venous thrombosis and evaluation of families with thrombophilia. In a Spanish study of 2,132 consecutive unselected patients with venous thromboembolism 12.9 % had an anticoagulant protein deficiency (7.3% of protein S, 3.2% of protein C, and 0.5% of antithrombin). Similar findings were noted in a series of 277 Dutch patients with deep venous thrombosis: 8.3% had an isolated deficiency of antithrombin, protein C, protein S, or plasminogen compared to 2.2% of controls subjects (Heijboer et al., 1990). In a study in 2001, five children from three Austrian families had a homozygous antithrombin deficiency type II affecting the heparin binding site (99 Leu → Phe mutation). Four children had severe spontaneous thromboembolic events (deep leg or caval vein thrombosis, ischemic stroke) at one week, 3 months, 13 and 14 years of age. The fifth patient, a 17 year-old boy, was asymptomatic (Kuhle et al., 2001).

The absolute risk of thrombosis among patients with inherited thrombophilia was evaluated by Martinelli et al. in 1998 in an Italian cohort study of 150 pedigrees consisting of 1,213 individuals. The study compared the risk for thrombosis in individuals with inherited thrombophilia due to factor V Leiden, antithrombin, protein C, and protein S deficiency (Martinelli et al., 1998). The lifetime probability of developing thrombosis compared to those with no defect was 8.5 times higher for carriers of protein S deficiency, 8.1 for type I antithrombin deficiency, 7.3 for protein C deficiency, and 2.2 for factor V Leiden. The selection of patients was not solely based on their registration at the thrombosis centers in Milan or Rome but also required individuals to provide clinical evidence of thrombotic events; hence, this fact increases the validity of the study.

5.2 Protein C deficiency

Protein C deficiency is less common than either the factor V Leiden or the prothrombin G20210A gene mutation with prevalence in Caucasians estimated to be 0.2–0.5% (Rosendaal, 1999). Protein C deficiency is inherited in an autosomal dominant manner and is associated with familial venous thrombosis. The gene for protein C is located on chromosome 2 (2q13–14) and appears to be closely related to the gene for factor IX (Foster et al., 1985). The primary effect of activated protein C (APC) is to inactivate coagulation factors Va and VIIIa, which are necessary for efficient thrombin generation and factor X activation (Clouse et al., 1986). The inhibitory effect of APC is markedly enhanced by protein S, another vitamin K-dependent protein. Two major subtypes of heterozygous protein C deficiency (Type I and Type II) have been delineated using immunologic and functional assays. Over 160 different gene abnormalities have been associated with the two subtypes (Reitsma et al., 1995).

Type I deficiency - The type I deficiency state is more common. Most affected patients are heterozygous, having a reduced plasma protein C concentration at approximately 50 percent of normal in both immunologic and functional assays (Broekmans et al., 1985). More than half of the mutations identified so far are missense and nonsense mutations. Other types of mutations include promoter mutations, splice site abnormalities. In frame deletions, frameshift deletions, in-frame insertions, and frameshift insertions (Reitsma et al., 1995). There is marked phenotypic variability among patients with heterozygous type I protein C deficiency. Similar mutations have been found among symptomatic and asymptomatic individuals. This finding suggests that the nature of the protein C gene defect alone does not explain the phenotypic variability.

Type II deficiency - Individuals with the type II deficiency state have normal plasma protein C antigen levels with decreased functional activity. A variety of different point mutations affecting protein function have been identified in this disorder (Reitsma et al., 1995).

Although the clinical manifestations of protein C are similar to those of antithrombin deficiency, there are some unique features of protein C deficiency. In a study of 11 infants in Denver (Colorado, U.S.), Manco-Johnson et al. suggested that homozygotes can develop a severe thrombotic tendency in infancy characterized as purpura fulminans (Manco-Johnson et al., 1988). Heterozygotes for protein C deficiency have an increased risk of developing warfarin-induced skin necrosis (Chan et al., 2000). Protein C deficiency has been implicated in adverse pregnancy outcomes such as deep venous thrombosis (DVT), preeclampsia, intrauterine growth restriction, and recurrent pregnancy loss (Greer, 2003). Family studies from the Netherlands and the US have shown that family members who are PC deficient are at an 8–10 fold increased risk of venous thrombosis, and, by age 40, 50% or more will have experienced a thrombotic event (Bovill et al., 1989); (Broekmans, 1985). The initial episode of venous thromboembolism in patients with protein C deficiency is apparently spontaneous in approximately 70 % of cases. The remainder of the cases suggests that other genetic or acquired factors are involved in the presentation of thrombotic events in this population. Further studies in the Netherlands showed that most patients are asymptomatic until their early twenties, with increasing numbers experiencing thrombotic events as they reach the age of 50 (Lensen et al., 1996). Lensen et al. concluded that the median age at onset for a thrombotic event and the risk of thrombosis is similar in both protein C deficiency and factor V Leiden (APC resistance). Approximately 60% of affected individuals develop recurrent venous thrombosis and about 40% have signs of pulmonary embolism.

The first case-control study looking at protein C deficiency was conducted by Heijboer et al. in 1990 that performed a study on 277 Dutch patients and 138 controls. The overall prevalence of protein C deficiency in the patients with venous thrombosis was 8.3% (23 of 277 patients) (95% CI 5.4–12.4), as compared with 2.2% in the controls (i.e. 3 of 138 subjects 95% CI 0.5–6.1; $P< 0.05$). Interestingly, the relative risk (RR) estimate for thrombosis given protein C deficiency was also close to 7 as in the case of the family studies in Netherlands.

Both the work done by Heijboer et al. and a subsequent study by Tait et al. estimated the population prevalence of heterozygous protein C deficiency at 0.2% (Tait et al., 1994). The relative risk for thrombosis among patients with protein C deficiency was also carried out by Koster et al. involving 474 consecutive outpatients at anticoagulation clinics who were excluded by age (older than 70) and known malignancy. The patients were asked to find their own controls by sex, age and no known thrombotic disorder. The study demonstrated the relative risk of thrombosis with protein C deficiency to be at least 3.1 (95% CI 1.4–7) with re-evaluation of patients with low levels increasing the RR to closer to 4 (Koster et al., 1993).

There is marked variability in risk among families with protein C deficiency that cannot be explained by the genetic defect itself. In severely affected families, as many as 75% of protein C-deficient individuals experience one or more thrombotic events (Broekmans et al., 1983); in other families, the thrombosis rate is much lower. A risk factor for more severe disease is the presence of a second thrombotic defect, particularly factor V Leiden as will be discussed in more detail later on in this chapter.

5.3 Protein S deficiency

Protein S serves as a cofactor for activated protein C. There are two homologous genes for protein S: PROS1 and PROS2, which both map to chromosome 3 (Schmidel et al., 1990). In 2000, Gandrille et al. identified 15 point mutations and 3 polymorphisms among 19 French patients affected of thrombosis; since then, mutations have been identified in 70% of protein S deficient probands and a database of known protein S gene mutations has been published (Gandrille et al., 2000). As in the case of other inherited thrombophilias, there seem to be few reports of large deletions causing the disorder. Three phenotypes of protein S deficiency have been defined on the basis of total protein S antigen concentrations, free protein S concentrations, and protein S functional activity:

Type I - The classic type of protein S deficiency is associated with a decreased level of total S antigen (approximately 50% of normal), and marked reductions in free protein S antigen and protein S functional activity (Simmonds et al., 1996).

Type II - This type of protein S deficiency is characterized by normal total and free protein S levels, but diminished protein S functional activity. Interestingly, all five mutations originally described in these patients were missense mutations located in the N-terminal end of the protein S molecule, which includes the domains that interact with activated protein C (Gandrille et al., 1995).

Type III - Also known as type IIa, this is characterized by total protein S antigen measurements in the normal range and selectively reduced levels of free protein S and protein S functional activity to less than approximately 40% of normal (Zoller et al., 1994). Interestingly, a case-control study by Zoller in 1995 involving 327 Swedish families showed that type I and type III are phenotypic variants of the same genetic disease.

Protein S deficiency is inherited in an autosomal dominant manner and is at least as common as antithrombin and protein C deficiency (Heijboer et al., 1990). The clinical manifestations are similar to those seen with antithrombin and protein C deficiency. Thrombosis occurs in heterozygotes whose levels of functional protein S are in the range of 15-50% of normal.

The prevalence of familial deficiency of protein S type I among Caucasians, estimated from a large cohort of healthy blood donors from the West of Scotland, is in the range of 0.03 to 0.13 percent (Dykes et al., 2001). The prevalence is much higher among individuals with established thrombophilia.

In a Spanish study of 2,132 consecutive unselected patients with venous thromboembolism, 7.3% had protein S deficiency (Mateo et al., 1997). Based on these and other studies, Martinelli et al. estimated that the life-time probability of developing thrombosis among carriers of protein S deficiency was 8.5 times higher compared to those without thrombosis events.

In 1987, Engesser and colleagues conducted a study on 12 Swedish families with 136 members and found 71 of them to be heterozygous for Type I protein S deficiency. 55% of those who carried the defect were found to have had a thrombotic event and 77% of those were recurrent. About half of the cases were precipitated by another condition. They also showed that in phenotypic protein S deficient families, the likelihood that affected family members remain thrombosis-free at 45 years of age was 35% to 50%. This study showed a difference in rates between men and women but was not able to provide an adequate explanation in terms of difference in risk factors between the two sexes (Engesser et al., 1987).

Another study examined the incidence of thrombosis in carriers in a Swedish family with a known missense mutation ($Gly^{295}Val$) (Simmonds et al., 1998). Simmonds studied 122 members in a family, with 44 of the members previously characterized for the specific gene defect in protein S. The study showed little thrombotic risk before the age of 15 years. On the other hand, the likelihood of being free of thrombosis by age 30 was only 50% compared to 97% in normal family members. The odds ratio for thrombosis in affected subjects was 11.5, and the study showed that measurement of free protein S antigen levels was predictive of the mutation and deficiency. In a UK based family study with 28 index patients with protein S deficiency, first degree relatives with the PROS1 gene defect had a five-fold higher risk of thrombosis than those with a normal gene and no other apparent thrombophilia (Makris et al., 2000).

Overall, both family and cohort studies demonstrate that like other thrombophilic disorders, heterozygous protein S deficiency usually manifests in adulthood with a thromboembolic event. When present with other thrombophilias or when present in the homozygous form, protein S usually presents in neonates with purpura fulminans (Mahasandana et al., 1996).

5.4 Factor V Leiden (F5) G1691A polymorphism

In 1994, Bertina et al. first described a defect in the factor V gene that makes it less susceptible to inactivation by activated protein C (APC) (Bertina et al., 1994). The following year, Kalafatis et al. showed that the mechanism of inactivation of the membrane bound profactor Va is an ordered event. Factor Va is sequentially cleaved at Arg^{506} and at Arg^{306} and Arg^{679} by activated protein C (Kalafatis et al., 1995). They suggested that the peptide bond cleavage at Arg^{506} facilitates the exposure of the subsequent cleavage sites at Arg^{306} and Arg^{679}. At around the same time, Shen and Dahlback et al. showed that factor V is also a cofactor in the inactivation of factor VIIIa by APC (Shen et al., 1994). The understanding of factor V inactivation was almost immediately followed by reports on how activated protein C in patients' plasma failed to prolong the activated partial thromboplastin time, hence the term "activated protein C resistance" was developed (Koster et al., 1993). Further studies have shown that most patients with activated protein C resistance have a factor V allele that is resistant to the proteolytic effect of protein C. A transition (guanine to adenine) at nucleotide 1691 (G1691) results in the replacement of arginine by glutamine. This gene product, called factor V Leiden, also known as factor V Q^{506} or $Arg^{506}Gln$, is named after the city in the Netherlands that it was first identified in. Factor V Leiden is a variant of the normal gene and is not susceptible to cleavage at position 506 by activated protein C. The consequence of this is a hypercoagulable state as more factors Va is available within the prothrombinase complex, thereby increasing the generation of thrombin. Factor V is also thought to be a cofactor, along with protein S, in supporting the role of activated protein C in the degradation of factors Va and VIIIa. Thus, lack of this cleavage product decreases the anticoagulant activity of activated protein C. Several mutations at the Arg^{306} residue in factor V have been described in patients with a history of thrombosis. These include replacement of Arg^{306} with threonine (factor V Cambridge) (Williamson et al., 1998) or with glycine (in Hong Kong Chinese) (Chan et al., 1998).

Occasionally, patients have been described who have heterozygous APC resistance due to the factor V Leiden mutation and type I factor V deficiency (Guasch et al., 1997). The plasma of these individuals manifests severe APC resistance in activated partial thromboplastin time assays, similar to that seen in patients with homozygous factor V Leiden. These patients appear to be more thrombosis prone than their heterozygous relatives with factor V Leiden alone, suggesting that the clinical phenotype is similar to patients who are homozygous for factor V Leiden.

5.4.1 Factor V Leiden mutation and risk of thrombosis

There are multiple studies showing evidence for factor V Leiden as a cause of deep vein thrombosis (DVT) among the Caucasian population. The major clinical manifestation is deep vein thrombosis with or without pulmonary embolism. There is also evidence that the factor V Leiden mutation, presumably due to thrombosis of placental vessels, may play a role in some cases of unexplained recurrent pregnancy loss (Ridker et al., 1997). Svennson and Dahlback et al. studied 34 families with the Factor V506 Arg to Gln mutation and found an increased lifetime risk of venous thrombosis. By age 50, at least 25% of those affected had experienced at least one thrombotic event.

The Leiden Thrombophilia Study by Koster et al. in the Netherlands provided a population-based case-control study to assess the prevalence of this disorder. APC resistance was found in 21% of those who had a history of thromboembolism compared with 5% of controls. Overall, the relative risk for a thromboembolic event was increased seven-fold in heterozygous individuals. They further studied individuals who were homozygous for factor V Leiden mutation and found an 80-fold increase in the lifetime risk for a thrombotic problem. It was subsequently estimated that homozygous individuals can be expected to experience at least one venous thromboembolic event in their lifetime (Koster et al., 1993). This is supported by a study of 306 family members from 50 Swedish families, which found 40% of homozygotes who had an episode of venous thrombosis by age 33, compared to 20% of heterozygotes and 8% of normals. Ridker et al. published a study in 1997 based on 4,047 American men and women The study found a 12% incidence of heterozygosity for the factor V Leiden mutation in patients with a first confirmed DVT or pulmonary embolism compared with 6% in controls (Ridker et al., 1997). The incidence reached 26% in men over the age of 60 with no identifiable precipitating factors.

In conclusion, Factor V Leiden seems to have a milder effect on the development of thrombosis in patients with APS compared with that seen in the general population due to the strong effect of aPL, but Factor V Leiden may in several patients increase the thrombogenic effect of aPL.

5.5 Prothrombin (F2) G20210A mutation

In 1996, Poort et al. described a single aminoacid genetic variation in the 3' untranslated region of the gene that codes for prothrombin. Prothrombin (factor II) is the precursor to thrombin, the end-product of the coagulation cascade. Prothrombin has procoagulant, anticoagulant and antifibrinolytic activities and thus a disorder involving prothrombin results in multiple imbalances in hemostasis. A report published in 1996 based on 28 families from the Netherlands with established venous thromboembolism identified a substitution of guanine to adenine at nucleotide 20210 in the 3'-UTR of the prothrombin gene (Poort et al., 1996). Linkage studies performed in 397 individuals from 21 Spanish families have provided further evidence that a quantitative trait locus (G20210) in the prothrombin gene influences prothrombin activity levels and susceptibility to thrombosis (Soria et al., 2000). The single base pair substitution in F2, termed F2 G20210A, is one of the most common genetic alterations described in thrombophilia. Its prevalence is higher in patients with venous thrombosis (6–18%) when compared with the general population (1–3%) (Poort et al., 1996).

5.5.1 Prothrombin gene mutation and risk of thrombosis

The prothrombin G20210A gene mutation is a common polymorphism associated with an elevated risk of deep venous thrombosis, although to a lesser degree than factor V Leiden is. The Leiden Thrombophilia Study, (a population-based study) demonstrated a prevalence of the prothrombin 20210A allele among healthy carriers of 6.2% among venous thrombosis patients and between 2% - 4% among healthy matched controls.

The initial studies did not show an increased risk of thrombosis related to the G20210A polymorphism in the prothrombin gene in APS patients of Caucassian (Bentolila et al., 1997); (Bertolaccini et al., 1998) or Mexican mestizo origin (Ruiz-Arguelles et al., 1999). However, from the first case of SLE-associated APS in a young female homozygous for the 20210A allele in the prothrombin gene who developed venous thrombosis while taking oral contraceptives (Sivera et al., 2000), several subsequent studies have demonstrated an association between the prothrombin G20210A polymorphim and thrombosis in APS patients. Torresan et al. found in 30 Brazilian patients with APS and thrombosis a higher prevalence of the 20210A allele of the prothrombin gene when compared with controls individuals (5% vs. 0,7%) (Torresan et al., 2000). Similarly, Forastiero et al. found in 105 Caucassian consecutive unselected patients with aPL grouped as having APS (n= 69) and not having APS (n= 36) that the 20210A allele was significantly more frequent in APS patients than in healthy controls subjects (8,7% vs. 2%) (Forastiero et al., 2001). Brouwer et al. in a cohort of 144 consecutive patients with SLE, found that the 20210A allele of the prothrombin gene was an independent risk factor for venous thromboembolism that when presented together with aPL and it increased the risk 30-fold (Brouwer et al., 2004).

Other studies, however, have shown no relationship between prothrombin G20210A polymorphim and thrombosis in APS. In this study of Galli et al. the prevalence of the G20210A polymorphim was evaluated in 145 Caucassian aPL-positive patients and they found no association between the 20210A allele with venous thrombosis (Galli et al., 2000). Similarly, in 157 aPL-positive patients (44% with previous thrombosis), the G20210A polymorphism was not associated with thrombosis (Chopra et al., 2002). Finally, in a recent study (Sallai et al., 2007) in 105 SLE patients, the prothrombin G20210A polymorphism was not associated with thrombosis risk.

6. Minor thrombophilia alterations in antiphospholipid syndrome

Several polymorphisms have been postulated to have the potential to modify the prothrombotic risk in aPL-positive patients. Some of these polymorphisms affect proteins directly related to aPLs, others are related to normal hemostasis components, and, finally, others are related to immune or inflammatory pathways.

6.1 Beta2-glycoprotein I gene polymorphisms

Among the targets of aPL, beta2-glycoprotein I (beta2-GPI), which bears the epitopes for aCL antibody binding, has been extensively studied. It is a glycoprotein of around 50 kDa, found in plasma at a concentration of approximately 200 μg/ml, which makes it one of the most abundant proteins in human serum, second only to fibrinogen among the plasma proteins involved in clotting (McNeil et al., 1990). A member of the short consensus-repeat protein family, beta2-GPI is characterized by five 'sushi-domains'. The fifth sushi-domain contains the binding site to phospholipid, and it attaches to activated cellular surfaces (Wurm, 1984). Although its physiological role is not known, 'in vitro' data suggest that beta2-GPI may play a role in coagulation. It binds to anionic phospholipids and inhibits the contact phase of the intrinsic blood coagulation pathway (Schousboe, 1985), adenosine diphosphate-dependent platelet aggregation (Nimpf et al., 1987), and the prothrombinase activity of human platelets (Nimpf et al., 1986). Although these data imply an anticoagulant role for beta2-GPI, deficiency of this protein is not a clear risk factor for thrombosis. The plasma level of this protein is under genetic control (Cleve, 1968). A study of familial thrombophilia demonstrated that heterozygous partial beta2-GPI deficiency is not associated with the risk of thrombosis (Bancsi et al., 1992). Patients with APS appear to have normal or somewhat elevated levels of beta2-GPI (De Benedetti et al., 1992); (Galli et al., 1992).

Neo- or cryptic- epitopes expressed on beta2-GPI as a result of the beta2-GPI/phopholipids interaction could be a potential antigenic target for the autoimmune type of aCL antibodies. The human beta2-GPI gene (ITGA2B) is mapped on chromosome 17q23-qter with four major polymorphisms (Ser^{88}/Asn, Leu^{247}/Val, Cys^{306}/Gly and Trp^{316}/Ser). Alterations in beta2-GPI properties related to these polymorphisms are not defined. The Leu^{247}/Val polymorphism locates in domain 5 of beta2-GPI which is a potential epitope site for anti-beta2-GPI antibodies (Ichikawa et al., 1994). As a result, polymorphisms on or near the phospholipid binding site or the antigenic site can affect autoantibody production. Hirose et al. (Hirose et al., 1999) found that the valine 247 allele was more frequently detected in Asian patients with APS than in matched normal individuals. Furthermore, it reported an association between the Val^{247}/Val homozygous genotype and the presence of anti-beta2GPI antibodies only among Asian patients with APS. The authors found no evidence of an increased risk of thrombosis in this Asian population. In this same line, we performed a study comparing the distribution of polymorphisms at codons 247 (Val^{247}Leu) and 316 (Trp^{316}Ser) of the β2-GPI gene in a Caucasian Spanish population of Primary APS patients and healthy controls subjects, and then making correlations with the development of anti-β2GPI antibodies and other aPL and associated clinical manifestations. In total, 57 primary APS patients and 100 control subjects were included in our study. In the analysis of Val^{247}Leu polymorphism, alleles (V and L) and genotypes (V/V, V/L, L/L) analyses were similarly distributed in PAPS patients and controls ($P= 0.66$ and $P= 0.22$, respectively).

Regarding $Trp^{316}Ser$ polymorphism, we found a higher percentage of patients with respect to controls subjects expressing S allele (11.4% vs. 5%, P= 0.02) and T/S genotype (22.8% vs. 10%, P= 0.02). However, when we compared T/T and T/S genotypes in primary APS patients, we found no differences regarding generation of anti-β2GPI antibodies, other aPLs and clinical manifestations favoring any genotype. Our findings suggest that among Spanish Caucasians, polymorphisms at codon 247 ($Val^{247}Leu$) do not seem to influence PAPS pathogenesis. On the contrary, polymorphisms at codon 316 ($Trp^{316}Ser$), by means of an increased S allele and T/S genotype presence in Spanish Caucasian patients, might play a role in the pathogenic development of primary APS, although it mechanism would not involve an increased production of anti-beta2-GPI antibodies and other aPLs (Pardos-Gea et al., 2011).

6.2 Tissue factor pathway inhibitor (TFPI T-33C; C-399T)

Several polymorphisms within the tissue factor pathway inhibitor gene (TFPI) may determine TFPI expression and increase the risk of venous thromboembolism (VTE) in predisposed individuals. Lincz et al. (Lincz et al., 2007) tested this hypothesis by comparing TFPI activity and the frequency of common TFPI polymorphisms (T-33C, C-399T and T-287C) or Factor V Leiden in patients with APS who had a history of VTE and compared them with those without VTE and also with normal control individuals. They found that only APS patients with a history of venous thrombosis had TFPI activity levels significantly different from control individuals (1.77 ± 0.60 vs. 0.77 ± 0.19 U/ml; p= 0.0001), and this was associated with inheritance of the TFPI -33C allele (1.70 ± 0.72 U/ml for TC/CC genotypes vs. 0.97 ± 0.56 U/ml for TT; p= 0.01). Multivariate analysis of APS and FVL patients revealed that the greatest independent contributor to VTE was TFPI activity, while inheritance of either the TFPI-33C or -399T alleles each increased the odds of VTE by nearly 13 times. These results indicate that the TFPI T-33C and C-399T polymorphisms are significantly associated with venous thrombosis in the presence of other risk factors, especially in APS, and may be clinically relevant in patients who are prone to hypercoagulability.

6.3 Methylenetetrahydrofolate-reductase (MTHFR) C677T/A1298C

The C677T methylenetetrahydrofolate reductase (MTHFR) polymorphism (thermolabile variant 677TT) has been shown to exert a potential effect on plasma homocysteine levels. At present, this polymorphism is not considered *per se* to be a risk factor for thrombosis (Bertina, 2001) and is recommended to exclude C677T MTHFR polymorphism from the analysis of multiple thrombophilic genotypes. In a series of 152 aPL-positive patients, Galli et al. (Galli et al., 2000) did not find an association between the C677T MTHFR polymorphism alone or in combination with either Factor V Leiden or G20210A prothrombin polymorphisms and thrombosis. Similar results were obtained by Torresan et al. (Torresan et al., 2000) in 30 patients with APS in whom no significant variation was found between the patient group and the controls regarding the prevalence of homozygotes for the mutated 677T allele (2.5% vs. 5.4%), and by Forastiero et al. (Forastiero et al., 2001) in 105 aPL- positive patients in whom the frequencies of the C677T MTHFR alleles were not different either between the aPL groups and normal controls or between APS and non-APS groups. In addition, cerebrovascular disease was not related to homozygous or heterozygous C677T MTHFR polymorphism in 44 primary APS patients (Kalashnikova et al., 2005). Finally, Ames et al. (Ames et al., 2001) also observed that the C677T MTHFR polymorphism was not related to venous thrombosis in 49 aPL-positive subjects, but the homozygous 677TT patients had lower mean age at first event and suffered an increased average number of events per person.

6.4 Thrombomodulin THMD Ala455Val

Thrombomodulin is an integral membrane protein of endothelial cells and monocytes. When thrombin binds to thrombomodulin, it loses its procoagulant activity, but becomes capable of activating PC. Therefore, a hereditary deficiency of thrombomodulin may very well play a role as a risk factor for thrombotic disease. A number of missense mutations are currently known in the thrombomodulin gene (THMD) of patients with venous thrombosis (Norlund et al., 1997). A particular aminoacid dimorphism, $Ala^{455}Val$, was found with frequencies of 0.81/0.18 in Caucasian patients who suffered from thrombophilia (van der Velden et al., 1991). The potential role of THMD mutations in myocardial infarction recently received further support from the documentation of a frame-shift mutation in a family with arterial disease (Kunz et al., 2000).

6.5 Protein C receptor (PROC), and endothelian (EPCR) (PROC 4031ins23)

The recently discovered endothelial protein C receptor (EPCR) on endothelial cells is another important regulator of the PC anticoagulant pathway. A 23-bp insertion at position 4,031 in exon 3 (4031ins23) of the gene encoding EPCR (PROCR) has been identified that may predispose patients to deep venous thrombosis (Biguzzi et al., 1998). Furthermore, mutations in PROCR and THMD have been associated with late fetal loss (Franchi et al., 2001). Given that EPCR plays a role in the anticoagulation system and in placental development, a study from Spain (Hurtado et al., 2004) hypothesized that anti-EPCR autoantibodies may be involved in clinical manifestations of APS and in fetal loss. They found that both IgM and IgG anti-EPCR serum levels were higher among APS patients than in controls (57 vs. 45 AU and 75 vs. 72 AU, respectively). They concluded that anti-EPCR autoantibodies could be detected in APS patients and constituted an independent risk factor for a first fetal death episode for anti-EPCR antibodies IgM (OR: 23; CI 2.0–266.3) and IgG (OR: 6.8; CI 1.2–38.4).

6.6 Polymorphisms in platelet glycoproteins

A Spanish study (Jiménez et al., 2008) analysed the genetic polymorphisms in platelet glycoproteins (GP) Ib-alpha (GP1BA), Ia/IIa (ITGA2) complex and IIb/IIIa (ITGA2B) complex and their correlation with the development of arterial thrombosis and preclinical atherosclerosis in patients with APS or with SLE. Thrombotic events were assessed clinically and confirmed by objective methods. They found a significant correlation between the 807 T/T genotype of ITGA2 and arterial thrombosis (22% in APS patients vs. 7% in controls, P= 0.04; OR: 3.59, CI 1.20–10.79). The variable number tamden repeat (VNTR) GP1BA and PIA1/2 ITGA2B polymorphisms were not associated with arterial thrombosis in patients with APS when they were individually analysed. The coexistence of both ITGA2 807T and ITGA2B PIA2 alleles increased the arterial thrombosis risk (28% vs. 7%, P=0.005; OR: 4.84, CI 1.67–13.96). Interestingly, the coexistence of ITGA2 807T and ITGA2B PIA2 was associated with the presence of carotid plaque (35% vs. 4%, P=0.002; OR: 12.92, CI 2.39–69.81). They concluded that the T/T genotype of the ITGA2 807C/T polymorphism may be an additional risk factor for the development of arterial thrombosis in APS.

6.7 Polymorphisms in platelet Fcγreceptor IIA

Platelet Fc gamma-receptor IIA (FcγRIIA; CD32) molecules are essential for the effect of aPL against beta2-GPI by causing platelet activation, thromboxane A2 generation, and granule release after their binding to the Fc fragments of aPL. Human FcγRIIA reacts best with IgG subclasses 1 and 3, but weakly with subclass 2, which includes the majority of the anti-beta2-GPI seen in autoimmune patients (Arvieux et al., 1994). The His^{131} allele of the $His^{131}Arg$ polymorphism of the FcγRIIA gene reacts much more efficiently than the Arg^{131} allele to IgG subclass 2. Carlsson & Atsumi et al. (Carlsson et al., 1998); (Atsumi et al., 1998) tested whether patients with the His131 allele of the FcγRIIA polymorphism may be at higher risk for developing thrombosis by this platelet activation mechanism. Carlsson et al. and Atsumi et al. studied 100 white patients with aPL and they found that none of the clinical manifestations of primary APS (arterial or venous thrombosis, recurrent pregnancy loss, and thrombocytopenia) was significantly correlated with the $His^{131}Arg$ FcγRIIA polymorphism. However, in a more recent meta-analysis (Karassa et al., 2003) a significant increase in Arg^{131} homozygosity was found in APS patients and the authors suggested a complex genetic background underlying the relationship between the FcγRIIA $Arg^{131}His$ polymorphism and APS as a composite of two different and opposing influences with regard to susceptibility. Unfortunately, the number of APS patients with specific clinical manifestations was too small to reliably assess the effect of the FcγRIIA polymorphism on the risk of vascular thromboses or other APS-related features. More recently (Schallmoser et al., 2005), the $Arg^{131}His$ FcγRIIA polymorphism was evaluated in 73 aPL-positive patients (47 with thrombosis) and an increased frequency of heterozygous patients was associated with thrombosis (OR: 6.76). In this study heterozygosity, rather than Arg^{131} homozygosity, was linked to the clinical manifestations of APS. The authors explained these data by the dual function of the FcγRIIA, namely binding of antibodies to platelets and thereby their activation, and, on the other hand, clearance of antibody-coated platelets by the phagocyte system.

6.8 Tissue plasminogen activator (PLAT) (Alu I/D) and Type-1 plasminogen activator inhibitor (SERPINE1 [4G/5G])

Impaired fibrinolytical outcomes may be one of the pathogenic factors for thrombotic events in patients with antiphospholipid antibodies (aPL). Yasuda et al. investigated the consequences of gene polymorphisms of tissue plasminogen activator (PLAT) and plasminogen activator inhibitor-1 (SERPINE1) in patients positive for aPL (Yasuda et al., 2002). Seventy-seven Japanese and 82 British patients with aPL were examined for an Alu-repeat insertion (I)/deletion (D) polymorphism of PLAT and for the 4G/5G polymorphism in the SERPINE1 promoter. Correlations between these polymorphisms and clinical symptoms of APS (arterial thrombosis, venous thrombosis, miscarriage) were analysed. No significant differences in the allele frequencies of these genes between patients and controls were found. There was no significant correlation between these gene polymorphisms and clinical symptoms of APS in patients with aPL antibodies. Therefore, polymorphisms of PLAT or SERPINE1 probably do not significantly influence the risk of arterial/venous thrombosis, or pregnancy morbidity in patients with aPL antibodies.

The effect of the 4G/5G polymorphism of SERPINE1 on the risk of venous thromboembolism (VTE) remains controversial. In a recent meta-analysis, Tsantes et al. investigated the association between the SERPINE1 4G/5G polymorphism and the risk of venous thromboembolism (VTE) in 18 papers; it included patients without another known risk factor, and comprised 2,644 cases and 3,739 controls. Based on their findings, the SERPINE1 4G allele appears to increase the risk of venous thrombosis, particularly in subjects with other genetic thrombophilic defects (Tsantes et al., 2007).

6.9 Coagulation factor XIII, A subunit (F13A1) (Val34Leu)

Diz-Kucukkaya et al. found that a polymorphism ($Val^{34}Leu$) in the factor XIIIA gene (F13A1) decreased the risk of both arterial and venous thrombosis (Diz-Kucukkaya et al., 2007). Nevertheless, the results showed that the F13A1 Leu^{34} allele had no protective effect in the development of thrombosis in patients with APS. On the contrary, De la Red et al. found that this polymorphism was associated with a higher risk of thrombosis in patients with the presence of both aPL antibodies and high fibrinogen levels (de la Red et al., 2009). They found no significant differences in F13A1 Leu^{34} allele frequencies between primary APS, APS/SLE, SLE-aPL and asymptomatic-aPL patients, or between patients with and without thrombosis. In this study, the F13A1 Leu^{34} allele seemed to have a protective effect on the development of thrombosis in patients with aPL antibodies, but only in those patients with high plasma fibrinogen values.

6.10 Annexin 5 (ANXA5 -1C – T)

Another study (de Laat et al., 2006) on the ANXA5 polymorphism (ANXA5 -1C–T) and the presence of antiannexin A5 antibodies in APS concluded that the detection of anti-annexin A5 antibodies does not seem relevant for estimating the risk for thrombosis or miscarriage in APS. The -1C–T mutation was an independent risk factor for miscarriage which is independent of APS.

6.11 P-selectin glycoprotein ligand-1 (SELPG) gene polymorphisms

Diz-Kucukkaya et al. studied the gene encoding P-selectin glycoprotein ligand-1 (SELPG) and showed that a variable number tandem repeats (VNTR) polymorphism on this gene is a significant determinant of thrombosis predisposition in patients with APS. Furthermore, this risk appears to correlate better with the combination of alleles inherited rather than with the presence of any particular allele (Diz-Kucukkaya et al., 2007).

6.12 CD40 ligand (CD154) gene polymorphisms

Increased levels of soluble CD154 have been described in various inflammatory disorders, particularly SLE. A polymorphic CA repeat sequence has been identified in the 3-UTR of the CD154 gene. The larger alleles of this CA repeat are more frequent in SLE patients and are also associated with a prolonged protein expression on T lymphocytes (Citores et al., 2004). In a recent study in 107 aPL-positive patients, Bugert et al. found than the CA repeat polymorphism in the 3-UTR of CD154 was associated with the development of arterial thrombosis (applying the dominant model and considering CD154 genotype exclusively containing alleles with 24 CA repeats, OR: 4.04) but not with venous thrombosis (Bugert et al., 2007).

6.13 TNF-alpha gene polymorphisms

Bertolaccini et al. explored in 83 Caucasoid patients with APS the possible involvement of the proinflammatory and prothrombotic cytokine tumor necrosis factor-alpha (TNF-α) and observed that the presence of the -238*A genotype in the promoter region of the TNF-alpha gene was more frequent in APS patients with arterial thrombosis and pregnancy loss than in controls (OR: 3.7 [95% CI 1.37-10.1], p= 0.007 and OR: 3.95 [95% CI 1.3-11.7], p= 0.01; respectively). HLA-DQB1*0303-DRB1*0701 haplotype was associated with TNFA -238*A in the control group (OR 96.0 [95% CI 9.6-959], p <0.0001) as well as in APS patient's group (OR 54.2 [95% CI 9.6-306.5], p <0.0001) (Bertolaccini et al., 2001).

6.14 Angiotensin-converting enzyme (ACE) gene polymorphisms

Evaluating the reported association between the D allele of the insertion (I)/deletion (D) polymorphism in the ACE gene and the occurrence of arterial thrombosis in coronary heart disease and stroke, Lewis et al. studied in 93 patients with APS whether this polymorphism could be an additional risk factor for arterial thrombosis. The distribution of the alleles was not significantly different between the patients with a history of arterial thrombosis and those without, although an unexpected skewing from DD to II was seen in patients older than 45 years in association with arterial thrombosis (Lewis et al., 2000).

6.15 Mannose-binding lectin (MBL) gene polymorphisms

Innate immunity is the first-line defense against pathogens. Among the components of innate immunity, mannose-binding lectin (MBL) and toll-like receptor 4 polymorphisms have been related to APS clinical manifestations. MBL is a liver-derived serum protein that binds to sugars on the surface of pathogenic microorganisms and triggers complement. Serum levels of MBL are associated with MBL gene polymorphisms. In 91 Caucassian patients with SLE MBL variant alleles were evaluated and a statistically significant association was found between the deficient homozygous 0/0 MBL genotype and the development of arterial thrombosis (OR: 5.8), but not venous thrombosis, mainly due to the strong association between this genotype and myocardial infarction (Ohlenschlaeger et al., 2004). However, MBL polymorphisms were not specifically evaluated in the APS subgroup. Font et al. studied MBL polymorphisms in a series of 114 Caucassian SLE patients (Font et al., 2007) and found that MBL-low genotypes showed a closer association with venous rather than arterial thrombosis. This fact probably is due to the different MBL alleles analyzed (0/XA and XA/XA were also included as deficient alleles) and/or to the varying prevalence of thrombotic events. In addition, in 53 patients with SLE, Seelen et al. reported that the presence of aCL was significantly associated with the variant alleles of MBL gene polymorphisms and they hypothesized that an enhanced production of autoantibodies may be related to disturbed clearance of apoptotic material due to impaired MBL function (Seelen et al., 2005). Additional contradictory results have been found in non-APS patients. In several different ethnic origin SLE patients, Calvo-Alen et al. found no differences in arterial thrombosis in patients homozygous for MBL-deficient alleles compared with non-SLE individuals (Calvo-Alen et al., 2006). Similar results were seen within ethnic groups, except for Caucassian patients in whom a statistically significant higher frequency of MBL-deficient alleles was found in those with cerebrovascular events. In a Japanese population, Takahashi et al. did not find a relationship between MBL alleles and the risk of arterial thrombosis. These results point out the need to bear in mind the importance of the differences in the genetic substrate among the ethnic group when evaluating the influence of genetic polymorphisms in APS clinical expression (Takahashi et al., 2005).

6.16 Toll-like receptor 4 (TLR4) polymorphisms

TLR4 belongs to the family of transmembrane receptors whose activation leads to induction of various genes and production of proinflammatory cytokines. Polymorphisms within TLR4 genes result in an altered susceptibility to infectious or inflammatory diseases. In 110 Caucassian patients with APS with arterial and/or venous thrombosis, Pierangeli et al. evaluated whether the two co-segregating TLR4 polymorphisms $Asp^{299}Gly$ and $Thr^{399}Ile$ are involved in aPL-mediated thrombosis. This study showed that the frequency of TLR4 Gly^{299} and Ile^{399} alleles in APS patients was significantly reduced in comparison to healthy controls (Pierangeli et al., 2007).

7. Limitations of genetics studies in antiphospholipid syndrome

Interpretation of the results from epidemiological and genetic studies in various ethnic populations is quite difficult for the following reasons:

1. Although the enzyme linked immunosorbent assay (ELISA) for aCL antibodies and LAC testing has been extensively standardised, significant variation between laboratories still remains. The precise cut-off points for positive/negative results vary among laboratories over the world.
2. Clinical heterogeneity: the clinical definition of APS has varied among studies. Some patients with APS also manifest SLE, and constitute a heterogeneous population, making it difficult to analyse the role of a single factor. With the publication of the Sapporo criteria for the preliminary classification criteria for definite APS this problem will be solved with studies done on more uniform patient groups.
3. Interethnic variation in the associations of aPL with thrombosis or pregnancy loss must also take into account the multiple risk factors that exist in most populations for these complications. Possibly, variation in such collateral risk factors—for example, drug use or genetic risk factors for thrombosis may influence complication rates associated with aPL in various populations. For instance, in Lebanon, a high prevalence of prothrombin G20210A and factor V Leiden mutations exist. These factors will increase the thrombotic risk, especially in patients with aPL.
4. Disease activity: the level of disease activity is an important factor to control for in future studies. In early studies in the African-American clinic population in New Orleans it was found that IgG aCL were present in 27% of patients with SLE during periods of disease activity, compared with only 5% of patients with SLE during periods of less active SLE (Wilson et al. 1988).
5. Geographical migration: with the current increasing geographical migration and intermingling across geographical and ethnic groups, it is important to consider these variables in the interpretation of future studies.

8. Future directions

One of the first questions that come to mind when a patient receives the diagnosis of APS is whether we can predict which patients with aPL antibodies will develop thromboembolic events or obstetric complications during her/him life-time as well an if there is an inherited predisposition to developing APS. There is obviously the most important question: "what is the course of the disease?" Identifying and understanding the causes of APS will likely lead to the identification of the major risk factors, the design of prevention strategies of thrombosis and obstetric complications and the development of targeted therapies with increased efficacy and minimal toxicity. No one knows the precise causes of APS (and there will likely be many that may differ among individuals), but there is strong evidence supporting a role for both genetics and infectious and non-infectious environmental factors. Current research has played an important role in the discovery of potential factors that influence its susceptibility. Ongoing research should lead to the further identification and understanding of both genetic and acquired factors that play a role in the development of APS. At this moment several 'Genome-Wide Association Studies' (GWAS) are underway in other autoimmune diseases such as systemic lupus erythematosus, rheumatoid arthritis, multiples sclerosis, Type 1 diabetes, and so on in which up to a million SNPs are tested in association studies. It is likely that these will add to the list of common and weak genetic risk factors. Individually, these risk factors have no clinical utility at all. It is possible; however, that comprehensive knowledge of all genetic risk factors in an individual may lead to relevant risks.

Nevertheless, it should be noted, that many acquired risk factors confer much higher risks that the genetic variants associated with thrombosis and obstetric complications in patients with APS. As these are often transient, they offer the best opportunity to reduce the burden of thrombosis and recurrent pregnancy losses by improved and individualized anticoagulant prophylaxis.

Family studies with GWAS using microsatellites are ongoing, and in the near future we will probably know which are the other DNA regions containing the susceptibility loci for APS.

The APS Clinical Research Task Force (CRTF) was one of the six Task Forces developed by the 13th International Congress on Antiphospholipid Antibodies organization committee recently held in Galveston, Texas, USA in April 2010 (Erkan et al., 2011) with the purpose of:

a. Evaluating the limitations of APS clinical research and developing guidelines for researchers to help improve the quality of APS research; and
b. Prioritizing the ideas for a well-designed multicenter clinical trial and discussing the pragmatics of getting such a trial done.

Following a systemic working algorithm, the Task Force identified five major issues that impede APS clinical research and the ability to develop evidence-based recommendations for the management of aPL-positive patients:

1. The aPLs detection has been based on partially or non-standardized tests, and clinical (and basic) APS research studies have included patients with heterogeneous aPL profiles with different clinical event risks;
2. Clinical (and basic) APS research studies have included a heterogeneous group of patients with different aPL-related manifestations (some controversial);
3. Thrombosis and/or pregnancy loss risk stratification and quantification are rarely incorporated in APS clinical research;
4. Most APS clinical studies include patients with single positive aPL results and/or low-titer aPLs ELISA results; furthermore, study designs are mostly retrospective and not

population based, with limited number of prospective and/or controlled population studies; and

5. Lack of the understanding of the particular mechanisms of aPL-mediated clinical events limits the optimal clinical study design.

The Task Force stated that there is an urgent need for a truly international collaboration approach to design and conduct well-designed prospective large-scale multicenter clinical trials of patients with persistent and clinically significant aPL profiles.

Notwithstanding the progress made over the last 15 years, APS remains poorly understood and have attracted the interest of many medical specialties including internal medicine, haematology, clinical immunology, rheumatology, and gynaecology.

9. Conclusions

APS is still seen as a rather obscure disease despite extensive research; this view is mainly the result of the unreliability of the current assays for detecting the presence of aPL. The consequences are a poor correlation between serological markers and clinical manifestations, and a lack of clarity about the pathogenetic mechanism causing the syndrome. Genetic susceptibility related to aPL and APS has been extensively examined during the last years. However, it has been difficult to determine genetic risk factors because of the heterogeneity in the antigen specificity and the pathogenesis of clinical manifestations related to APS. It is becoming increasingly clear that interactions between more than one genetic abnormality or between a genetic factor and environment components determine whether and when an individual will suffer from thrombosis. Given the fact that APS is characterized mainly by the presence of thromboembolic events, it seems perfectly plausible that several genetic factors may also be involved in its pathophysiology. Genome-wide linkage analysis and larger cohort cases-controls association studies, as well as multicenter international collaborations, would be useful to obtain a better understanding of the genetic predisposition which produces aPL and leads to the development of the clinical features of APS. As more genes responsible for these effects can be identified, a clearer understanding of the pathogenesis of this syndrome will be achieved, which undoubtedly will lead to more useful and safer therapeutic strategies.

10. References

Ahmed, S.A., & Verthelyi, D. (1993). Antibodies to cardiolipin in normal C57BL/6J mice: induction by estrogen but not dihydrotestosterone. *J Autoimmun* 6, 265-279.

Ames, P.R., Margaglione, M., Tommasino, C., Bossone, A., Iannaccone, L., & Brancaccio, V. (2001). Impact of plasma homocysteine and prothrombin G20210 A on primary antiphospholipid syndrome. *Blood Coagul Fibrinolysis* 12, 699-704.

Arnett, F.C., Olsen, M.L., Anderson, K.L., & Reveille, J.D. (1991). Molecular analysis of major histocompatibility complex alleles associated with the lupus anticoagulant. *J Clin Invest* 87, 1490-1495.

Arvieux, J., Roussel, B., Ponard, D., & Colomb, M.G. (1994). IgG2 subclass restriction of anti-beta 2 glycoprotein 1 antibodies in autoimmune patients. *Clin Exp Immunol* 95, 310-315.

Asherson, R.A., Doherty, D.G., Vergani, D., Khamashta, M.A., & Hughes, G.R. (1992). Major histocompatibility complex associations with primary antiphospholipid syndrome. *Arthritis Rheum* 35, 124-125.

Atsumi, T., Caliz, R., Amengual, O., Khamashta, M.A., & Hughes, G.R. (1998). Fcgamma receptor IIA H/R131 polymorphism in patients with antiphospholipid antibodies. *Thromb Haemost* 79, 924-927.

Atsumi, T., Tsutsumi, A., Amengual, O., Khamashta, M.A., Hughes, G.R., Miyoshi, Y., Ichikawa, K., & Koike, T. (1999). Correlation between beta2-glycoprotein I valine/leucine247 polymorphism and anti-beta2-glycoprotein I antibodies in patients with primary antiphospholipid syndrome. *Rheumatology (Oxford)* 38, 721-723.

Bancsi, L.F., van der Linden, I.K., & Bertina, R.M. (1992). Beta 2-glycoprotein I deficiency and the risk of thrombosis. *Thromb Haemost* 67, 649-653.

Bentolila, S., Ripoll, L., Drouet, L., Crassard, I., Tournier-Lasserve, E., & Piette, J.C. (1997). Lack of association between thrombosis in primary antiphospholipid syndrome and the recently described thrombophilic 3'-untranslated prothrombin gene polymorphism. *Thromb Haemost* 78, 1415.

Bertina, R.M. (2001). Genetic approach to thrombophilia. *Thromb Haemost* 86, 92-103.

Bertina, R.M., Koeleman, B.P., Koster, T., Rosendaal, F.R., Dirven, R.J., de Ronde, H., van der Velden, P.A., & Reitsma, P.H. (1994). Mutation in blood coagulation factor V associated with resistance to activated protein C. *Nature* 369, 64-67.

Bertolaccini, M.L., Atsumi, T., Caliz, A.R., Amengual, O., Khamashta, M.A., Hughes, G.R., & Koike, T. (2000). Association of antiphosphatidylserine/prothrombin autoantibodies with HLA class II genes. *Arthritis Rheum* 43, 683-688.

Bertolaccini, M.L., Atsumi, T., Hunt, B.J., Amengual, O., Khamashta, M.A., & Hughes, G.R. (1998). Prothrombin mutation is not associated with thrombosis in patients with antiphospholipid syndrome. *Thromb Haemost* 80, 202-203.

Bertolaccini, M.L., Atsumi, T., Lanchbury, J.S., Caliz, A.R., Katsumata, K., Vaughan, R.W., Kondeatis, E., Khamashta, M.A., Koike, T., & Hughes, G.R. (2001). Plasma tumor necrosis factor alpha levels and the -238*A promoter polymorphism in patients with antiphospholipid syndrome. *Thromb Haemost* 85, 198-203.

Bertolaccini, M.L., & Khamashta, M.A. (2006). Laboratory diagnosis and management challenges in the antiphospholipid syndrome. *Lupus* 15, 172-178.

Biguzzi, E., Mozzi, E., Alatri, A., Taioli, E., Moia, M., & Mannucci, P.M. (1998). The post-thrombotic syndrome in young women: retrospective evaluation of prognostic factors. *Thromb Haemost* 80, 575-577.

Bovill, E.G., Bauer, K.A., Dickerman, J.D., Callas, P., & West, B. (1989). The clinical spectrum of heterozygous protein C deficiency in a large New England kindred. *Blood* 73, 712-717.

Broekmans, A.W. (1985). Hereditary protein C deficiency. *Haemostasis* 15, 233-240.

Broekmans, A.W., Bertina, R.M., Reinalda-Poot, J., Engesser, L., Muller, H.P., Leeuw, J.A., Michiels, J.J., Brommer, E.J., & Briet, E. (1985). Hereditary protein S deficiency and venous thrombo-embolism. A study in three Dutch families. *Thromb Haemost* 53, 273-277.

Broekmans, A.W., Veltkamp, J.J., & Bertina, R.M. (1983). Congenital protein C deficiency and venous thromboembolism. A study of three Dutch families. *N Engl J Med* 309, 340-344.

Brouwer, J.L., Bijl, M., Veeger, N.J., Kluin-Nelemans, H.C., & van der Meer, J. (2004). The contribution of inherited and acquired thrombophilic defects, alone or combined with antiphospholipid antibodies, to venous and arterial thromboembolism in patients with systemic lupus erythematosus. *Blood* 104, 143-148.

Bugert, P., Pabinger, I., Stamer, K., Vormittag, R., Skeate, R.C., Wahi, M.M., & Panzer, S. (2007). The risk for thromboembolic disease in lupus anticoagulant patients due to pathways involving P-selectin and CD154. *Thromb Haemost* 97, 573-580.

Caliz, R., Atsumi, T., Kondeatis, E., Amengual, O., Khamashta, M.A., Vaughan, R.W., Lanchbury, J.S., & Hughes, G.R. (2001). HLA class II gene polymorphisms in antiphospholipid syndrome: haplotype analysis in 83 Caucasoid patients. *Rheumatology (Oxford)* 40, 31-36.

Calvo-Alen, J., Alarcon, G.S., Tew, M.B., Tan, F.K., McGwin, G., Jr., Fessler, B.J., Vila, L.M., & Reveille, J.D. (2006). Systemic lupus erythematosus in a multiethnic US cohort: XXXIV. Deficient mannose-binding lectin exon 1 polymorphisms are associated with cerebrovascular but not with other arterial thrombotic events. *Arthritis Rheum* 54, 1940-1945.

Carlsson, L.E., Santoso, S., Baurichter, G., Kroll, H., Papenberg, S., Eichler, P., Westerdaal, N.A., Kiefel, V., van de Winkel, J.G., & Greinacher, A. (1998). Heparin-induced thrombocytopenia: new insights into the impact of the FcgammaRIIa-R-H131 polymorphism. *Blood* 92, 1526-1531.

Chan, W.P., Lee, C.K., Kwong, Y.L., Lam, C.K., & Liang, R. (1998). A novel mutation of Arg306 of factor V gene in Hong Kong Chinese. *Blood* 91, 1135-1139.

Chan, Y.C., Valenti, D., Mansfield, A.O., & Stansby, G. (2000). Warfarin induced skin necrosis. *Br J Surg* 87, 266-272.

Chopra, N., Koren, S., Greer, W.L., Fortin, P.R., Rauch, J., Fortin, I., Senecal, J.L., Docherty, P., & Hanly, J.G. (2002). Factor V Leiden, prothrombin gene mutation, and thrombosis risk in patients with antiphospholipid antibodies. *J Rheumatol* 29, 1683-1688.

Citores, M.J., Rua-Figueroa, I., Rodriguez-Gallego, C., Durantez, A., Garcia-Laorden, M.I., Rodriguez-Lozano, C., Rodriguez-Perez, J.C., Vargas, J.A., & Perez-Aciego, P. (2004). The dinucleotide repeat polymorphism in the 3'UTR of the CD154 gene has a functional role on protein expression and is associated with systemic lupus erythematosus. *Ann Rheum Dis* 63, 310-317.

Cleve, H. (1968). [Genetic studies on the deficiency of beta 2-glycoprotein I of human serum]. *Humangenetik* 5, 294-304.

Clouse, L.H., & Comp, P.C. (1986). The regulation of hemostasis: the protein C system. *N Engl J Med* 314, 1298-1304.

De Benedetti, E., Reber, G., Miescher, P.A., & de Moerloose, P. (1992). No increase of beta 2-glycoprotein I levels in patients with antiphospholipid antibodies. *Thromb Haemost* 68, 624.

de la Red, G., Tassies, D., Espinosa, G., Monteagudo, J., Bove, A., Plaza, J., Cervera, R., & Reverter, J.C. (2009). Factor XIII-A subunit Val34Leu polymorphism is associated with the risk of thrombosis in patients with antiphospholipid antibodies and high fibrinogen levels. *Thromb Haemost* 101, 312-316.

de Laat, B., Derksen, R.H., Mackie, I.J., Roest, M., Schoormans, S., Woodhams, B.J., de Groot, P.G., & van Heerde, W.L. (2006). Annexin A5 polymorphism (-1C-->T) and the presence of anti-annexin A5 antibodies in the antiphospholipid syndrome. *Ann Rheum Dis* 65, 1468-1472.

De Stefano, V., Finazzi, G., & Mannucci, P.M. (1996). Inherited thrombophilia: pathogenesis, clinical syndromes, and management. *Blood* 87, 3531-3544.

Diz-Kucukkaya, R., Inanc, M., Afshar-Kharghan, V., Zhang, Q.E., Lopez, J.A., & Pekcelen, Y. (2007). P-selectin glycoprotein ligand-1 VNTR polymorphisms and risk of thrombosis in the antiphospholipid syndrome. *Ann Rheum Dis* 66, 1378-1380.

Dykes, A.C., Walker, I.D., McMahon, A.D., Islam, S.I., & Tait, R.C. (2001). A study of Protein S antigen levels in 3788 healthy volunteers: influence of age, sex and hormone use, and estimate for prevalence of deficiency state. *Br J Haematol* 113, 636-641.

Engesser, L., Broekmans, A.W., Briet, E., Brommer, E.J., & Bertina, R.M. (1987). Hereditary protein S deficiency: clinical manifestations. *Ann Intern Med* 106, 677-682.

Erkan, D., Derksen, R., Levy, R., Machin, S., Ortel, T., Pierangeli, S., Roubey, R., & Lockshin, M. (2011). Antiphospholipid Syndrome Clinical Research Task Force report. *Lupus* 20, 219-224.

Exner, T., Barber, S., Kronenberg, H., & Rickard, K.A. (1980). Familial association of the lupus anticoagulant. *Br J Haematol* 45, 89-96.

Font, J., Ramos-Casals, M., Brito-Zeron, P., Nardi, N., Ibanez, A., Suarez, B., Jimenez, S., Tassies, D., Garcia-Criado, A., Ros, E., Sentis, J., Reverter, J.C., & Lozano, F. (2007). Association of mannose-binding lectin gene polymorphisms with antiphospholipid syndrome, cardiovascular disease and chronic damage in patients with systemic lupus erythematosus. *Rheumatology (Oxford)* 46, 76-80.

Forastiero, R., Martinuzzo, M., Adamczuk, Y., Varela, M.L., Pombo, G., & Carreras, L.O. (2001). The combination of thrombophilic genotypes is associated with definite antiphospholipid syndrome. *Haematologica* 86, 735-741.

Ford, P.M., Brunet, D., Lillicrap, D.P., & Ford, S.E. (1990). Premature stroke in a family with lupus anticoagulant and antiphospholipid antibodies. *Stroke* 21, 66-71.

Foster, D.C., Yoshitake, S., & Davie, E.W. (1985). The nucleotide sequence of the gene for human protein C. *Proc Natl Acad Sci U S A* 82, 4673-4677.

Franchi, F., Biguzzi, E., Cetin, I., Facchetti, F., Radaelli, T., Bozzo, M., Pardi, G., & Faioni, E.M. (2001). Mutations in the thrombomodulin and endothelial protein C receptor genes in women with late fetal loss. *Br J Haematol* 114, 641-646.

Freitas, M.V., da Silva, L.M., Deghaide, N.H., Donadi, E.A., & Louzada-Junior, P. (2004). Is HLA class II susceptibility to primary antiphospholipid syndrome different from susceptibility to secondary antiphospholipid syndrome? *Lupus* 13, 125-131.

Galeazzi, M., Sebastiani, G.D., Tincani, A., Piette, J.C., Allegri, F., Morozzi, G., Bellisai, F., Scorza, R., Ferrara, G.B., Carcassi, C., Font, J., Passiu, G., Smolen, J., Papasteriades, C., Houssiau, F., Nebro, A.F., Ramon Garrido, E.D., Jedryka-Goral, A., & Marcolongo, R. (2000). HLA class II alleles associations of anticardiolipin and anti-beta2GPI antibodies in a large series of European patients with systemic lupus erythematosus. *Lupus* 9, 47-55.

Galli, M., Cortelazzo, S., Daldossi, M., & Barbui, T. (1992). Increased levels of beta 2-glycoprotein I (aca-Cofactor) in patients with lupus anticoagulant. *Thromb Haemost* 67, 386.

Galli, M., Finazzi, G., Duca, F., Norbis, F., & Moia, M. (2000). The G1691 --> A mutation of factor V, but not the G20210 --> A mutation of factor II or the C677 --> T mutation of methylenetetrahydrofolate reductase genes, is associated with venous thrombosis in patients with lupus anticoagulants. *Br J Haematol* 108, 865-870.

Gandrille, S., Borgel, D., Eschwege-Gufflet, V., Aillaud, M., Dreyfus, M., Matheron, C., Gaussem, P., Abgrall, J.F., Jude, B., Sie, P., & et al. (1995). Identification of 15 different candidate causal point mutations and three polymorphisms in 19 patients with protein S deficiency using a scanning method for the analysis of the protein S active gene. *Blood* 85, 130-138.

Gandrille, S., Borgel, D., Sala, N., Espinosa-Parrilla, Y., Simmonds, R., Rezende, S., Lind, B., Mannhalter, C., Pabinger, I., Reitsma, P.H., Formstone, C., Cooper, D.N., Saito, H., Suzuki, K., Bernardi, F., & Aiach, M. (2000). Protein S deficiency: a database of mutations--summary of the first update. *Thromb Haemost* 84, 918.

Goel, N., Ortel, T.L., Bali, D., Anderson, J.P., Gourley, I.S., Smith, H., Morris, C.A., DeSimone, M., Branch, D.W., Ford, P., Berdeaux, D., Roubey, R.A., Kostyu, D.D., Kingsmore, S.F., Thiel, T., Amos, C., & Seldin, M.F. (1999). Familial antiphospholipid antibody syndrome: criteria for disease and evidence for autosomal dominant inheritance. *Arthritis Rheum* 42, 318-327.

Goldberg, S.N., Conti-Kelly, A.M., & Greco, T.P. (1995). A family study of anticardiolipin antibodies and associated clinical conditions. *Am J Med* 99, 473-479.

Greer, I.A. (2003). Inherited thrombophilia and venous thromboembolism. *Best Pract Res Clin Obstet Gynaecol* 17, 413-425.

Guasch, J.F., Lensen, R.P., & Bertina, R.M. (1997). Molecular characterization of a type I quantitative factor V deficiency in a thrombosis patient that is "pseudo homozygous" for activated protein C resistance. *Thromb Haemost* 77, 252-257.

Hashimoto, Y., Kawamura, M., Ichikawa, K., Suzuki, T., Sumida, T., Yoshida, S., Matsuura, E., Ikehara, S., & Koike, T. (1992). Anticardiolipin antibodies in NZW x BXSB F1 mice. A model of antiphospholipid syndrome. *J Immunol* 149, 1063-1068.

Heijboer, H., Brandjes, D.P., Buller, H.R., Sturk, A., & ten Cate, J.W. (1990). Deficiencies of coagulation-inhibiting and fibrinolytic proteins in outpatients with deep-vein thrombosis. *N Engl J Med* 323, 1512-1516.

Hirose, N., Williams, R., Alberts, A.R., Furie, R.A., Chartash, E.K., Jain, R.I., Sison, C., Lahita, R.G., Merrill, J.T., Cucurull, E., Gharavi, A.E., Sammaritano, L.R., Salmon, J.E., Hashimoto, S., Sawada, T., Chu, C.C., Gregersen, P.K., & Chiorazzi, N. (1999). A role for the polymorphism at position 247 of the beta2-glycoprotein I gene in the generation of anti-beta2-glycoprotein I antibodies in the antiphospholipid syndrome. *Arthritis Rheum* 42, 1655-1661.

Hoffman, R. (2000). Hematology: Basic Principles and Practice, Churchill Livingstone.

Horita, T., & Merrill, J.T. (2004). Genetics of antiphospholipid syndrome. *Curr Rheumatol Rep* 6, 458-462.

Hurtado, V., Montes, R., Gris, J.C., Bertolaccini, M.L., Alonso, A., Martinez-Gonzalez, M.A., Khamashta, M.A., Fukudome, K., Lane, D.A., & Hermida, J. (2004). Autoantibodies against EPCR are found in antiphospholipid syndrome and are a risk factor for fetal death. *Blood* 104, 1369-1374.

Ichikawa, K., Khamashta, M.A., Koike, T., Matsuura, E., & Hughes, G.R. (1994). beta 2-Glycoprotein I reactivity of monoclonal anticardiolipin antibodies from patients with the antiphospholipid syndrome. *Arthritis Rheum* 37, 1453-1461.

Iguchi, S., Kazama, J.J., Ito, S., Shimada, H., Nishi, S., Gejyo, F., Higuchi, W., & Fuse, I. (2002). Combined Ala601-Thr-type dysplasminogenaemia and antiphospholipid antibody syndrome in a patient with recurrent thrombosis. *Thromb Res* 105, 513-517.

Jimenez, S., Tassies, D., Espinosa, G., Garcia-Criado, A., Plaza, J., Monteagudo, J., Cervera, R., & Reverter, J.C. (2008). Double heterozygosity polymorphisms for platelet glycoproteins Ia/IIa and IIb/IIIa increases arterial thrombosis and arteriosclerosis in patients with the antiphospholipid syndrome or with systemic lupus erythematosus. *Ann Rheum Dis* 67, 835-840.

Kalafatis, M., Bertina, R.M., Rand, M.D., & Mann, K.G. (1995). Characterization of the molecular defect in factor VR506Q. *J Biol Chem* 270, 4053-4057.

Kalashnikova, L.A., Dobrynina, L.A., Patrusheva, N.L., Kovalenko, T.F., Patrushev, L.I., Aleksandrova, E.N., Berkovskii, A.L., Sergeeva, E.V., & Nasonov, E.L. (2005). [Mutations of genes associated with thromboses in ischemic stroke in patients with primary antiphospholipid syndrome]. *Ter Arkh* 77, 49-53.

Karassa, F.B., Bijl, M., Davies, K.A., Kallenberg, C.G., Khamashta, M.A., Manger, K., Michel, M., Piette, J.C., Salmon, J.E., Song, Y.W., Tsuchiya, N., Yoo, D.H., & Ioannidis, J.P. (2003). Role of the Fcgamma receptor IIA polymorphism in the antiphospholipid syndrome: an international meta-analysis. *Arthritis Rheum* 48, 1930-1938.

Khan, S., & Dickerman, J.D. (2006). Hereditary thrombophilia. *Thromb J* 4, 15.

Koster, T., Rosendaal, F.R., de Ronde, H., Briet, E., Vandenbroucke, J.P., & Bertina, R.M. (1993). Venous thrombosis due to poor anticoagulant response to activated protein C: Leiden Thrombophilia Study. *Lancet* 342, 1503-1506.

Kuhle, S., Lane, D.A., Jochmanns, K., Male, C., Quehenberger, P., Lechner, K., & Pabinger, I. (2001). Homozygous antithrombin deficiency type II (99 Leu to Phe mutation) and childhood thromboembolism. *Thromb Haemost* 86, 1007-1011.

Kunz, G., Ireland, H.A., Stubbs, P.J., Kahan, M., Coulton, G.C., & Lane, D.A. (2000). Identification and characterization of a thrombomodulin gene mutation coding for an elongated protein with reduced expression in a kindred with myocardial infarction. *Blood* 95, 569-576.

Lane, D.A., Mannucci, P.M., Bauer, K.A., Bertina, R.M., Bochkov, N.P., Boulyjenkov, V., Chandy, M., Dahlback, B., Ginter, E.K., Miletich, J.P., Rosendaal, F.R., & Seligsohn, U. (1996). Inherited thrombophilia: Part 1. *Thromb Haemost* 76, 651-662.

Lensen, R.P., Rosendaal, F.R., Koster, T., Allaart, C.F., de Ronde, H., Vandenbroucke, J.P., Reitsma, P.H., & Bertina, R.M. (1996). Apparent different thrombotic tendency in patients with factor V Leiden and protein C deficiency due to selection of patients. *Blood* 88, 4205-4208.

Lewis, N.M., Katsumata, K., Atsumi, T., Sanchez, M.L., Romero, F.I., Bertolaccini, M.L., Funke, A., Amengual, O., Khamashta, M.A., & Hughes, G.R. (2000). An evaluation of an angiotensin-converting enzyme gene polymorphism and the risk of arterial thrombosis in patients with the antiphospholipid syndrome. *Arthritis Rheum* 43, 1655-1656.

Lincz, L.F., Adams, M.J., Scorgie, F.E., Thom, J., Baker, R.I., & Seldon, M. (2007). Polymorphisms of the tissue factor pathway inhibitor gene are associated with venous thromboembolism in the antiphospholipid syndrome and carriers of factor V Leiden. *Blood Coagul Fibrinolysis* 18, 559-564.

Lulli, P., Sebastiani, G.D., Trabace, S., Passiu, G., Cappellacci, S., Porzio, F., Morellini, M., Cutrupi, F., & Galeazzi, M. (1991). HLA antigens in Italian patients with systemic lupus erythematosus: evidence for the association of DQw2 with the autoantibody response to extractable nuclear antigens. *Clin Exp Rheumatol* 9, 475-479.

Mackworth-Young, C., Chan, J., Harris, N., Walport, M., Bernstein, R., Batchelor, R., Hughes, G., & Gharavi, A. (1987). High incidence of anticardiolipin antibodies in relatives of patients with systemic lupus erythematosus. *J Rheumatol* 14, 723-726.

Mahasandana, C., Veerakul, G., Tanphaichitr, V.S., Suvatte, V., Opartkiattikul, N., & Hathaway, W.E. (1996). Homozygous protein S deficiency: 7-year follow-up. *Thromb Haemost* 76, 1122.

Makris, M., Leach, M., Beauchamp, N.J., Daly, M.E., Cooper, P.C., Hampton, K.K., Bayliss, P., Peake, I.R., Miller, G.J., & Preston, F.E. (2000). Genetic analysis, phenotypic diagnosis, and risk of venous thrombosis in families with inherited deficiencies of protein S. *Blood* 95, 1935-1941.

Manco-Johnson, M.J., Marlar, R.A., Jacobson, L.J., Hays, T., & Warady, B.A. (1988). Severe protein C deficiency in newborn infants. *J Pediatr* 113, 359-363.

Martinelli, I., Mannucci, P.M., De Stefano, V., Taioli, E., Rossi, V., Crosti, F., Paciaroni, K., Leone, G., & Faioni, E.M. (1998). Different risks of thrombosis in four coagulation defects associated with inherited thrombophilia: a study of 150 families. *Blood* 92, 2353-2358.

Mateo, J., Oliver, A., Borrell, M., Sala, N., & Fontcuberta, J. (1997). Laboratory evaluation and clinical characteristics of 2,132 consecutive unselected patients with venous thromboembolism--results of the Spanish Multicentric Study on Thrombophilia (EMET-Study). *Thromb Haemost* 77, 444-451.

May, K.P., West, S.G., Moulds, J., & Kotzin, B.L. (1993). Different manifestations of the antiphospholipid antibody syndrome in a family with systemic lupus erythematosus. *Arthritis Rheum* 36, 528-533.

McGhee-Harvey, A.a.S., LE (1966). Connective tissue disease and the chronic biologic false-positive test for syphilis (BFP reaction). *The Medical Clinics of North America* 50, 1271-1279.

McNeil, H.P., Simpson, R.J., Chesterman, C.N., & Krilis, S.A. (1990). Anti-phospholipid antibodies are directed against a complex antigen that includes a lipid-binding inhibitor of coagulation: beta 2-glycoprotein I (apolipoprotein H). *Proc Natl Acad Sci U S A* 87, 4120-4124.

Miyakis, S., Lockshin, M.D., Atsumi, T., Branch, D.W., Brey, R.L., Cervera, R., Derksen, R.H., PG, D.E.G., Koike, T., Meroni, P.L., Reber, G., Shoenfeld, Y., Tincani, A., Vlachoyiannopoulos, P.G., & Krilis, S.A. (2006). International consensus statement on an update of the classification criteria for definite antiphospholipid syndrome (APS). *J Thromb Haemost* 4, 295-306.

Nimpf, J., Bevers, E.M., Bomans, P.H., Till, U., Wurm, H., Kostner, G.M., & Zwaal, R.F. (1986). Prothrombinase activity of human platelets is inhibited by beta 2-glycoprotein-I. *Biochim Biophys Acta* 884, 142-149.

Nimpf, J., Wurm, H., & Kostner, G.M. (1987). Beta 2-glycoprotein-I (apo-H) inhibits the release reaction of human platelets during ADP-induced aggregation. *Atherosclerosis* 63, 109-114.

Norlund, L., Zoller, B., & Ohlin, A.K. (1997). A novel thrombomodulin gene mutation in a patient suffering from sagittal sinus thrombosis. *Thromb Haemost* 78, 1164-1166.

Ohlenschlaeger, T., Garred, P., Madsen, H.O., & Jacobsen, S. (2004). Mannose-binding lectin variant alleles and the risk of arterial thrombosis in systemic lupus erythematosus. *N Engl J Med* 351, 260-267.

Pardos-Gea, J., Castro-Marrero, J., Cortes-Hernandez, J., Balada, E., Pedrosa, A., Vilardell-Tarres, M., & Ordi-Ros, J. (2011). Beta2-glycoprotein I gene polymorphisms Val247Leu and Trp316Ser in Spanish patients with primary antiphospholipid syndrome. *Rheumatol Int* DOI 10.1007/s00296-010-1726-5,

Picard, V., Dautzenberg, M.D., Villoutreix, B.O., Orliaguet, G., Alhenc-Gelas, M., & Aiach, M. (2003). Antithrombin Phe229Leu: a new homozygous variant leading to spontaneous antithrombin polymerization in vivo associated with severe childhood thrombosis. *Blood* 102, 919-925.

Pierangeli, S.S., Vega-Ostertag, M.E., Raschi, E., Liu, X., Romay-Penabad, Z., De Micheli, V., Galli, M., Moia, M., Tincani, A., Borghi, M.O., Nguyen-Oghalai, T., & Meroni, P.L. (2007). Toll-like receptor and antiphospholipid mediated thrombosis: in vivo studies. *Ann Rheum Dis* 66, 1327-1333.

Poort, S.R., Rosendaal, F.R., Reitsma, P.H., & Bertina, R.M. (1996). A common genetic variation in the 3'-untranslated region of the prothrombin gene is associated with elevated plasma prothrombin levels and an increase in venous thrombosis. *Blood* 88, 3698-3703.

Reitsma, P.H., Bernardi, F., Doig, R.G., Gandrille, S., Greengard, J.S., Ireland, H., Krawczak, M., Lind, B., Long, G.L., Poort, S.R., & et al. (1995). Protein C deficiency: a database of mutations, 1995 update. On behalf of the Subcommittee on Plasma Coagulation Inhibitors of the Scientific and Standardization Committee of the ISTH. *Thromb Haemost* 73, 876-889.

Reitsma, P.H., & Rosendaal, F.R. (2007). Past and future of genetic research in thrombosis. *J Thromb Haemost* 5 Suppl 1, 264-269.

Ridker, P.M., Miletich, J.P., Hennekens, C.H., & Buring, J.E. (1997). Ethnic distribution of factor V Leiden in 4047 men and women. Implications for venous thromboembolism screening. *Jama* 277, 1305-1307.

Rosendaal, F.R. (1999). Venous thrombosis: a multicausal disease. *Lancet* 353, 1167-1173.

Roubey, R.A. (1996). Immunology of the antiphospholipid antibody syndrome. *Arthritis Rheum* 39, 1444-1454.

Ruiz-Arguelles, G.J., Garces-Eisele, J., Ruiz-Delgado, G.J., & Alarcon-Segovia, D. (1999). The G20210A polymorphism in the 3'-untranslated region of the prothrombin gene in Mexican mestizo patients with primary antiphospholipid syndrome. *Clin Appl Thromb Hemost* 5, 158-160.

Sallai, K.K., Nagy, E., Bodo, I., Mohl, A., & Gergely, P. (2007). Thrombosis risk in systemic lupus erythematosus: the role of thrombophilic risk factors. *Scand J Rheumatol* 36, 198-205.

Sanchez, M.L., Katsumata, K., Atsumi, T., Romero, F.I., Bertolaccini, M.L., Funke, A., Amengual, O., Kondeatis, E., Vaughan, R.W., Cox, A., Hughes, G.R., & Khamashta,

M.A. (2004). Association of HLA-DM polymorphism with the production of antiphospholipid antibodies. *Ann Rheum Dis* 63, 1645-1648.

Schallmoser, K., Rosin, C., Knittelfelder, R., Sailer, T., Ulrich, S., Zoghlami, C., Lehr, S., Pabinger, I., & Panzer, S. (2005). The Fc gammaRIIa polymorphism R/H131, autoantibodies against the platelet receptors GPIb alpha and Fc gammaRIIa and a risk for thromboembolism in lupus anticoagulant patients. *Thromb Haemost* 93, 544-548.

Schmidel, D.K., Tatro, A.V., Phelps, L.G., Tomczak, J.A., & Long, G.L. (1990). Organization of the human protein S genes. *Biochemistry* 29, 7845-7852.

Schousboe, I. (1985). beta 2-Glycoprotein I: a plasma inhibitor of the contact activation of the intrinsic blood coagulation pathway. *Blood* 66, 1086-1091.

Sebastiani, G.D., Galeazzi, M., Tincani, A., Scorza, R., Mathieu, A., Passiu, G., Morozzi, G., Piette, J.C., Cervera, R., Houssiau, F., Smolen, J., Fernandez Nebro, A., De Ramon, E., Goral, A.J., Papasteriades, C., Ferrara, G.B., Carcassi, C., Bellisai, F., & Marcolongo, R. (2003). HLA-DPB1 alleles association of anticardiolipin and anti-beta2GPI antibodies in a large series of European patients with systemic lupus erythematosus. *Lupus* 12, 560-563.

Seelen, M.A., van der Bijl, E.A., Trouw, L.A., Zuiverloon, T.C., Munoz, J.R., Fallaux-van den Houten, F.C., Schlagwein, N., Daha, M.R., Huizinga, T.W., & Roos, A. (2005). A role for mannose-binding lectin dysfunction in generation of autoantibodies in systemic lupus erythematosus. *Rheumatology (Oxford)* 44, 111-119.

Shen, L., & Dahlback, B. (1994). Factor V and protein S as synergistic cofactors to activated protein C in degradation of factor VIIIa. *J Biol Chem* 269, 18735-18738.

Shoenfeld, Y., Meroni, P.L., & Cervera, R. (2008). Antiphospholipid syndrome dilemmas still to be solved: 2008 status. *Ann Rheum Dis* 67, 438-442.

Simmonds, R.E., Ireland, H., Kunz, G., & Lane, D.A. (1996). Identification of 19 protein S gene mutations in patients with phenotypic protein S deficiency and thrombosis. Protein S Study Group. *Blood* 88, 4195-4204.

Simmonds, R.E., Ireland, H., Lane, D.A., Zoller, B., Garcia de Frutos, P., & Dahlback, B. (1998). Clarification of the risk for venous thrombosis associated with hereditary protein S deficiency by investigation of a large kindred with a characterized gene defect. *Ann Intern Med* 128, 8-14.

Sivera, P., Bosio, S., Bertero, M.T., Demaestri, M., Mazza, U., & Camaschella, C. (2000). G20210A homozygosity in antiphospholipid syndrome secondary to systemic lupus erythematosus. *Haematologica* 85, 109-110.

Smolen, J.S., Klippel, J.H., Penner, E., Reichlin, M., Steinberg, A.D., Chused, T.M., Scherak, O., Graninger, W., Hartter, E., Zielinski, C.C., & et al. (1987). HLA-DR antigens in systemic lupus erythematosus: association with specificity of autoantibody responses to nuclear antigens. *Ann Rheum Dis* 46, 457-462.

Soria, J.M., Almasy, L., Souto, J.C., Tirado, I., Borell, M., Mateo, J., Slifer, S., Stone, W., Blangero, J., & Fontcuberta, J. (2000). Linkage analysis demonstrates that the prothrombin G20210A mutation jointly influences plasma prothrombin levels and risk of thrombosis. *Blood* 95, 2780-2785.

Tait, R.C., Walker, I.D., Perry, D.J., Islam, S.I., Daly, M.E., McCall, F., Conkie, J.A., & Carrell, R.W. (1994). Prevalence of antithrombin deficiency in the healthy population. *Br J Haematol* 87, 106-112.

Takahashi, R., Tsutsumi, A., Ohtani, K., Wakamiya, N., & Sumida, T. (2005). Lack of relationship between mannose-binding lectin variant alleles and risk of arterial thrombosis in Japanese patients with systemic lupus erythematosus. *Mod Rheumatol* 15, 459-460.

Torresan, M., Machado, T.F., Siqueira, L.H., Ozelo, M.C., Arruda, V.R., & Annichino-Bizzacchi, J.M. (2000). The impact of the search for thrombophilia risk factors among antiphospholipid syndrome patients with thrombosis. *Blood Coagul Fibrinolysis* 11, 679-682.

Tsantes, A.E., Nikolopoulos, G.K., Bagos, P.G., Rapti, E., Mantzios, G., Kapsimali, V., & Travlou, A. (2007). Association between the plasminogen activator inhibitor-1 4G/5G polymorphism and venous thrombosis. A meta-analysis. *Thromb Haemost* 97, 907-913.

Van Cott, E.M., & Laposata, M. (1998). Laboratory evaluation of hypercoagulable states. *Hematol Oncol Clin North Am* 12, 1141-1166, v.

van der Velden, P.A., Krommenhoek-Van Es, T., Allaart, C.F., Bertina, R.M., & Reitsma, P.H. (1991). A frequent thrombomodulin amino acid dimorphism is not associated with thrombophilia. *Thromb Haemost* 65, 511-513.

Vargas-Alarcon, G., Granados, J., Bekker, C., Alcocer-Varela, J., & Alarcon-Segovia, D. (1995). Association of HLA-DR5 (possibly DRB1*1201) with the primary antiphospholipid syndrome in Mexican patients. *Arthritis Rheum* 38, 1340-1341.

Williamson, D., Brown, K., Luddington, R., Baglin, C., & Baglin, T. (1998). Factor V Cambridge: a new mutation (Arg306-->Thr) associated with resistance to activated protein C. *Blood* 91, 1140-1144.

Wilson, W.A., Gharavi, A.E., Koike, T., Lockshin, M.D., Branch, D.W., Piette, J.C., Brey, R., Derksen, R., Harris, E.N., Hughes, G.R., Triplett, D.A., & Khamashta, M.A. (1999). International consensus statement on preliminary classification criteria for definite antiphospholipid syndrome: report of an international workshop. *Arthritis Rheum* 42, 1309-1311.

Wurm, H. (1984). beta 2-Glycoprotein-I (apolipoprotein H) interactions with phospholipid vesicles. *Int J Biochem* 16, 511-515.

Yasuda, S., Tsutsumi, A., Atsumi, T., Bertolaccini, M.L., Ichikawa, K., Khamashta, M.A., Hughes, G.R., & Koike, T. (2002). Gene polymorphisms of tissue plasminogen activator and plasminogen activator inhibitor-1 in patients with antiphospholipid antibodies. *J Rheumatol* 29, 1192-1197.

Zoller, B., Svensson, P.J., He, X., & Dahlback, B. (1994). Identification of the same factor V gene mutation in 47 out of 50 thrombosis-prone families with inherited resistance to activated protein C. *J Clin Invest* 94, 2521-2524.

Section 3

Antiphospholipid Antibodies Detection, Clinical Manifestation and Treatment

4

Antiphospholipid Antibodies – Detection and Clinical Importance

Jakub Swadzba[1] and Jolanta Kolodziejczyk[2]
[1]*Jagiellonian University Medical College*
[2]*Diagnostyka Sp. ZO.O.*
Poland

1. Introduction

Antiphospholipid syndrome (APS) is a common and very devastating disease. It is an autoimmune disease, which differs from most other systemic autoimmune illnesses by its propensity to develop thrombosis. APS is defined as the co-occurrence of antiphospholipid antibodies (aPL) with the characteristic clinical symptoms. The problem exists on the laboratory side of the diagnosis which is important to estimate the risk of further thrombosis or pregnancy complications. The diagnosis has to be made based on the presence of aPL, which are very complex entities. The main objective of this chapter is to review the methods of the aPL determinations and the clinical utility of their presence. The aPL pathogenic mechanism will be shortly discussed with an emphasis on the relation between thrombosis and inflammation.

2. The short history of the research in the field of aPL

APL with the ability to prolong *in vitro* phospholipid depending coagulation times were discovered in 1952 (Conley & Hartmann, 1952) in patients suffering from systemic lupus erythematosus (SLE). Only much later, it was discovered that *in vivo* they do not act as anticoagulants (Bowie et al. 1963) and can be found not only in SLE patients but also in apparently healthy subjects. The term "lupus anticoagulant" (LA) was used for the first time in 1972 by Feinstein and Rapaport (Feinstein & Rapaport, 1972). In 1980s, it became clear that LA belongs to a group of autoantibodies directed against negatively charged phospholipids and anticardiolipin antibodies (aCL) were determined for the first time using radioimmunoassay (Harris et al., 1983). The presence of aPL was associated with many different clinical signs and symptoms. Finally for the first time a definition of APS was established in 1987 (Harris, 1987). Then, in the 1990s, antibodies to antiphospholipid protein cofactors - beta2 glycoprotein I (aβ_2GPI) and prothrombin were discovered (Bevers et al., 1991; Galli et al., 1990; Mc Neil et al., 1990).

A set of guidelines for the detection of LA were published in 1991 and 1995 and then revised in 2009 (Exner et al., 1991; Brand et al., 1995; Pengo et al., 2009). Similar efforts were started from the beginning to standardize enzyme-immunoassays to detect aCL (Pierangeli & Harris, 2008). In 1999, first changes (e.g. exclusion of thrombocytopenia) were introduced to the definition of APS (Wilson et al., 1999) and then the definition was modified in 2006 (Miyakis et al., 2006). Since the last modification aβ_2GPI are one of the laboratory criteria of APS.

3. LA phenomenon – The most clinically relevant aPL

LA was the first discovered aPL antibody, and until now, it has been known as the most clinically relevant. Although sensitive and quantitative ELISA-based methods were developed to detect antiphospholipid antibodies, LA detected by coagulometric tests has been shown to be more associated with thrombosis (Galli et al., 2003). From the beginning, LA together with aCL were included among laboratory criteria of the APS (Harris, 1987).

The term LA is a double misnomer because these antibodies are present mainly in patients without *lupus erythematosus* and *in vivo* react as procoagulant (Jamrozik et al., 1993). The name "anticoagulant" was given because *in vitro* in phospholipid-dependent liquid-phase assays they prolong these tests acting as anticoagulants.

The detection of LA is founded on a wide range of clot-based tests and according to the guidelines three-step procedure is required. The laboratory diagnosis should be based on prolongation of a phospholipid dependent clotting tests, lack of correction of the prolonged clotting time by addition of a small amount of normal plasma and correction by the presence of the higher concentration of phospholipids.

The detection of LA is delicate and sometimes impossible when the patient is already treated with oral anticoagulants. Pre-analytical variables (e.g. quality of sample collection, centrifugation, temperature of storage) strongly influence final results. The specimen is sodium citrate anticoagulated blood which requires immediate, quick, double centrifugation. If the test is not immediately performed, the sample needs to be frozen in a deep freeze. Moreover, one of the extremely important aspects ensuring the good test results is the process of the blood collection. The smooth blood flow prevents activation of the coagulation processes.

In the past, many different tests were used in the process of LA detection, e.g.: kaolin clotting time (KCT) (Galli et al., 1995), silica clotting time (SCT) (Dragoni et al., 2001), diluted prothrombin time (dPT) (Liestøl et al., 2002), activated partial thromboplastin time sensitive/insensitive ratio (aPTT ratio) (Ames et al., 2001), Textarin/Ecarin clotting time (Triplett et al., 1993). Recently, only two following tests have been recommended for LA detection based on practicality and global experience: diluted Russell viper venom time (dRVVT) and aPTT. The use of other tests has been discouraged mainly due to the limited experience rather than their poor performance (Pengo et al., 2009). Interestingly, according to one systematic literature review, the risk of thrombosis appeared to be independent of the laboratory tests used for LA identification (Horbach et al., 1996).

Our clinical research results show a comparable performance of the LA tests based on aPTT and dRVVT as recommended by the latest guidelines for LA detection with the other tests (Swadzba et al., 2011 a). Our study group that was used consisted of 336 subjects suffering from various autoimmune diseases. We used aPTT, dRVVT and dPT tests for LA detection together with a ratio between sensitive and insensitive aPTT reagents. All LA tests performed were associated with a previous episode of thrombosis (ORs range: 3,5 to 8,4). Diluted PT dependent LA showed stronger association with the history of thrombosis than aPTT or dRVVT dependent LAs (OR = 6,0 vs. 5,0 and 4,3 respectively). On the other hand, LA based on the ratio between sensitive and insensitive aPTT reagents showed weaker association with APS clinical symptoms than other LA tests.

Furthermore, it has been shown that aβ_2GPI are better predictors of thrombotic complications than antibodies directed against prothrombin (Swadzba et al., 1997). For this reason, various attempts have been made to specifically detect β_2GPI dependent LAs. Two methods of β_2GPI dependent LA identification were described (Pengo et al., 2004; Simmelink et al., 2003). The first studies indicate that the β_2GPI dependent LAs show superior association with thrombotic complications than LAs caused by other antibodies (De Laat et al., 2004, 2001). It was confirmed recently in our study (Swadzba et al., 2011 a). The highest odds ratio for thrombosis was found for aβ_2GPI dependent LA (OR= 8,3; specificity/sensitivity=98%/15%). Because of high specificity (98%) but low sensitivity (15%) aβ_2GPI dependent LA was suggested to be the second line assay to choose the patients with the highest risk of thrombosis.

In the recent guidelines only two tests were selected because if more tests were performed the percentage of false positive results could be too high. In our study even only two tests were used the odds ratio for both (and/or) was lower than for each one separate test. LA tested by aPTT and/or dRVVT (at least one out of two positive tests), as it was recommended by the published guidelines, was associated less strongly with the history of thrombosis (OR=4,1) than any of these tests separately (OR=5,0 and 4,3 respectively). The advantage of the latter (aPTT and/or dRVVt) lies only in their higher sensitivity (45% vs. 43% for aPTT dependent LA and 32% for dRVVT dependent LA). When both tests were positive ("double LA positivity") the association with thrombosis was stronger (OR=6,5) than when only one test was positive. Double LA positivity detected by all tests performed was firmly associated with the history of thrombosis.

We agree with the recommendation, that two tests should be performed and the number of positive tests should be given and commented on the final result. The results with two positive LA tests could be named as "double LA positive" and possibly point to the patients with the highest risk of thrombosis.

LA detection is troublesome, poorly standardized, and its laboratory accuracy and clinical utility varies, igniting a lot of controversies. As a consequence several national and international inter-laboratory surveys have shown unacceptable differences in LA test results between various participating laboratories (Arnout et al., 1999; Pengo et al., 2007b). The rates of false positive and false negative results remained relatively high. In the future the differences among laboratories should be less pronounced, because the new guidelines gave more strict recommendations about blood collection requirements, choice of the tests, mixing studies (1:1 proportion), confirmatory tests, interpretation, expressing and reporting the results.

However there is still a need to conduct more research to answer a lot of questions, e.g.: how identify the most clinically relevant LA, how to define the presence of strong LA as opposed to the weak ones. From a clinical point of view, any LA results should always be considered in the context of a full laboratory aPL profile comprising of aCL and aβ_2GPI, because isolated LA positivity may be frequently found in subjects without any clinical symptoms (Pengo et al., 2007a).

4. ACL – The most sensitive aPL test

ACL were firstly detected by radioimmunoassay but just after ELISA based format replaced the former tests (Loizou et al., 1985). It is well known that basic performance of aCL assays is determined by various factors including the type of microtiterplate, the source of cardiolipin, the solvents, the usage of cofactor (De Groot et al., 2008). There were a lot of efforts to standardize the aCL tests (Wong et al., 2005, Wong & Favaloro, 2008). However it is not easy because the aCL ELISA does not detect aCL, but antibodies to proteins which bind to cardiolipin coated on the surface of microtiterplate. β_2GPI is present in the microtiterplate wells from the patient serum (tested), bovine serum (solvent) or sometimes β_2GPI is extra added to aCL tests. β_2GPI can bind to cardiolipin coated on the plate and later aβ_2GPI bind to the complex β_2GPI-cardiolipin. However the cardiolipin on microtiterplate can be bound also to prothrombin and other proteins. For this reason an aCL test is not purely aβ_2GPI test, but, in fact, there are detected antibodies against different proteins which bind to anionic phospholipids. This is probably the reason why ELISAs to detect anticardiolipin antibodies are more sensitive but less specific tests than aβ_2GPI ELISAs.

Proper and stable calibrators are very important for conducting aCL tests. Almost since the beginning one source of human polyclonal calibrators from patients samples was applied (Louisville calibrators) (Harris et al., 1987). These widely used calibrators helped produce comparable results between laboratories and introduce international units (GPL and MPL units) (Harris, 1990). The Louisville calibrators were used for many years in spite of the problems with batch to batch variations (Favaloro & Wong, 2011). Some years ago monoclonal antibodies to β_2GPI became available and they started to be used as the calibrators both for β_2GPI ELISA and aCL ELISA (Ichikawa et al., 1999). Even though a great progress has been made, there is no consensus for internationally accepted aCL calibrators.

The other important issue in aCL testing is associated with choosing an optimal cut-off point. In the first studies, the 95th percentile of healthy population was used (Musial et al., 1997), but from the beginning it was well known that low positive results were less important than high positives. In the Sapporo APS criteria, only medium or high titer of aCL were considered as serological criterion of APS (Wilson et al., 1999). In the newest, updated criteria, aCL are regarded as positive if exceed the 99th percentile or 40 GPL/MPL units (Miyakis et al., 2006). There is an inconsistence in offering two different, alternative values to identify the presence of aCL in a meaningful, pathological levels (Swadzba et al., 2007). In our in-house method the value of the 99th percentile of a normal population corresponded to 26 GPL and 27 MPL, respectively. Obviously, the sensitivity was higher for a lower cut-off value (99th percentile), specificity - for the higher one (above 40 GPL/MPL), but overall, relative risk for thrombosis was quite similar (3,71 vs. 3,72) (Swadzba et al., 2007).

However, until generally accepted international standard is developed, any arbitrarily chosen cut-off value will leave doubts about its validity. It seems reasonable to have only one threshold value when comparisons between different methods and laboratories are required. In our opinion, the 99th percentile of the healthy population offers by far the better threshold value that could be generally accepted (Swadzba & Musial, 2009).

Nevertheless, one needs to remember that lower levels of both aCL and aβ_2GPI can be associated with significant (but low) risk of clinical complications (Swadzba et al., 2007). Even if it is persistent positivity, one low positive result could be neglected, but when two or more aPL are present in low titer the situation can be different. We can speculate that in the recently developed definition of the "triple positivity" maybe even low positive antibodies could be enough to register as positive (when at least one kind of antibodies is highly positive).

On the contrary, patients with very high levels of antibodies, especially of the IgG class, are at particularly high risk of thrombosis. This has been clearly reflected in our study by a group of patients with anticardiolipin antibodies level above 80 GPL/MPL who had the highest number of thrombosis in the past (Swadzba et al., 2007). In our opinion, this finding requires and calls for an objective, clinically important and uniformly accepted definition of "high levels" of aPL.

It should be emphasized that the class of anticardiolipin antibodies is crucial for determining the risk of APS clinical symptoms. It was shown in many studies that IgG class of antibodies correlates much better with the history of thrombosis than IgM type (Swadzba et al., 2007). It is of concern that the updated criteria do not separate IgG and IgM classes. We propose to grouped separately IgG and IgM antibodies and introduce the thrombosis risk score in which IgG antibodies will be more important than IgM. Some other authors even think that IgM antibodies should be abandoned from the criteria of APS (Galli et al., 2008).

The value of IgA antibodies in diagnosis of APS is still uncertain. According to the latest guidelines this class of antibodies does not add clinically important information (Miyakis et al., 2006).

5. Anti β_2GPI – The most "real" aPL test?

β_2GPI is a 50-kDA phospholipid binding protein present in plasma in concentrations of approximately 200 mcg/ml. The function of β_2GPI is not clear until now however it was regarded as natural anticoagulant. The genetic deficiency of β_2GPI appears to be not involved with any diseases (Matsuura et al., 2010). It has been found recently that β_2GPI can play an important role in the immunity (De Groot & Meijers, 2011). There is no evidence that any of *β_2GPI* polymorphism is connected with the presence aβ_2GPI antibodies or APS (Swadzba et al., 2006).

Antibodies against β_2GPI were discovered in 1990 and it is well documented nowadays that β_2GPI is the main important antigen in APS pathophysiology. It was demonstrated that the mice injected with β_2GPI produce aCL as well as aβ_2GPI (Gharavi et al. 1992). From the pathophysiological point of view, inclusion of β_2GPI antibodies to existing criteria seems to be well-founded. It is generally accepted that domain I of β_2GPI serves as a major antigen for pathological aPL (Ioannou & Rahman, 2010). Aβ_2GPI IgG antibodies are strongly associated with clinical complications of APS. This further justifies inclusion aβ_2GPI into the APS laboratory classification criteria.

It is noted, that the presence of aβ_2GPI was closely associated with the presence of other aPL. For this reason, addition of aβ_2GPI to the diagnostic armamentarium changed only slightly the risk prediction of clinical complications based on the presence of LA and aCL. In our study their inclusion added 5 extra patients diagnosed with APS, who otherwise would be missed (less than 5% of the APS population) (Swadzba et al., 2007). Overall, the addition of aβ_2GPI to the classification criteria might slightly limit the number of the so-called "seronegative APS" patients; a relatively small group of subjects with very suggestive clinical features and negative LA and/or aCL determinations.

Aβ_2GPI, especially of the IgG class, appeared in our patients less frequently than aCL (Swadzba et al., 2007). For this reason, being more specific, they showed quite low sensitivity, as it was already reported by others (Favaloro & Wong, 2011). Overall odds ratios for thrombosis and pregnancy loss is similar to the aCL ones.

The proposed single method of establishing an upper limit of normal values for aβ_2GPI introduced by the updated APS criteria would certainly help to compare results between laboratories. The choice of 99th percentile as a suggested cut-off value seems valid and very well-supported. For example in our research studies, patients tested positive for aβ_2GPI based on a cut-off set at 99th percentile were at a higher relative risk for thrombosis than those considered positive when the cut-off value was set at 95th percentile. However, quite low sensitivity of the test (in our study for aβ_2GPI IgG - 24%) seems to qualify it rather as a risk stratification test or a second test identifying population at the highest risk among APS patients (Swadzba et al., 2007). As a screening test or as a test served in a "triple positivity" the cut-off value that lies in the 95th percentile may be better and it needs further studies.

6. Non classical aPL

The spectrum of autoantibodies associated with APS is likely to extend beyond tests known from APS criteria. From the very beginning it was known that cardiolipin is not the only one but only one out of the many possible phospholipids served in the tests for detecting aPL. It was unlikely that cardiolipin could serve as real antigen for aPL and even that *in vivo* it is a surface for the proteins because cardiolipin is situated only in the inner side of mitochondria membranes.

Other phospholipids were proposed as the antigens. From a pathophysiological point of view the phosphatidylserine was very attractive as phospholipid that exists in the cellular membranes and flip-flops to the outer side during the cell activation. In fact in our studies, the correlation with APS clinical symptoms did not differ between phosphatidylserine antibodies and aCL. The correlation between two methods was very high (r=0,8) (Musial et al., 2003). Antibodies against other phospholipids were tested less extensively (e.g. antibodies against phosphatidylinositol) but similar results were obtained. Due to high cross reactivity there was only a little additional clinical information leading to the conclusion that there is no need any additional ELISA tests against anionic phospholipids other than aCL. The special attention was drawn to antibodies against phosphatidylethanolamine (aPE). Phosphatidylethanolamine is a zwitterionic phospholipid normally present in the outer leaflet of cell membranes, and it plays a role in reactions of protein C pathway. Antibodies can react with the complexes of aPE with high and low molecular weight kininogens (HMWK, LMWK), factor XI and prekallikrein (Sugi & McIntyre, 2001). There were some studies conducted that show aPE as the only antibody in a limited number of APS patients (Karmochkine et al., 1992).

The method using the mixture of different phospholipids was proposed as an alternative to cardiolipin tests and it was called "the real antiphospholipid test". The concept of the test was similar to LA (detecting antibodies against different antigens) and the aPL ELISA from

Louisville in some studies showed better sensitivity and specificity than aCL (Pierangeli & Harris, 2008). However, most of the studies used cardiolipin as the antigen that was easier to standardize and compare between laboratories than tests with different mixtures of different antiphospholipids.

As mentioned early, in 1991 antibodies to the prothrombin (aPT) were discovered (Bevers et al., 1991). In the clinical studies aPT were found to be less clinically important than other aPL antibodies (Swadzba et al., 1997). However the group of researchers developed a new test recognizing clinically relevant aPT. They coated prothrombin on phosphatidylserine (PS/PT test) causing new structure configuration of prothrombin. The complex of prothrombin and phosphatidylserine is probably showing epitopes which bind clinically relevant antibodies. These antibodies rather than antibodies against phrothrombin alone are closely associated with APS and LA (Atsumi et al., 2000).

Test for the presence of anti annexin V antibodies is one of the new tests especially used in obstetrical APS. Annexin V plays a significant role as an anticoagulant shield on the surface of the trophoblast. In some studies, the presence of anti annexin V antibodies correlates positively with a history of pregnancy losses (Iaccarino et al., 2011).

Anti β_2GPI - domain I antibodies were tested recently. In contrast to antibodies recognizing other domains of β_2GPI, anti-domain I antibodies are found to be highly associated with APS clinical symptoms, however their sensitivity is very low (De Laat & de Groot, 2011).

7. New trends in aPL determination

ELISA method is state-of-the-art for aCL and aβ_2GPI determination. It is a manual or semi-manual technology and inter-assay reproducibility is difficult to obtain. Manufacturers put a lot of effort to develop new methods. There are some new automated assays for diagnosis of the antiphospholipid syndrome on the market (De Moerloose et al., 2010; Persijn et al., 2011). These assays are two-step immunoassays consisting of paramagnetic particles coated with cardiolipin and/or human β_2GPI. Sensitivity, specificity, agreement and the odds ratios when predicting a thrombotic or obstetric event gave comparable results with the ELISA methods.

Western blot is the other technique used recently in aPL determination (Egerer et al., 2011). It was published that it gives similar results as ELISA, although the results are only qualitative.

High avidity aβ_2GPI was associated with thrombosis and APS, while in the low avidity aβ_2GPI group non-APS (predominantly SLE) patients prevailed (Cucnik et al., 2011). Controversies concerning the role of antibody avidity may be attributed mainly to the absence of suitable detection methods.

We proposed to use ROC (Receiver Operating Curve) methodology to establish retrospectively optimal cut-off point for each clinical symptom, each type of the antiphospholipid antibodies and to determine the test with the best clinical accuracy (Musial et al., 2003). The comparison between tests based on ROC plot analysis is independent of any particular threshold values. The calculation of the area under the ROC curve (AUC) gives the information about the clinical accuracy. The area of 1,0 means that the test perfectly separates subjects with a given APS clinical symptom from those without it (an ideal situation - 100% sensitivity and 100% specificity). When the area is < 0,5 the test does not separate such two groups of patients at all. ROC plot analysis is further used to find threshold values for aPL which discriminate the best between the patients who experienced an APS clinical symptom in the past from those do did not. The optimum the cut-off point is the nearest point to the left upper corner on the graph of ROC curve. Such calculated cut-off value provides the optimum trade-off between the specificity and sensitivity of the test towards a particular clinical symptom.

8. APS definition and aPL clinical utility

Classification criteria for the antiphospholipid syndrome were proposed for the first time by Harris in 1987 (Harris, 1987). In the definition, he emphasized the co-existence of typical clinical complications and laboratory test abnormalities. Among laboratory tests, he listed the presence of LA and aCL, which were discovered four years earlier (Harris et al., 1983). Typical clinical manifestations included venous and arterial thrombosis, thrombocytopenia and obstetrical complications. These criteria were slightly modified during the Conference in Sapporo in 1999 (Wilson et al., 1999). Thrombocytopenia was removed as being not specific, obstetrical criteria were revised and their very detailed description was given. At the beginning of the 1990's, β_2GPI was shown to be a major antigen for aPL. For this reason, although aCL and aβ_2GPI often coexist, aβ_2GPI were added to the criteria (Miyakis et al., 2006). Subsequently, it was shown that aβ_2GPI were more specific, but less sensitive than aCL as markers of clinical complications of APS. Based on the updated criteria, it is recommended to divide patients into classes according to the type and number of antibodies present. Patients should be classified into class I when they possess more than one type of antibody. In our study, this group did not differ in terms of thrombosis risk from patients with the presence of only one type of aPL (Swadzba et al., 2007). Only groups with all three types of antibodies (LA + aCL + aβ_2GPI) were connected with the higher risk. Class II comprises patients with the presence of only one type of antibody (IIa-LA, IIb-aCL and IIc-aβ_2GPI). For thrombosis in general, and especially for venous thrombosis, the presence of LA (class IIa) brings the higher risk than groups IIb and IIc (Swadzba et al., 2007). APS patients are not routinely connected with the groups because it did not clearly differ by the risk of thrombosis or pregnancy loss.

It was shown that not only the presence of antibodies is important but also the coexistence of different antibodies can increase the risk of thrombosis. The term "triple positivity" for the presence of all classic aPL was given (Pengo et al., 2010). It is connected with high risk of thrombosis. The other high risk factors of APS clinical symptoms have been recently discovered: anti domain 1 antibodies, beta2 GPI dependent LA and double positive LA.

It is concerning, that the updated criteria do not separate IgG from IgM class of antibodies. The group of patients with combined: LA and aCL IgG or LA and aβ_2GPI IgG, can have similar risk of thrombosis as the patients with triple positivity: LA and two IgM antibodies (aCL and aβ_2GPI). We agree that there is little evidence demonstrating significant association between IgM aβ_2GPI and aCL but still there are some patients with only high IgM positive antibodies and clinical manifestations of APS. It could be too preliminary to exclude IgM antibodies completely, so we rather suggest to make a clear distinction between antibodies of the IgG and IgM class as the high and low risk antibodies until prospective studies remove any doubts that antibodies of the IgM class, even in very high titers bring negligible risk of thrombosis.

Undoubtedly, laboratory criteria that define the antiphospholipid syndrome require modification because the two different possible cut-off values for discrimination between positive and negative aCL (>99th percentile and >40 GPL). In 90 aCL-positive APS patients it was shown that the values defining 99th percentile of the normal population (17,4 GPL and 26,8 MPL) were significantly lower than 40 GPL (Swadzba et al., 2007); this finding was already reported by our group about some years earlier (26 GPL and 27 MPL, respectively) (Musial et al., 2003). We suggest to change the criteria and start using the 99th percentile as the only accepted cut-off value (as for anti-β_2GPI antibodies). Interestingly, Ruffatti (Ruffatti et al., 2008) proposed: one criterion to be used for thrombosis (40 GPL) and the other (99th percentile) for pregnancy complications. In group of their patients the mean value of aCL IgG was higher in thrombosis than in the group with obstetrical complications. It was concluded that lower titers can provoke obstetrical complications and are not enough for stimulating thrombosis. In our group of patients, the results were quite different. Using ROC curves the best cut-off for thrombosis was 17,2 and for recurrent fetal loss slightly higher 18,4 (Wu et al., 2008). A certain percentile of healthy population is the objective method for determination cut-offs regardless of the test used. It is important because there are many debates related to what percentile (i.e., 95th, 97,5th or 99th) is the best to use. This is the problem of optimal sensitivity/specificity ratio. The ROC curve methodology can show the best cut-off to reach optimum ratio between sensitivity and specificity and the highest OR for clinical symptoms connected with positive values of the tests. In 2003 we published cut-offs based on ROC curves for different antiphospolipid antibodies. Optimal cut-off for aCL IgG was slightly lower than 99th percentile (26 GPL) and far lower than 40 GPL. We regard it as correct that 99th percentile should be included in the criteria of APS but 95th percentile can be used as for a group with doubtful antibodies or in triple positivity when two others antibodies are positive.

Another radical proposition is to abandon aCL determinations completely, which is bringing up the argument of high specificity of aβ_2GPI for clinical APS symptoms. However we should not forget about sensitivity, which is quite low for these antibodies. Also, it has not been proven beyond any doubts that aCL antibodies directed against other proteins than β_2GPI are with no clinical importance. ACL like LA measure a cocktail of antibodies against different proteins and epitopes. From a practical point of view, aCL tests are much cheaper, better known by the clinicians and give similarly important clinical information.

APL positive patients with no APS clinical symptoms are at present excluded from the diagnosis of APS syndrome. We agree that the term "syndrome" is connected with any clinical symptom. If we agree that "triple positivity" gives high risk for thrombosis even if there were no clinical APS symptoms we should consider to develop a new definition. The proposition could be aPL dependent thrombophilia. LA and persistently high titers of all groups of aPL antibodies in IgG class probably are connected with even higher risk of thrombosis than moderate aCL of IgM class in women with one pregnancy loss in the history.

9. APL – A pathogenic mechanism, the role of inflammation in thrombosis

The coexistence of aPL and clinical signs of APS is obvious but causative role of aPL is not certain. There are some theories how aPL can cause thrombosis or abortions. Most of them are connected with prothrombotic and antifibrinolytic mechanisms. Relations between thrombosis and inflammation are researched recently.

Tumor necrosis factor alpha (TNF-α) is a cytokine which shares proinflammatory and prothrombotic actions, while a soluble form of interleukin-2 receptor (sIL-2R) is considered as a typical marker of (auto)immune inflammation with not known direct links to thrombosis. The differences in the pathogenesis of APS as compared to other autoimmune diseases might be connected with different serum levels of both mediators (Swadzba et al., 2011 b).

APS was characterized in our study by the highest levels of TNF-α. Moreover, patients with *lupus anticoagulant* or elevated levels of IgG anticardiolipin or IgG anti-β_2-glycoprotein I antibodies had higher TNF-α levels than patients without the presence of any type of antiphospholipid antibodies. The presence of aPL is associated with higher TNF-α level, whereas increased level of sIL-2R is rather connected with definite SLE where inflammatory processes prevail. It might be hypothesized that TNF-α plays a major role in pathogenesis of APS thrombotic phenomena.

In general, systemic inflammation is a potent prothrombotic stimulus. Inflammatory mechanisms upregulate procoagulant factors, downregulate natural anticoagulants and inhibit fibrinolytic activity (Esmon, 2003). Endotoxin, tumor necrosis factor alpha and interleukin-1α (IL-1α) induce tissue factor (TF) expression, primarily on endothelial cells and monocytes/macrophages, promoting blood coagulation (Bevilaqua et al., 1986). Activation of the complement C5b-C9 complex changes the cell surface to a more procoagulant phenotype by the shift of negatively charged phospholipids from the inner to the outer membrane (Sims et al., 1988). Inflammatory reaction is also accompanied by the increase in fibrinogen and C-reactive protein (CRP) blood levels. CRP itself increases TF and decreases TF pathway inhibitor (TFPI) concentrations, what may be important in pathogenesis of arterial thrombosis and myocardial infarction (Wu et al., 2008). Of the natural anticoagulants, protein C pathway appears to be the most strongly influenced by inflammation with thrombomodulin (TM) and the endothelial cell protein C receptor (EPCR) being both downregulated by TNF-α (Conway & Rosenberg, 1988).

On the other hand, thrombotic processes enhance inflammatory reactions, mainly through the action of TF and thrombin (Chu, 2005). Activation of platelets leads to the release of CD40 ligand, which in turn induces TF expression and increases interleukin 6 (IL-6) levels (Miller et al., 1993). Thrombin also augments leukocyte adhesion and activation, stimulates endothelial cells to produce platelet activating factor (PAF) and increases an expression of P-selectin (Pierangeli et al., 2001).

A common inhibitory pathway for thrombosis and inflammation also exists. Activated protein C (APC) acting directly as an anticoagulant, functions also as an anti-inflammatory and cytoprotective agent through specific receptors: EPCR and protease activated receptor-1 (PAR-1) (Crawley & Efthymiou, 2008).

It is possible that TNF-α is a proinflammatory cytokine with the strongest prothrombotic action. TNF-α stimulates monocyte and neutrophil adhesion to endothelium, inhibits protein C system, impairs fibrinolysis and increases TF expression on the cell surface (Esmon, 2003). Produced mainly by activated monocytes, macrophages, and T lymphocytes, this cytokine has been found to be elevated in patients suffering from both SLE (Studnicka-Benke et al., 1996) and APS (Forastiero et al., 2005). We hypothesized that TNF-α might be more elevated in APS patients, with thrombosis as its prominent feature, than in those with other autoimmune diseases where immune mediated inflammation prevails.

10. Conclusion

In summary, an updated list of APS classification criteria and a revision of LA guidelines represent a step forward for better detection of clinically important aPL. However, many problems still need to be addressed and an additional research in this field followed by new modifications in definitions and criteria seems to be necessary. The important issue is to find optimal methods for high risk aPL detection. This may lead to the development of an effective primary and secondary prophylaxis of clinical APS complications, which constitutes a major goal and challenge for the future.

11. References

Ames, P., Iannaccone, L., de Lasio, R., & Brancacio, V. (2001). Improved confirmation of weak lupus anticoagulants by employing sensitive and insensitive reagents to the lupus anticoagulant. *Blood Coagulation & Fibrynolisis*. Vol. 12, pp. 563-567, ISSN 0957-5235

Arnout, J., Meijer, P., & Vermylen, J. (1999). Lupus anticoagulant testing in Europe: an analysis of results from the first European Concerted Action on Thrombophilia (ECAT) survey using plasmas spiked with monoclonal antibodies against human beta2-glycoprotein I. *Journal of Thrombosis and Haemostasis*. Vol. 81, pp. 929-934. ISSN 1538-7836

Atsumi, T., Ieko, M., Bertolaccini, M., Ichikawa, K., Tsutsumi, A., Matsuura, E., & Koike, T. (2000). Association of autoantibodies against the phosphatidylserine-phrothrombin complex with manifestation of the antiphospholipid syndrome and with the presence of lupus anticoagulant. *Arthritis & Rheumatism*. Vol. 43, No. 9, pp. 1982-1993, ISSN 1529-0131

Bevers, E., Galli, M., Barbui, T., Comfurius, P., & Zwall R. (1991). Lupus anticoagulant IgG's (LA) are not directed to phospholipids only, but to a complex of lipid bound human prothrombin. *Thrombosis & Haemostasis*. Vol. 66, pp. 629-632, ISSN 0340-6245

Bevilaqua, M., Pober, J., Majeau, G., Fiers, W., Cotran, R., & Gimbrone, M. (1986). Recombinant tumor necrosis factor induces procoagulant activity in cultured human vascular endothelium: Characterization and comparison with the actions of interleukin 1. *Proceedings of the National Academy of Sciences of the United States of America*. Vol. 83, pp. 4533-4537, ISSN 0027-8424.

Bowie, E., Thompson, J., Pascuzzi, C., & Owen, C. (1963). Thrombosis in systemic lupus erythematosus despite circulating anticoagulants. *Clinical Chemistry and Laboratory Medicine*. Vol. 62, pp. 416-430, ISSN 1434-6621

Brandt, J., Triplett, D., Alving, B., & Scharer, I. (1995). Criteria for diagnosis of lupus anticoagulants: an update. On behalf of the Subcommittee on Lupus Anticoagulant/Antiphospholipid Antibody of the Scientific and Standardisation Committee of the ISTH. *Thrombosis & Haemostasis*. Vol. 74, pp. 1185-1190, ISSN 0340-6245

Chu, A. (2005).Tissue factor mediates inflammation. *Archives of Biochemistry and Biophysics*. Vol. 400, pp. 123-132, ISSN 0003-9861

Conley, C. & Hartmann, R. (1952). A haemorrhage disorder caused by circulating anticoagulant in patients with disseminated lupus erythematosus. *Journal of Clinical Investigation*, Vol. 31, pp. 621-622, ISSN 00219738

Conway, E., & Rosenberg, R. (1988). Tumor necrosis factor suppresses transcription of the trombomodulin gene in endothelial cells. *Molecular and Cellular Biology*. Vol. 8, pp. 5588-5592, ISSN 1098-5549

Crawley, J., & Efthymiou, M. (2008). Cytoprotective effect of activated protein C: specificity of PAR-1 signaling. *Journal of Thrombosis and Haemostasis*. Vol. 6, pp. 951-953, ISSN 1538-7836

Cucnik, S., Kveder, T., Ulcova-Gallova, Z., Swadzba, J., Musial, J., Valesini, G., Avcin, T., Rozman, B., & Bozic, B. (June 2011). Avidity of anti-ss2-glycoprotein I antibodies in patients with or without antiphospholipid syndrome: a collaborative study in the frame of the European forum on antiphospholipid antibodies. In: *Lupus*. 28.06.2011. Available from: http://lup.sagepub.com/content/early/2011/07/31/0961203311406308

De Groot, P., Derksen, R. & de Laat B. (2008). Twenty two years of failure to set-up undisputed assays to detect patients with the antiphospholipid antibodies. *Seminars in Thrombosis and Haemostasis*. Vol. 34, No. 4, pp. 347-55, ISSN 00946176

De Groot, P., & Meijers, J. (2011). β(2)-glycoprotein I: evolution, structure and function. *Journal of Thrombosis and Haemostasis*. Vol. 9, No. 7, pp. 1275-84, ISSN 1538-7836

De Laat, B., & de Groot, P. (2011). Autoantibodies directed against domain I of beta2-glycoprotein I. *Current Rheumatology Reports*. Vol. 13, No. 4, pp. 70-76, ISSN 1523-3774.

De Laat, B., Derksen, R., Reber, G., Musial, J., Swadzba, J., Bozic, B., Cucnic, S., Regnault, V., Forastiero, R., Woodhams, B., & de Groot, P. (2011). An international multicentre-laboratory evaluation of a new assay to detect specifically lupus anticoagulants dependent on the presence of anti-beta2-glycoprotein autoantibodies. *Journal of Thrombosis and Haemostasis*. Vol. 9, pp. 149-153, ISSN 1538-7836

De Laat, B., Derksen, R., Urbanus, R., Roest, M., & de Groot, P. (2004). Beta2 glycoprotein-I – dependent lupus anticoagulant highly correlates with thrombosis in the antiphospholipid syndrome. *Blood*. Vol. 104, pp. 3598-3602, ISSN 0006-4971

De Moerloose, P., Reber, G., Musial, J., & Arnout, J. (2010). Analitycal and clinical performance of a new, automated assay panel for the diagnosis of antuphospholipid syndrome. *Journal of Thrombosis and Haemostasis*. Vol. 8, pp. 1540-1546, ISSN 1538-7836

Dragoni, F., Minotti, C., Palumbo, G., Faillace, F., Redi, R., Bongarzoni, V., & Avvisati, G. (2001). As compared to kaolin clotting time, silica clotting time is a specific and sensitive automated method for detecting lupus anticoagulant. *Thrombosis Research*. Vol. 101, pp. 45-51, ISSN 0049-3848

Egerer, K., Roggenbuck, D., Buettner, T., Lehmann, B., Kohn. A., von Landenberg, P., Hiemann. R., Feist, E., Burmester, G., & Dorner, T. (2011). Single-step autoantibody profiling in antiphospholipid syndrome using a Multi-line dot assay. *Arthritis research & Therapy*. Vol. 13, No. 4, pp. 118, ISSN 1478-6354

Esmon C. (2003). Inflammation and thrombosis. *Journal of Thrombosis and Haemostasis*. Vol. 1, pp.1343-1348, ISSN 1538-7836

Exner, T., Triplett, D., Taberner, D., & Machin, S. (1991). Guidelines for testing and revised criteria for lupus anticoagulants. *Thrombosis & Haemostasis.* Vol. 65,pp. 320-322, ISSN 0340-6245

Favaloro, E., & Wong, R. (2011). Laboratory testing for the antiphospholipid syndrome: making sense of antiphospholipid antibody assays. *Clinical Chemistry and Laboratory Medicine.* Vol. 49, No. 3, pp. 447-461, ISSN 1434-6621

Feinstein, D., & Rapaport, S. (1972). Acquired inhibitors of blood coagulation. *Progress in Haemostasis and Thrombosis.* Vol. 1, pp. 75-95

Forastiero, R., Martinuzzo, M., & de Larranaga, G. (2005). Circulating levels of tissue factor and proinflammatory cytokines in patients with primary antiphospholipid syndrome or leprosy related antiphospholipid antibodies. *Lupus.* Vol. 14, pp. 129-136, ISSN 0961-2033

Galli, M., Comfurius, P., Maassen, C., Hemker, H., De Baets, M., van Breda-Vriesman, P., Barbui, T., Zwaal, R., & Bevers E. (1990). Anticardiolipin antibodies (ACA) directed not to cardiolipin but to plasma protein cofactor. *Lancet.* Vol. 335, pp. 1544-1547, ISSN 0140-6736

Galli, M., Finazzi, G., Bevers, E., & Barbui T. (1995). Kaolin clotting time and dilute Russell viper venom time distinguish between prothrombin dependent and beta-2 glycoprotein-I - dependent antiphospholipid antibodies. *Blood.* Vol. 86, pp. 617-623, ISSN 0006-4971

Galli, M., Luciani, D., Bertollini, G., & Barbui, T. (2003). Lupus anticoagulants are stronger risk factors for thrombosis than anticardiolipin antibodies in the antiphospholipid syndrome: a systemic review of the literature. *Blood.* Vol. 101, pp. 1827-1832, ISSN 0006-4971

Galli, M., Reber. G., de Moerloose, P., & de Groot, P. (2008). Invitation to a debate on the serological criteria that define the antiphospholipid syndrome. *Journal of Thrombosis and Haemostasis.* Vol. 6, pp. 399-401, ISSN 1538-7836

Gharavi, A., Sammaritano, L., Wen, J., & Elkon K. (1992). Induction of antiphospholipid autoantibodies by immunization with β_2-glycoprotein I (apolipoprotein H). *Journal of clinical Investigation.* Vol. 90, pp. 1105-1109, ISSN 00219738

Harris, E. (1987). Syndrome of the black swan. *British Journal of Rheumatology.* Vol. 26, pp. 324-326, ISSN 0263-7103

Harris, E. (1990). The second international anti-cardiolipin standardization workshop/the Kongston Antiphospholipid Antibody study (KAPS) group. *American Journal of Clinical Pathology.* Vol. 94, No. 4, pp. 476-484, ISSN 0002-9173

Harris, E., Gharavi, A., Boey, M., Patel, B., Loizou, S., & Hughes, G. (1983). Anticardiolipin antibodies: detection by radioimmunoassay and association with thrombosis in lupus erythematosus. *Lancet.* Vol. 2, pp. 1211-1214, ISSN 0140-6736

Harris, E., Gharavi, A.E., Patel, S. & Hughes, G.R.V. (1987). Evaluation of the anti-cardiolipin antibody test: Report of an international workshop held April 4 1986. *Clinical & Experimental Immunology,* Vol. 68, pp. 215-22, ISSN 1365-2249

Horbach, D., van Oort, E., Donders, C., Derksen, R., & de Groot, P. (1996). Lupus anticoagulant is a strongest risk factor for both venous and arterial thrombosis in patient with systemic lupus erythematosus. Comparison between different assays for the detection of antiphospholipid antibodies. *Thrombosis & Haemostasis.* Vol. 76, pp. 916-924, ISSN 0340-6245

Iaccarino, L., Ghirardello, A., Canova, M., Zen, M., Bettio, S., Nalotto, L., Punzi, L., & Doria, A. (2011). Anti-annexins autoantibodies: their role as biomarkers of autoimmune diseases. *Autoimmunity Reviews*. Vol. 10, No. 9, pp. 553-8, ISSN 1568-9972

Ichikawa, K., Tsutsumi, A., Atsumi, T., Matsuura, E., Kobayashi, S., Hughes, G., Kamashta, M., & Koike, T. (1999). A chimeric antibody with the human gammal constant region as a putative standard for assays to detect IgG beta2-glycoprotein I-dependent aticardiolipin and anti-beta2-glycoprotein I antibodies. *Arthritis & Rheumatism*. Vol. 42, No. 11, pp. 2461-70, ISSN 1529-0131

Ioannou, Y., & Rahman, A. (2010). Domain I of β_2-glycoprotein I: its role as an epitope and the potential to be developed as a specific target for the treatment of the antiphospholipid syndrome. *Lupus*. Vol. 19, pp. 400-405, ISSN 0961-2033

Jamrozik, J., Jankowski, M., Partyka, L., Skowiniak, A., & Swadzba, J. (1993). Lupus antykoagulant -- tajemniczy pro koagulant. *Polskie Archiwum Medycyny Wewnętrznej*. Vol. 90, pp. 348-355, ISSN 0032-3772

Karmochkine, M., Cacoub, P., Piette, J., Godeau, P., & Boffa M. (1992). Antiphosphatidylethanoloamine antibody as a sole antiphospholipid antibody in systemic lupus erythematosus with thrombosis. *Clinical and Experimental Rheumatology*. Vol. 10, pp. 603-605, ISSN 1593-098X

Liestøl, S., Jacobsen, E., & Wisløff, F. (2002). Dilute prothrombin time-based lupus ratio test. Integrated LA testing with recombinant tissue thromboplastin. *Thrombosis Research*. Vol. 15, No. 105, pp. 177-82, ISSN 0049-3848

Loizou, S., McCrea, L., Rudge, A., Reylnolds, R., Boyle, C., & Harris, E. (1985). Measurement of anti-cardiolipin antibodies by an enzyme-linked immunosorbent assai (ELISA). *Clinical & Experimental Immunology*. Vol. 62, pp. 738-45, ISSN 1365-2249

Matsuura, E., Shen, L., Matsunami, Y., Quan, N., Makarova, M., Geske F., Boisen, M., Yasuda S., & Kobayashi K. (2010). Pathopysiology of β_2-glycoprotein I in antiphospholipid syndrome. *Lupus*. Vol. 19, No. 4, pp. 379-384, ISSN 0961-2033

Mc Neil, H., Simpson, R., Chesterman, C., & Krilis S. (1990). Anti-phospholipid antibodies are directed against a complex antigen that includes the lipid binding inhibitor of coagulation: β2-glycoprotein I (apolipoprotein H). *Proceedings of the National Academy of Sciences of the United States of America*. Vol. 87, pp. 4120-4124, ISSN 0027-8424

Miller, D., Yaron, R., & Yellin, M. (1993). CD40L-CD40 interaction regulate endothelial cell surface tissue factor and thrombomodulin expression. *Journal of Leukocyte Biology*. Vol. 63, pp. 373-379, ISSN 0741-5400

Miyakis, S., Lockshin, M., Atsumi, T., Branch, D., Brey, R., Cervera, R., Derksen, R., de Groot, P., Koike, T., Meroni, P., Reber, G., Shoenfeld, Y., Tincani. A., Vlachoyiannopoulos, P., & Krilis S. (2006). International consensus statement on an update of the classification criteria for definite antiphospholipid syndrome (APS). *Journal of Thrombosis and Haemostasis*. Vol. 4, pp. 295-306, ISSN 1538-7836

Musial, J., Swadzba, J., Jankowski, M., Grzywacz, M., Bazan-Socha, S., & Szczeklik, A. (1997). Thrombin generation measured *ex vivo* following microvascular injury is increased in SLE patients with antiphospholipid-protein antibodies. *Thrombosis & Haemostasis*. Vol. 78, pp. 1173-1177, ISSN 0340-6245

Musial, J., Swadzba, J., Motyl, A., & Iwaniec, T. (2003). Clinical significance of antiphospholipid protein antibodies. Receiver operating characteristics plot analysis. *The Journal of Rheumatology*. Vol. 30, pp. 723-730, ISSN 0315-162X

Pengo, J., Biasiolo, A., Gresele, P., Marongiu, F., Erba, N., Veschi, F., Ghirarduzzi, A., Barcellona, D., & Tripodi, A. (2007 a). A comparison of lupus anticoagulant positive patients with clinical picture of antiphospholipid syndrome and those without. *Arteriosclerosis, Thrombosis and Vascular Biology*. Vol. 27, pp. 309-310, ISSN 1079-5642

Pengo, J., Biasiolo, A., Pegoraro, C., & Iliceto, S. (2004). A two-step coagulation test to indentify anti beta2-glycoprotein I lupus anticoagulants. *Thrombosis & Haemostasis*. Vol. 2, pp. 702-707, ISSN 0340-6245

Pengo, V., Banzato, A., Bison, E., Denas, G., Padayatti Jose, S., & Ruffatti, A. (2010). Antiphospholipid syndrome: critical analysis of the diagnostic path. *Lupus*. Vol. 19, No. 4, pp. 428-431, ISSN 0961-2033

Pengo, V., Biasiolo, A., Gresele, P., Marongiu, F., Erba, N., Veschi, F., Ghirarduzzi, A., de Candia, E., Montaruli, B., Testa, S., Barcellona, D., & Tripodi, A. (2007 b). Survey on lupus anticoagulant diagnosis by central evaluation of positive plasma samples. *Thrombosis & Haemostasis*. Vol. 5, pp. 925-930, ISSN 0340-6245

Pengo, V., Tripodi, A., Reber, G., Rand, J., Ortel, T., Galli, M., & de Groot, P. (2009). Update of the guidelines for lupus anticoagulant detection. *Journal of Thrombosis and Haemostasis*. Vol. 7, pp. 1737-1740, ISSN 1538-7836

Persijn, L., Decavele, A., Schouwers, S., & Devreese, K. (May 2011). Evaluation of a new set of automated chemiluminescense assays for anticardiolipin and anti-beta2-glycoprotein I antibodies in the laboratory diagnosis of the antiphospholipid syndrome. In: *Thrombosis Research*. 06.05.2011. Available from: http://www.ncbi.nlm.nih.gov/pubmed?term=Persijn%20decavele%20evaluation

Pierangeli, S., & Harris E. (2008). A quarter of a century in anticardiolipin antibody testing and attempted standardization has led us tu here, which is? *Seminars in Thrombosis and Haemostasis*. Vol. 34, No. 4, pp. 313-28, ISSN 00946176

Pierangeli, S., Espinola, R., Liu, X., & Harris E. (2001). Thrombogenic effects of antiphospholipid antibodies are mediated by intracellular adhesion molecule-1, vascular cell adhesion molecule-1 and P-selectin. *Circulation Research*. Vol. 88, pp. 245-50, ISSN 00097330

Ruffatti, A., Olivieri, S., Tonello, M., Bortolati, M., Bison, E., Salvan, E., Facchinetti, M., & Pengo, V. (2008). Influenece of different IgG anticardiolipin antibody cut-off values on antiphospholipid syndrome classification. *Journal of Thrombosis and Haemostasis*. Vol. 6, pp. 1693-1696, ISSN 1538-7836

Simmelink, M., Derksen, R., Arnout, J., & de Groot, P. (2003). A simple method to discriminate between beta2-glycoprotein I and prothrombin dependent lupus anticoagulants. *Journal of Thrombosis and Haemostasis*. Vol. 1, pp. 740-747. ISSN 1538-7836

Sims, P., Faioni, P., Wiedmer, T., & Shattil, S. (1988). Complement proteins C5b-9 cause release of membrane vesicles from the platelet surface that are enriched in the membrane receptor for coagulation factor Va and express prothrombinase activity. *The Journal of Biological Chemistry*. Vol. 263, pp. 18205-18212, ISSN 0021-9258

Studnicka-Benke, A., Steiner, G., Petera, P., & Smolen, J. (1996). Tumor necrosis factor alpha and its soluble receptors parallel clinical disease and autoimmune activity in systemic lupus erythematosus. *British Journal of Rheumatology*. Vol. 35, pp. 1067-1074, ISSN 0263-7103

Sugi, T., & McIntyre, J. (2001). Certain autoantibodies to phosphatidyletanolaminae (aPE) recognize factor XI and prekallikrein independently or in addition to the kininogens. *The Journal of Immunology*. Vol. 17, pp. 207-214, ISSN 0022-1767

Swadzba, J., & Musial, J. (2009). More on: the debate on antiphospholipid syndrome classification criteria. *Journal of Thrombosis and Haemostasis*. Vol. 7: pp. 501-502. ISSN 1538-7836

Swadzba, J., de Clerck, L., Stevens, W., Bridts, C., van Cotthem, K., Musial, J., Jankowski, M., & Szczeklik, A. (1997). Anticardiolipin antibodies, anti-β2-glycoprotein I, antiprothrombin antibodies and lupus anticoagulant in patients with systemic lupus erythematosus with a history of thrombosis. The *Journal of Rheumatology*. Vol. 24, pp. 1710-1715, ISSN 0315-162X

Swadzba, J., Iwaniec, T., & Musial, J. (2011 b). Increased level of tumour necrosis factor-α in patients with antiphospholipid syndrome - marker not only of inflammation but also of the prothrombotic state. *Rheumatology International*. Vol. 31, pp. 307-313. ISSN 0172-8172

Swadzba, J., Iwaniec, T., Szczeklik, A., & Musial, J. (2007). Revised classification criteria for antiphospholipid syndrome and the thrombotic risk in patients with autoimmune diseases. *Journal of Thrombosis and Haemostasis*. Vol. 5, pp. 1883-1889, ISSN 1538-7836

Swadzba, J., Sanak, M., Iwaniec, T., Dziedzina S., & Musial J. (2006). Valive/leucine 247 polymorphism of $\beta_2 GPI$ in patients with antiphospholipid syndrome: lack of association with anti- β_2GPI antibodies. *Lupus*. Vol. 15, pp. 218-222, ISSN 0961-2033

Swadzba, J., Iwaniec, T., Pulka, M., de Groot, P., & Musial, J. (2011 a). Lupus anticoagulant: performance of the tests as recommended by the latest ISTH guidelines. *Journal of Thrombosis and Haemostasis*. Vol. 9, No. 9, pp. 1776-1783, ISSN 1538-7836

Triplett, D., Stocker, K., Unger, G., & Barna, L. The (1993). Textarin/Ecarin ratio: a confirmatory test for lupus anticoagulants. *Thrombosis & Haemostasis*. Vol. 70, pp. 925-931, ISSN 0340-6245

Wilson, W., Gharavi, A., Koike, T., Lockshin, M., Branch, D., Piette, J-C., Brey, R., Derksen, R., Harris, E., Hughes, G., Triplett, D., & Khamashta, A. (1999). International consensus statement on preliminary classification criteria for definite antiphospholipid syndrome. *Arthritis & Rheumatism*. Vol. 42, pp. 1309-11, ISSN 1529-0131

Wong, R., & Favaloro, E. (2008). A consensus approach to the formulation of guidelines for laboratory testing and reporting of anti-pgospholipid antibody assays. *Seminars in Thrombosis and Haemostasis*. Vol. 34, No. 4, pp. 61-372, ISSN 00946176

Wong, R., Adelstein, S., Gillis, D. & Favaloro, E. (2005). Development of consensus guidelines for anticardiolipin and lupus anticoagulant testing. *Seminars in Thrombosis and Haemostasis*. Vol. 31, No. 1, pp. 39-48, ISSN 00946176

Wu, J., Stevenson, M., Brown, J., Grunz, E., Strawn, T., & Fay, W. (2008). C-reactive protein enhances tissue factor expression by vascular smooth muscle cells. *Arteriosclerosis, Thrombosis and Vascular Biology*. Vol. 28, pp. 698-704, ISSN 1079-5642

5

Presence of Antibodies Against *Mycoplasma penetrans* in Patients with Antiphospholipid Syndrome

Elizabeth Herrera-Saldivar[1], Antonio Yáñez[2,6,7,8], David Bañuelos[3], Constantino Gil[4,8] and Lilia Cedillo[4,5,7]

[1]*Posgrado en Ciencias Ambientales, Instituto de Ciencias, Benemérita Universidad Autónoma de Puebla (B.U.A.P.)*
[2]*Facultad de Estomatología, B.U.A.P.*
[3]*Centro Médico Nacional Gral. Manuel Ávila Camacho, Instituto Mexicano del Seguro Social I.M.S.S. Hospital de Especialidades San José, Puebla*
[4]*Centro de Investigaciones en Ciencias Microbiológicas del Instituto de Ciencias, B.U.A.P.*
[5]*Vicerrectoría de Extensión y Difusión de la Cultura, B.U.A.P.*
[6]*Cuerpo Académico de Ciencias Básicas*
[7]*Profesor con Perfil Deseable PROMEP*
[8]*Programa Integral de Fortalecimiento Institucional PIFI*
México

1. Introduction

The etiology of autoimmune diseases is multifactorial. The degree to which genetic and environmental factors influence susceptibility to autoimmune diseases is not fully understood. The antiphospholipid syndrome (APS) is characterized by vascular thrombosis, and/or pregnancy morbidity associated with anticardiolipin (aCL), anti-β2-glycoprotein-I (anti-β2-GPI) and lupus anticoagulant (LAC). [Levy et al., 2006].

1.1 Antiphospholipid syndrome

Antiphospholipid syndrome (APS), first described between 1983 to 1986, is characterized by a wide variety of hemocytopenic and vaso-occlusive manifestations and is associated with antibodies directed against negatively charged phospholipids. Features of APS include hemolytic anemia, thrombocytopenia, venous and arterial occlusions, livedo reticularis, pulmonary manifestations, recurrent fetal loss, neurologic manifestations (stroke, transverse myelitis, Guillain-Barré syndrome); and a positive Coombs test, anticardiolipin antibodies, or lupus anticoagulant activity. The factor(s) causing production of the antiphospholipid antibodies in primary antiphospholipid syndrome (PAPS) remain unidentified. [Hughes, 1993; Asherson et al., 1994; Yáñez et al., 1999].

2. Mycoplasmas

Mycoplasmas are eubacteria included within the Class Mollicutes, which comprises the smallest self-replicating bacteria, showing distinctive features such as: a) lack of a rigid cell wall envelope, b) sterol incorporation into their own plasma membrane, and c) reduced cellular (0.3 - 0.8 μm diameter) and genome sizes (0.58-2.20 Mb). [Bove, 1993; Razin et al., 1998]. Due to their reduced genome sizes, mycoplasmas exhibit restricted metabolic and physiological pathways for replication and survival [Razin et al., 1998]. Thus it is evident why these bacteria display strict dependence to their hosts for acquisition of aminoacids, nucleotides, lipids and sterols as biosynthetic precursors. [Baseman & Tully, 1997; Razin et al., 1998]. Currently, there are more than 200 species allocated into four orders, five families and eight genera within the Class Mollicutes [Brown et al., 2007]. All species of Mycoplasmataceae are obligate parasites and host specificity is quite strict for hosts including humans, rodents and birds. Mycoplasmal infections are most frequently associated with disease in the urogenital or respiratory tracts and, in most cases, mycoplasmas infect the host persistently. Like other parasites, many mycoplasma species display antigenic diversity, which has been noted in a variety of protein profiles or colony immunoblotting. [Sasaki, 2002].

2.1 Immune response against mycoplasmas

Host defense in mycoplasmal disease is dependent on both innate and humoral immunity. [Waites & Atkinson, 2009]. Molecular mimicry, survival within cells and phenotypic plasticity (antigenic variation) are the major mechanisms by which mycoplasmas evade the immune response [Chambaud et al, 1999; Razin et al., 1998; Rottem & Naot, 1998]. Association between immunodeficiency and mycoplasmal infections has been reported since the mid 1970s. Mycoplasmas can disseminate from localized infections and cause invasive diseases, especially in hypogammaglobulinemic subjects. [Cassell et al., 1994]. Antigenic variation is considered to be a strategy for persistence in the face of immune responses by the host. [Sasaki, 2002].

2.2 Diagnostic procedures

Many mycoplasmal diseases are quite different than those for fast-growing bacteria. It is noteworthy that mycoplasmal etiology of respiratory diseases is considered only after failure of diagnosis of other common bacterial etiologies. In addition, there are few specialized or reference laboratories and skilled personnel [Cassell et al., 1994; Waites & Atkinson, 2009]. PCR testing for species-specific mycoplasmal infection is suitable for clinical diagnosis. A culture enhanced PCR approach has also been suggested to overcome the effect of inhibitors in the amplification process [Abele-Horne et al., 1998].

2.3 Treatment

Due to absence of the cell wall envelope, mycoplasmas are insensitive to β-lactam antibiotics. However, antibiotics targeting protein synthesis or DNA modification molecules are highly effective against these bacteria. Macrolides, tetracyclines and fluoroquinolones eliminate mycoplasmas efficiently both *in vivo* and *in vitro* [Cassell et al., 1994; Waites & Atkinson, 2009].

3. Mycoplasma penetrans

Mycoplasma penetrans infects humans in the urogenital and respiratory tracts. A typical feature of *Mycoplasma penetrans* is its penetration into human cells. Internalization of the organisms into the urothelium was detected in autopsy samples from an acquired immunodeficiency syndrome (AIDS) patient [Lo, et al., 1992]. Intracellular replication and persistence for at least 6 months has been observed in cultured cells. [Dallo, et al., 2000].

Mycoplasma penetrans was first isolated from urine of homosexual men infected with (HIV), but not from healthy age-matched subjects. Subsequent studies suggested an association of this mycoplasma with Kaposi's sarcoma, but later findings did not confirm such association. [Baseman & Tully, 1997].

In humans, *Mycoplasma penetrans* is associated mainly with HIV-1 infection, particularly in adults among the homosexual population in Europe and the USA, and among both homosexual and heterosexual males in South America. Anti- *Mycoplasma penetrans* antibodies are found even in asymptomatic HIV carriers and in patients in the process of developing AIDS [Lo, S.C. et al., 1992; Cordova, et al., 1999; Grau, et al. 1995; Lo, et al. 1991; Lo, et al. 1992, Lo, et al. 1993; Wang, et al. 1992; Wang, et al., 1993]. Both the rapid decline in CD4-positive lymphocyte counts in *Mycoplasma penetrans* -seropositive HIV-infected individuals and the mitogenic effects of this organism on lymphocytes imply a contribution of persistent *Mycoplasma penetrans* infection to the deterioration of the immune system in HIV infection. [Grau, et al. 1998; Sasaki, et al., 1995]

On the other hand, *Mycoplasma penetrans* infection has also been suggested to be a primary cause of human disease in non-HIV-related urethritis and respiratory disease. [Cordova, et al, 1999; Yáñez et al. 1999] The *Mycoplasma penetrans* HF-2 strain was isolated from a previously healthy HIV-negative patient suffering from severe respiratory distress caused by *Mycoplasma penetrans* infection-associated systemic disease. [Yáñez et al. 1999]

The *Mycoplasma penetrans* HF-2 strain possesses a 1.3 Mb genome, which is the largest among the Mycoplasmataceae species thus far analyzed. Sasaki et al., identified 1038 putative coding DNA sequences (CDSs), among which 463 are *Mycoplasma penetrans* specific. The relatively large *Mycoplasma penetrans* genome compared with other mycoplasma genomes may be accounted for a probably rich core proteome. This data should be of great use for understanding the mechanism of *Mycoplasma penetrans* infection of humans and will also provide new insights into the regulation of virulence factors in *Mycoplasma penetrans* as well as other Mycoplasmataceae. [Sasaki, 2002].

4. Objective

The aim of this study was to determine the presence of antibodies against *Mycoplasma penetrans* in patients with antiphospholipid Syndrome.

5. Material and methods

5.1 Subjects

Eighty-eight patients at the Rheumatology Service of the "Hospital Manuel Avila Camacho del Instituto Mexicano del Seguro Social" in Puebla City, Mexico were included in the study.

A rheumatologist examined the patients and all fulfilled the American College Rheumatology criteria. Eighteen patients were diagnosed with Primary Antiphospholipid Syndrome, 26 patients with Secondary Antiphospholipid Syndrome and 44 patients with Systemic Lupus Erythematosus (SLE).

Forty four women without any autoimmune or infectious disease were included in the study as healthy women. Healthy women were not under antibiotic or drug treatment. The ethics committee of the Hospital approved this study and informed patient consent was obtained.

5.2 Specimens

Peripheral whole blood samples from patients and healthy women were collected in order to detect IgG, IgM and IgA antibodies against cardiolipin and β2 glycoprotein I using a ELISA Test. Immunoglobulin M and G against *Mycoplasma penetrans* were also investigated using ELISA and Western blot assays. Blood samples were collected in tubes without anticoagulant and stored at -20^{0}C until use.

5.3 Detection of antibodies anticardiolipin using ELISA test

Antibodies anticardiolipin and anti-β2 glycoprotein I were tested in all patients and healthy persons. Diagnostic Automation Inc. ELISA test was used to detect IgG, IgA and IgM against cardiolipin and β2 glycoprotein I.

5.4 Detection of antibodies against *Mycoplasma penetrans* by ELISA test

Mycoplasma penetrans HF strain was cultured in E media, centrifuged at 12,000 rpm for 40 min and suspended in PBS (0.015 M pH 7.4). This procedure was repeated 3 times until the suspension was adjusted to an OD_{600} = 1 using a carbonate buffer (0.1M pH 9.6). This suspension was considered the antigen. Two hundred microliters of antigen was added to each well of the plate. The plates were covered and incubated at 37°C for two hours. The plates were kept at 4°C for 4 days before use and antigen excess was removed. The plates were washed five times with PBS and then dried. Two hundred microliters of 2 % skim milk diluted in PBS-Tween 0.05% were added to each well of the plate. Plates were covered and kept at 4°C for one night, then, excess skim milk was removed. Two hundred microliters of patient´s sera diluted 1:200 in PBS-Tween 0.05% were added to each well plate and incubated at room temperature during night. Antihuman IgM or IgG alkaline-phosphatase conjugates diluted 1:1000 were added and incubated at room temperature for one hour. The conjugate was removed and the plates were washed five times with PBS/Tween (0.05 %). Two hundred microliters of alkaline phosphatase substrate was added to each well. These plates were incubated in the dark until a yellow color was visible and reaction was stopped adding 20 microliters of Na OH 1N in each well. Plates were read at 405 nm in a multiscan ELISA meter. Positive and negative controls were tested.

5.5 Detection of antibodies against *Mycoplasma penetrans* using Western Blot tests

Mycoplasma penetrans HF whole cell was used as an antigen. The bacteria was cultured in E media, centrifuged at 12,000 rpm for 40 min and suspended in PBS (0.015 M pH 7.4). This procedure was repeated 3 times until the suspension was adjusted to an OD_{600} =1 using PBS and 750 microliters of this solution was mixed with 250 microliters of sample buffer (40 % glycerol, 240 mM Tris/HCl pH 6.8, 0.04% bromophenol blue, 5 % β-mercaptoethanol and boiled during 10 minutes. A 14 % PAGE-SDS gel was used in order to separate proteins using 100 volts for 3 hours. The proteins were transferred to nitrocellulose (0.45 nm pore). Transfers were done using a semidry chamber at 15 volts for 15 minutes. Membranes were stained using amido black to verify proteins transference. The membranes were blocked using a 2% skim milk solution for 1 hour at room temperature. The IgM and IgG antibodies against *Mycoplasma penetrans* were detected using 2 nitrocellulose 5 mm wide strips in each patient's serum diluted 1:50 in PBS. The strips were stirred constantly for 1 hour at room temperature and washed 5 times with PBS-Tween (0.05%). Each strip was in contact with the alkaline phosphatase conjugate (anti-human IgM or IgG) for 1 hour at room temperature. The strips were washed five times with PBS-Tween (0.05%) and presence of antibodies was detected with a mixture of 66 microliters of nitro blue tetrazolium (NTB), 33 microliters of 5-bromo-4-cloro-3-indolilphosphate (BCIP), and 10 microliters of alkaline phosphatase buffer.

5.6 Environmental data collection

Patients and healthy people were questioned about environmental factors (living conditions, presence of pets at home, presence of rivers, garbage dumps or standing water, use of insecticide, presence of preeclampsia, infectious diseases and their medical history).

6. Results

Eighty eight patients were included in the study, 18 patients were diagnosed with Primary Antiphospholipid Syndrome (APS), 26 patients with Secondary Antiphospholipid Syndrome and 44 patients with Systemic Lupus Erythematosus. All patients were females whose age ranged from 13 to 64 years old.

6.1 Anticardiolipin antibodies

Five patients with Primary APS tested positive for anticardiolipin and anti-β2 glycoprotein I (5/18), five patients with Secondary APS tested positive (5/26) in remained 13 Primary APS and 21 Secondary APS patients, lupus anticoagulant were present. Two patients with SLE (2/44), none of the healthy persons were positive (0/44) for anticardiolipin and anti-β2 glycoprotein I antibodies. X^2 was calculated and it showed an association between anticardiolipin antibodies and primary APS (p= 0.006)

6.2 Detection of antibodies against *Mycoplasma penetrans* by ELISA

Antibodies against *Mycoplasma penetrans*	Primary APS	Secondary APS	SLE	Healthy Persons
Ig G	8/18 (44 %)	20/26 (77%)	20/44 (45%)	2/44 (4%)
Ig M	14/18 (78%)	22/26 (85%)	33/44 (75%)	2/44 (4%)

X^2 was calculated, there was an association between presence of both Ig G and IgM antibodies with Secondary APS

6.3 Detection of antibodies against *Mycoplasma penetrans* using Western Blot

Antibodies against *Mycoplasma penetrans*	Primary APS	Secondary APS	SLE	Healthy Persons
Ig G	13/18 (72%)	11/19 (55%)	13/24 (54%)	2/44 (4%)
Ig M	13/18 (72%)	13/19 (68%)	16/24 (67%)	2/44 (4%)

X^2 was calculated $p>0.05$. There was no association between the development of antibodies and disease.

We performed first the detection of antibodies using ELISA test and then using Western Blot test. Unfortunately we did not have enough serum from 7 patients with Secondary APS and 20 patients with SLE and we could not contact them to get more sample.

6.4 Presence of antibodies in patients and controls

Antibody	Primary APS	Secondary APS	SLE	Healthy persons
Anticardiolipin and Anti-β2 glycoprotein I	6/18 (33%)	5/26 (19%)	2/44 (4%)	0/44 (0%)
IgG vs *Mycoplasma penetrans* (ELISA)	8/18 (44%)	20/26 (77%)	20/44 (45%)	2/44 (4%)
IgM vs *Mycoplasma penetrans* (ELISA)	14/18 (78%)	22/26 (85%)	33/44 (75%)	2/44 (4%)
IgG vs. *Mycoplasma penetrans* (Western blot)	3/18 (72%)	11/19 (55%)	13/24 (54%)	2/44 (4%)
IgM vs. *Mycoplasma penetrans* (Western blot)	3/18 (72%)	13/19 (68%)	16/24 (67%)	2/44 (4%)

X^2 was calculated $p<0.0007$. There was an association between presence of antibodies only in patients with APS and SLE.

6.5 Presence of environmental factors

Environmental Factors	Primary APS	Secondary APS	SLE	Healthy Persons
Lack of running water, electricity and sewage system	1/18 (5%)	5/26 (19%)	1/44 (2%)	3/44 (7%)
More than 3 people sleeping in the same room	1/18 (5%)	3/26 (11%)	11/44 (25%)	8/44 (18%)
Presence of pets (dogs, cats and birds) at home	11/18 (61%)	13/26 (50%)	30/44 (68%)	30/44 (68%)
Presence of rivers, garbage dumps or standing water near their houses	8/18 (44%)	12/26 (46%)	22/44 (50%)	15/44 (34%)
Frequent use of insecticide	6/18 (33%)	11/26 (42%)	13/44 (30%)	16/44 (36%)

Environmental Factors	Primary APS	Secondary APS	SLE	Healthy Persons
Preeclampsia	1/18 (5%)	4/26 (15%)	6/44 (14%)	6/44 (14%)
Common presence of infectious diseases	8/18 (44%)	8/26 (31%)	23/44 (52%)	1/44 (2%)
Seasonal aggravation of symptoms	13/18 (72%)	12/26 (46%)	32/44 (72%)	0/44 (0%)
Family medical history of rheumatic diseases	3/18 (17%)	10/26 (38%)	18/44 (41%)	3/44 (7%)

X^2 was calculated $p<0.0001$. There was an association between presence of some environmental factors and disease.

7. Discussion

The etiology and pathogenesis of most autoimmune diseases, including the APS, remain unclear, with the involvement of infectious, autoimmune, and auto inflammatory pathways possibly being implicated. Infection may initiate a disease, although it is the combination of genetic regulation in the host, the interplay between virus or bacteria persistence, and autoimmunity that produces the later phases of disease, the antigenic determinants responsible for inducing autoimmune disease, and the pathogenic effector mechanisms. [Garcia-Carrasco et al., 2009].

Cervera et al., analyzed the clinical characteristics of 100 patients with antiphospholipid syndrome (APS) associated with infections. The main clinical manifestations of APS included: pulmonary involvement (39%), skin involvement (36%), and renal involvement (35%); nine with renal thrombotic microangiopathy. The main associated infections and agents included skin infection (18%), HIV (17%), pneumonia (14%), hepatitis C (13%), and urinary tract infection (10%). They concluded that various different infections can be associated with thrombotic events in patients with APS, including the potentially lethal subset termed catastrophic APS. [Cervera et al., 2004].

Infectious agents can play a dual role in the etiopathogeny of APS, acting as the initial trigger of the production of antibodies cross-reacting with β2 glycoprotein I (β2GPI) and infectious peptides, and also inducing an inflammatory response. This is the so-called "two-hit theory" in which pathogenic anti-β2GPI antibodies act as the first hit and inflammatory responses as the second. [Amital et al. 2008; García-Carrasco et al. 2009].

Antiphospholipid antibodies (aPL) may be demonstrated during the course of many infections in addition to occurring in conditions such as Systemic Lupus Erythematosus (SLE), APS, and a wide variety of other rheumatic diseases. Syphilis was the first infection to be linked with aPL: one of the components of the VDRL reagent (cardiolipin) being responsible for the original finding that antibodies thought initially to be directed against cardiolipin were, in fact, pivotal in the pathogenesis and for the diagnosis of the APS. [Asherson, R.A., & Shoenfield, Y., 2003].

Interestingly, it has been reported that a substantial number of patients with *Mycoplasma pneumoniae*-induced respiratory disease have anticardiolipin antibodies. Furthermore, many clinical criteria for APS have also been well documented in patients with *M. pneumoniae* infection, including Guillain-Barré-like illness and other central nervous system manifestations, hemolytic anemia, positive Coombs test, thrombocytopenia, and arthritis. [Asherson et al., 1994; Snowden et al., 1990; Yáñez et al., 1999].

Snowden et al. (1990) found antiphospholipid antibodies in more than 50% of patients with *M. pneumoniae* pneumonia, especially those with severe infections requiring hospitalization. Catteau et al., described two cases of Stevens-Johnson syndrome associated with *M. pneumoniae* infection and the presence of antiphospholipid antibodies. [Snowden et al., 1990; Catteau et al., 1995].

In a previous work, *Mycoplasma penetrans* was isolated from the blood and throat of a previously healthy non-HIV-infected 17-year-old woman sexually inactive who had an acute onset of arthritis, fever, and hemolytic anemia. Upon hospital admission, she developed respiratory distress, severe hemolytic anemia, leukocytosis, and thrombocytopenia. Blood and bone marrow smears did not show a neoplasic process. She was treated with methylprednisolone and trimethoprim/sulfamethoxazole on day 2, but her condition deteriorated. On day 3, the antibiotic treatment was changed to ceftazidime. On day 4 severe respiratory distress and hypoxemia developed, and the patient was admitted to the intensive care unit. Venereal Disease Research Laboratory (VDRL) tests were negative as were tests for Systemic Lupus Erythematosus. The patient was shown to have anti-dsDNA antibodies but positive anticardiolipin antibodies by ELISA test. Respiratory secretions were culture-negative and were shown to be negative by immunofluorescence for respiratory syncytial virus, adenovirus, influenza A, influenza B, parainfluenza 1,2,3, and *Chlamydia*. Serologic analysis indicated that the patient had no antibodies against HIV, hepatitis B or C virus. No acid-fast bacilli or other bacteria were observed on blood and tracheal aspirate smears. In addition, thoracic radiography showed only bilateral diffuse pulmonary infiltrates. On day 2 of hospital admission, blood and throat samples were cultured for aerobic flora and mycoplasma. *Mycoplasma penetrans* was isolated in a pure culture from the patient's blood (isolate HF-1) and throat (isolate HF-3). Later *Mycoplasma penetrans* was isolated from tracheal aspirate in pure culture (isolate HF-2). Treatment was initiated on day 6 with clindamycin and vancomycin. The patient also received transfusion of two units of washed red blood cells. After 3 days of treatment, the patient improved clinically and was released from the intensive care unit on day 9; thoracic radiographs were clear. [Yáñez et al., 1999].

Mycoplasma penetrans infection was detected in the APS patient's specimens prior to culture and was confirmed by specific polymerase chain reaction (PCR). Similar results were obtained by another pair of PCR primers also within the 16S rRNA gene and designed for the specific detection of *Mycoplasma penetrans*. Samples from both original specimens and broth cultures were tested by PCR for other human mycoplasmas, but none were detected. This finding was the basis of our present study, where the main purpose was to determine if the presence of *Mycoplasma penetrans* is a casual event or the bacteria may play a role in the pathogenesis of APS and SLE. [Yáñez et al., 1999].

Since autoimmune diseases may be influenced by environmental factors, we questioned patients about the presence of these factors. Some aspects about the epidemiology and pathogenesis of *Mycoplasma penetrans* infections remain unknown, so some questions try to search for the primary habitat of the bacteria and others about the contact of the patients with some environmental factors that may influence the development of APS and SLE. [Yáñez et al., 1999].

Mycoplasmas are the smallest free living microorganisms and also defined as fastidious bacteria because of their nutritional requirements that is why the detection used immunological techniques to determine if the presence of antibodies anti- *Mycoplasma penetrans* are common in patients with APS and SLE but they are absent or in a low proportion of healthy people. IgG and IgM antibodies were detected suggesting a recent infection in the patient and/or a permanent contact of the bacteria with the host. Most patients were under corticosteroid or immunosuppressive therapy. These treatments may favor the persistence of *Mycoplasma penetrans* in patients with APS and SLE. [Yáñez et al., 1999].

The presence of *Mycoplasma penetrans* may not be casual and it could favor the development of APS or SLE. *Mycoplasma penetrans* is able to produce Phospholipase A2. This enzyme degrades the phospholipids of the host membrane and helps *Mycoplasma penetrans* in the penetration to the host cell [Salman, et al., 1998; Rottem, S., 2003]. It is well known that mycoplasmas induce autoimmune diseases in appropriate hosts. [Baseman & Tully, 1997; Waites & Atkinson, 2009]. Previous studies suggest that mycoplasmas may induce antiphospholipid antibodies [Snowden, et al., 1990; Yáñez et al., 1999]. Although there was an association between common presence of infectious diseases and seasonal aggravation of symptoms and/or APS and SLE, more studies need to be done. It was not possible to establish an association between the presence of an environmental factor and APS and SLE.

8. Conclusion

Mycoplasma penetrans was first reported in 1993 as an emerging infectious agent. Yáñez et al., 1999 reported the first of *Mycoplasma penetrans* isolation in a non-HIV-infected patient with APS. The mycoplasma strain isolated from the APS patient exhibited typical morphologic features of *Mycoplasma penetrans,* which are unique among mycoplasmas isolated from humans. The lack of *Mycoplasma penetrans* strong humoral response in the APS patient was a factor in favor of dissemination of the mycoplasma, hence its isolation from the blood. A possible association between *Mycoplasma penetrans* and APS should be considered.

Antibodies against *Mycoplasma penetrans* in a high proportion of APS or SLE patients suggest that the presence of the bacteria is not casual and mycoplasmas may play a role in the development of these diseases.

9. Acknowledgment

Authors want to thank Dr. Antonio Rivera Tapia for his help in the study and Elliot Heilman for his valuable review of the manuscript.

10. References

Abele-Horn, M.; Busch, U.; Nitschko, H.; Jacobs, E.; Bax, R.; Pfaff, F.; Schaffer, B. & Heesemann, J. (1998). Molecular Approaches to Diagnosis of Pulmonary Diseases

Due to *Mycoplasma pneumoniae. Journal of Clinical Microbiology,* Vol. 36, No. 2 (February 1998), pp. 548–551, ISSN 0095-1137.

Amital, H.; Govoni, M.; Maya, R.; Meroni; P.L.; Ori, B.; Shoenfeld, F.; Tincani, A.; Trotta, F.; Sarzi-Puttini, P. & Atzeni, F. (2008). Role of the infectious agents in systemic rheumatic diseases. *Clinical Experimental Rheumatology.* Vol. 26. Suppl. 48, pp. S27-S32, ISSN 1593-098X.

Asherson, R.A. & Cervera, R. (1994). "Primary"," secondary", and other variants of the antiphospholipid syndrome. *Lupus* Vol. 3 pp. 293-8, ISSN 0961-2033.

Asherson, R.A. & Shoenfeld, Y. (2003). Human immunodeficiency virus infection, antiphospholipid antibodies, and the antiphospholipid syndrome (Editorial). *Journal of Rheumatology.* Vol. 30, pp. 214-219, ISSN 0315-162X.

Baseman, J.B. & Tully, J.G. (1997). *Mycoplasmas*: Sophisticated Reemerging and Burdened by Their Notoriety. *Emerging Infectious Diseases,* Vol. 3, No. 1 (January-March 1997), pp. 21-32, ISSN 1080-6040.

Bové, J.M. (1993). Molecular features of *Mollicutes. Clinical Infectious Diseases,* Vol. 17, Supplement 1 (August 1993), pp. S10-S31, ISSN 1058-4838

Brown, D.R.; Whitcomb, R.F. & Bradbury, J.M. (2007). Revised Minimal Standards for Description of New Species of the Class *Mollicutes* (Division Tenericutes). *International Journal of Systematic and Evolutionary Microbiology,* Vol. 57, No. 11 (November 2007), pp. 2703–2719. ISSN 1466-5026

Cassell, G.H.; Blanchard, A.; Duffy, L.; Crabb, D. & Waites, K.B. (1994). *Mycoplasmas*, In: *Clinical and Pathogenic Microbiology,* B.J. Howard, J.F. Keiser, A.S. Weissfeld, T.F. Smith, & R.C. Tilton (Eds), pp. 491-502, Mosby, Boston, USA, ISBN 978-0801664267.

Catteau, B.; Delaporte, E.; Hachulla, E.; Piette, F. & Bergoend, H. (1995). Infection à mycoplasme avec syndrome de Stevens-Johnson et anticorps antiphospholipides: à propos de deux cas. *Revue de Medicine Interne,* Vol. 16, pp. 10-14, ISSN 0248-8663.

Cervera, R.; Asherson, R.A.; Acevedo, M.L.; Gómez-Puerta, J.A.; Espinosa, G.; G de la Red, G.; Gil, V.; Ramos-Casals, M.; García-Carrasco, M.; Ingelmo, M. & Font, J. (2004). Antiphospholipid syndrome associated with infections: clinical and microbiological characteristics of 100 patients. *Annals of Rheumatic Diseases,* Vol. 63, pp. 1312-1317, ISSN 0003-4967.

Chambaud, I.; Wroblewski, H. & Blanchard, A. (1999). Interactions between Mycoplasma Lipoproteins and the Host Immune System. *Trends in Microbiology,* Vol. 7, No. 12 (December 1999), pp. 493-499, ISSN 0966-842X

Cordova, C.M.; Takei, K.; Rosenthal, C.; Miranda, M.A.; Vaz, A.J. & da Cunha, R.A. (1999) Evaluation of IgG, IgM and IgA antibodies to Mycoplasma penetrans detected by ELISA and immunoblot in HIV-1-infected and STD patients, in São Paulo, Brazil. *Microbes and Infection,* Vol. 1, pp. 1095–1101, ISSN 1286-4579.

Dallo, S.J. & Baseman, J.B. (2000). Intracellular DNA replication and long term survival of the pathogenic mycoplasmas. Microbial Pathogenesis. Vol. 29 pp. 301-309, ISSN 0882-4010.

García-Carrasco, M.; Galarza-Maldonado, C.; Mendoza-Pinto, C. & Escarcega, R.O. (2009). Infections and the Antiphospholipid Syndrome. *Clinical Reviews in Allergy & Immunology,* Vol. 36, pp. 104-108, ISSN 1559-0267.

Grau, O.; Slizewicz, B.; Tuppin, P.; Launay, V.; Bourgeois, E.; Sagot, N.; Moynier, M.; Lafeuillade, A.; Bachelez, H.; Clauvel, J.P.; Blanchard, A.; Bahraoui, E. &

Montagnier, L. (1995) Association of Mycoplasma penetrans with HIV infection. *Journal of Infection*, Vol. 172, pp. 672–681, ISSN 0300-8126.

Grau, O.; Tuppin, P.; Slizewicz, B.; Launay, V.; Goujard, C.; Bahraoui, E.; Delfraissy, J.F. & Montagnier, L. (1998) A longitudinal study of seroreactivity against Mycoplasma penetrans in HIV-infected homosexual men: association with disease progression. *AIDS Research Human Retroviruses,* Vol. 14, pp. 661–667, ISSN 0889-2229.

Hughes, G.R.V. (1993). The antiphospholipid syndrome ten years on. *The Lancet* Vol. 342, pp. 341-4, ISSN 0140-6736.

Levy, Y.; Almong, O.; Gorshtein, A. & Shoenfeld, Y. (2006). The environment and antiphospholipid syndrome. *Lupus*, Vol. 15, pp. 784-790, ISSN 0961-2033.

Lo, S.C.; Hayes, M.M.; Wang, R.Y.; Pierce, P.F.; Kotani, H. and Shih, J.W. (1991) Newly discovered mycoplasma isolated from patients infected with HIV. *The Lancet*, Vol. 338, pp. 1415–1418, ISSN 0140-6736.

Lo, S.C.; Hayes, M.M.; Tully, J.G.; Wang, R.Y.; Kotani, H.; Pierce, P.F.; Rose, D.L. & Shih, J.W. (1992) Mycoplasma penetrans sp. nov., from the urogenital tract of patients with AIDS. *International Journal of Systematic Bacteriology*, Vol. 42, pp. 357–364, ISSN 0020-7713.

Lo, S.C.; Hayes, M.M.; Kotani, H.; Pierce, P.F.; Wear, D.J.; Newton, P.B.,III; Tully, J.G. & Shih, J.W. (1993) Adhesion onto and invasion into mammalian cells by Mycoplasma penetrans: a newly isolated mycoplasma from patients with AIDS. *Modern Pathology*, Vol. 6, pp. 276–280, ISSN 0893-3952.

Razin, S.; Yoguev, D. & Naot, Y. (1998). Molecular Biology and Pathogenicity of Mycoplasmas. *Microbiology and Molecular Biology Reviews,* Vol. 62, No. 4 (December 1998), pp. 1094-1156, ISSN 1092-2172.

Rottem, S. & Naot, Y. (1998). Subversion and Exploitation of Host Cells by Mycoplasmas. *Trends in Microbiology*, Vol 6, No. 11 (November 1998), pp. 436-440.

Rottem, S. (2003). Interaction of mycoplasmas with host cells. *Physiological Reviews*, Vol. 83, pp. 417-432, ISSN 0031-9333.

Salman, M.; Borovsky, Z. & Rottem, S. (1998). Mycoplasma penetrans infection of Molt-3 lymphocytes induces changes in the lipid composition of host cells. *Microbiology*, Vol. 144, pp. 3447-3454, ISSN 1350-0872.

Sasaki, Y.; Blanchard, A.; Watson, H.L.; Garcia, L.S.; Dulioust, A.; Montagnier, L. & Gougeon, M.L. (1995) In vitro influence of Mycoplasma penetrans on activation of peripheral T lymphocytes from healthy donors or human immunodeficiency virus-infected individuals. *Infection and Immunity*, Vol. 63, pp. 4277–4283, ISSN 1098-5522.

Sasaki, Y.; Ishikawa, J.; Yamashita, A.; Oshima, K.; Kenri, T.; Furuya, K.; Yoshino, C.; Horino, A.; Shiba, T.; Sasaki, T. & Hattori, M. (2002). The complete genomic sequence of Mycoplasma penetrans, an intracellular bacterial pathogen in humans *Nucleic Acids Research*, 30(23):5293-5300, ISSN 1362-4962.

Snowden, N.; Wilson, P.B.; Longson, M. & Pumphrey, R.S.H. (1990). Antiphospholipid antibodies and Mycoplasma pneumonia infection. *Postgraduate Medical Journal*, Vol. 66, pp. 356-62, ISSN 0032-5473.

Waites, K.B. & Atkinson, T.P., (2009). The role of Mycoplasma in upper respiratory infections. *Current Infectious Diseases Reports*, Vol. 11, pp. 198-206, ISSN 1523-3847.

Wang, R.Y.; Shih, J.W.; Grandinetti, T.; Pierce, P.F.; Hayes, M.M.; Wear, D.J.; Alter, H.J. & Lo, S.C. (1992) High frequency of antibodies to Mycoplasma penetrans in HIV-infected patients. *The Lancet*, Vol. 340, pp. 1312–1316, ISSN 0140-6736 .

Wang, R.Y.; Shih, J.W.; Weiss, S.H.; Grandinetti, T.; Pierce, P.F.; Lange, M.; Alter, H.J.; Wear, D.J.; Davies, C.L.; Mayur, R.K. & Lo, S.C. (1993) Mycoplasma penetrans infection in male homosexuals with AIDS: high seroprevalence and association with Kaposi's sarcoma. *Clinical Infectious Diseases*, Vol. 17, pp. 724–729, ISSN 1058-4838.

Yáñez, A.; Cedillo, L.; Neyrolles, O.; Alonso, E.; Prévost, M.C.; Rojas, J.; Watson, H.L.; Blanchard, A. & Cassell, G.H. (1999). *Mycoplasma penetrans* Bacteremia and Primary Antiphospholipid Syndrome. *Emerging Infectious Diseases*, Vol. 5, No. 1 (January-February 1999), pp. 164-167, ISSN: 1080-6059

6

Antiphospholipid Antibodies and Their Association with Atherosclerotic Changes in Patients with Systemic Lupus Erythematosus – Review of Literature and Own Experiences

Katarzyna Fischer, Jacek Fliciński and Marek Brzosko
Department of Rheumatology and Internal Diseases,
Pomeranian Medical University in Szczecin
Poland

1. Introduction

Systemic lupus erythematosus (SLE) is a chronic autoimmune and inflammatory disease. There are many tissues and organs involved in the course of the disease: skin, joints, kidneys, serous membranes, and haematopoetic, nervous and cardiovascular systems as well. The course of the disease is characterized by periods of exacerbations and remissions (Bombardier et al., 1992).

The crucial role in SLE pathogenesis plays dysregulation of both the innate and adaptive immune systems. Defective function of T cells and overactivation of B cells as well as defective clearance of apoptotic debris cause the production of autoantibodies, formation and deposition of immune complexes and, consequently, systemic tissue and organ damage (Shoenfeld et al., 1999; Muñoz et al., 2010).

On the other hand, an involvement of both innate and adaptive immunity in atherosclerosis pathogenesis is well documented and recent data clearly characterize atherosclerosis as an inflammatory and autoimmune disease. The presence of monocytes/macrophages transformed into lipid loaded foam cells, natural killer cells, dendritic cells, mast cells and immunoglobulins within the plaque has been documented. Various autoantibodies have been reported to associate with atherosclerosis including anti-heat shock protein 60/65, anti-oxidized low density lipoprotein (aoxLDL) and selected antiphospholipid antibodies (aPL) (George et al., 2000; Gordon et al., 2001; Doria et al., 2005).

There is also a growing bulk of evidence on the strength of association between systemic connective tissue diseases, such SLE and premature and accelerated atherosclerosis development (Fischer, 2008; Doria et al., 2003) and atherosclerotic cardiovascular events are considered a leading cause of mortality in those patients (Borchers, 2004). Because traditional risk factors alone fail to fully account for accelerated atherosclerosis in SLE (Esdaile et al., 2001; Lee et al., 2010), it has been attributed to complex interactions between traditional risk factors and factors associated with the disease process and its treatment (Svenungsson et al., 2001; Bruce et al., 2000).

The purpose of this chapter was to review the risk of atherosclerotic disorders development in SLE as well as antiphospholipid syndrome (APS) patients, and to analyze the role of selected immune mechanisms in atherosclerosis pathogenesis, including potential role of autoantibodies, especially aPL.

2. Atherosclerosis in systemic lupus erythematosus – The background

Initial reports on the development of early atherosclerotic lesions in patients with SLE came from autopsy examinations performed by Bulkley and Roberts in 1975 (Bulkley & Roberts, 1975). A year later, these observations were confirmed by other investigators, who developed a bimodal pattern of causes of mortality in this patient group, indicating that the first mortality peak applies to patients with active SLE, concurrent renal involvement, and recurrent infections, who were treated with high dose glucocorticosteroids. The second mortality peak was observed in patients with inactive SLE, who had been treated with glucocorticosteroids for many years and had previous myocardial infarction (Urowitz et al., 1976).

Study performed at the University of Pittsburgh Medical Centre from 1980 to 1993 showed that women with SLE in the 35- to 44-year age group were more than 50 times more likely to have myocardial infarction than women of similar age in the Framingham offspring cohort. Overall, risk of myocardial infarction in SLE female patients was 6-fold higher in comparison with the general population. Of note, two thirds of all first cardiac events occurred in women younger than 55 years old (Manzi et al., 1997). Similar data demonstrated cohort study at Toronto lupus clinic. The rate of myocardial infarction in lupus patients was 5 per 1000 persons in comparison with 1 per 1000 persons in the general population from 1993 to 1994 and the mean age of first cardiac episode was 49 years in SLE patients compared with the peak incidence in the general population aged 65 to 74 years (Bruce et al., 2000).

Furthermore, the report from the Toronto SLE cohort study showed among 10.9% of 1087 patients at least one atherosclerotic vascular event either cardiac, cerebrovascular or peripheral vascular. The prevalence of coronary events was as follows: myocardial infarction - 2.2%, angina - 7.2% and sudden death - 0.3% (Urowitz et al., 2007). Comparable results provided large lupus cohorts studies in Pittsburgh and Baltimore showing the occurrence of clinical symptoms of coronary artery disease in 6.6% and 8.3% patients respectively (Manzi et al, 1997; Petri et al, 1992).

Study performed in 129 SLE patients at Department of Rheumatology and Internal Diseases Pomeranian Medical University, which focused on prevalence and selected risk factors of ischemic heart disease and myocardial infarction, demonstrated ischemic heart disease in 20 (15.5%) SLE patients and myocardial infarctions in 9 (6.97%). Ischemic heart disease and myocardial infarction were related to high activity of SLE, odds ratio (OR): 7.18; $p = 0.012$ and OR: 27.3; $p = 0.006$ respectively. Ischemic heart disease was significantly more common in older patients (52.8 years versus 42.2 years; $p = 0.0008$), in patients with hypertension ($p < 0.05$) and with impaired glucose tolerance (OR: 8.44; $p = 0.03$). Myocardial infarction was significantly associated with high uric acid level (OR: 5.01; $p = 0.052$) and impaired glucose tolerance (OR: 7.42; $p = 0.047$) (Ostanek et al., 2006a).

Our next study was aimed at the assessment of cardiovascular abnormalities in SLE patients in echocardiographic examination. The following pathologies were significantly more frequent in SLE patients: pericardial involvement (58%), organic changes of the mitral valve cusps (54%), organic changes of the aortic valve cusps (36%), widening of the aortal lumen (35%), enlargement of the atrium (18%), hypokinenesis of the left ventricle myocardial muscle (15%). Moreover, pericarditis was marker of high activity of the disease (OR: 3.89; 95% confidence interval (CI): 1.05-14.40; p = 0.042) and enlargement of the left atrium was significantly associated with the low level of HDL-cholesterol (OR: 6.94; 95%CI: 1.17-40.9; p = 0.033) (Ostanek et al., 2006b).

These data clearly show that cardiac involvement is a frequent and early systemic complication in the course of SLE. Cardiovascular disorders are often associated with high activity of the disease and classic risk factors are poorly related to these manifestations.

Additionally, many reports on subclinical atherosclerosis development in SLE patients have been published in recent years. Early diagnosis of subclinical changes can be established using noninvasive imaging techniques, which enable to assess atherosclerotic lesions on different stages of their development. The subclinical atherosclerosis was reported in 30% to 67% of SLE patients (Manzi et al., 1999; Fischer, 2008).

Endothelial dysfunction is a widespread phenomenon which represents an early stage of atherogenesis and it is established as a precursor and denominator of atherosclerotic events (Celermajer et al., 1992). Techniques designed to assess endothelial function are based on measurement of brachial artery reactivity in response to changes in blood-flow caused by passive congestion (flow-mediated vasodilatation, which is dependent on endothelial function) (Corretti et al., 2002). Studies performed in SLE patients documented an impaired endothelial function and this fact was attributed to reduced nitric oxide bioavailability resulting from increased oxidative stress in the course of SLE (El-Magadmi et al., 2004; Kiss et al., 2006; Wright et al., 2006). Furthermore, impairment of endothelial function remained significant even after adjustment for other classic atherosclerosis risk factors and the authors suggested that SLE is an independent risk factor for endothelial dysfunction (El-Magadmi et al., 2004). Interestingly, study completed in young females with SLE (mean age 29.4 years) disclosed vasomotor dysfunction of the coronary arteries, thus indicating the presence of subclinical coronary artery disease in these patients (Hirata et al., 2007).

Early stage of atherosclerosis can be also defined as a reduction of vascular elasticity. Measurement of pulse wave velocity is the most commonly used approach to assess stiffness of the large arteries (Tanaka et al.; 1998). Evaluation of aortal wall elasticity in patients with SLE was the subject of numerous clinical studies. They all documented increased aorta stiffness in SLE patients and its relationship to a higher risk of cardiovascular events (Selzer et al., 2001; Bjarnegård et al., 2006) and its association with active inflammation in analyzed patient groups (Roman et al., 2005).

Ankle-brachial index measurement enables to identify atherosclerotic lesions in the arteries of the lower extremities. Because of its simplicity and low cost it is recommended for use in routine diagnostic evaluation especially to detect asymptomatic atherosclerotic lesions. Furthermore, this test is used in the stratification of overall cardiovascular risk (Graham et al., 2007). Clinical studies confirmed the usefulness of ankle-brachial index in detecting early atherosclerotic changes in SLE patients (Theodoridou et al., 2003).

Measurement of carotid intima-media thickness (CIMT) with B-mode ultrasound is a surrogate marker of atherosclerosis. The utility of CIMT in the evaluation of subclinical atherosclerosis in SLE patients has been well documented (Svenungsson et al., 2001; Doria et al., 2003; Fischer, 2008). This method is often used in epidemiological studies (Denarié et al., 2000; Sun et al., 2002) and also in assessing total cardiovascular risk (Ebrahim et al., 1999). Emphasis is put on a correlation between CIMT and the development of coronary artery disease (O'Leary et al., 1999; Takashi et al., 2002) and cerebrovascular manifestations (Chambless et al., 2000; Touboul et al., 2005). These findings were supported by our study, which also disclosed association between high cumulative dose of glucocorticosteroids and CIMT as well as carotid plaques development and confirmed less significance of classic risk factors for atherosclerosis in SLE patients (Fischer, 2008).

We also showed the clinical usefulness of vascular resistance assessment in SLE patients. Our study conducted in 92 patients was based on high resistance index measurement, which was calculated from Doppler spectrum of the popliteal arteries. Significantly lower values of high resistance index were observed in SLE patients, especially those with coexistence of APS, compared with the controls. This indicates that high resistance index measurement can be used to evaluate early, subclinical lesions in vessels in the course of SLE (Walecka et al., 2004).

The detailed analysis of noninvasive imaging techniques and their usefulness in early, subclinical atherosclerotic changes detection in SLE patients is reviewed elsewhere (Fischer & Brzosko, 2009). However, from this short description it can be concluded that lupus patients are at high risk of atherosclerosis as well as cardiovascular disorders development. Atherosclerotic lesions at an initial stage can be detected by means of increasingly sophisticated diagnostic tools, which allow evaluating systemic atherosclerosis, and they should represent an essential component of the diagnostic evaluation of SLE that is necessary to implement appropriate preventive and therapeutic procedures.

Furthermore, studies performed in children and adolescents with SLE strongly evidenced the premature atherosclerosis development in the course of the disease. On the other hand, they also suggest necessity of vascular testing with different imaging methods (Schanberg et al., 2009; Boros et al., 2011). Moreover, the authors emphasized a significant impact of applied treatment on atherosclerotic lesions development (Schanberg et al., 2009) and lipids' metabolism (Boros et al., 2011) in pediatric SLE. Traditional risk factors predictive of increased atherosclerotic risk, similarly like in adult SLE patients, had limited clinical significance (Schanberg et al., 2009).

Understanding risk factors in the development of atherosclerosis in the course of SLE, especially those associated with the disease process, and early identification of patients at risk will enable to avoid irreversible cardiovascular damage, which represents the primary cause of morbidity and mortality in SLE patients.

3. Association between atherosclerosis and antiphospholipid antibodies in systemic lupus erythematosus – Related mechanisms

3.1 Antiphospholipid antibodies and lupus-related atherosclerosis – Clinical studies

Accelerated atheromatosis is a well recognized clinical problem in SLE patients. Systemic lupus erythematosus has been considered an independent risk factor for endothelial dysfunction, an early stage in atherogenesis (El-Magadmi et al., 2004), and an increased CIMT (Colombo et al., 2007). Because the cardiovascular risk factors in SLE significantly differ from those in the general population, many clinical as well as experimental studies investigated the role of SLE-related immune and inflammatory mechanisms of cardiovascular involvement.

The analysis of preclinical vascular disease in SLE and primary antiphospholipid syndrome (PAPS) patients showed higher prevalence of carotid plaque in SLE patients with coexistent APS than in patients with PAPS. However, the relationship with aPL (anticardiolipin antibodies - aCL and lupus anticoagulant - LA) was not found (Jiménez et al., 2005). On the other hand, the study performed in 200 SLE patients focused on evaluation of classic and lupus-related factors associated with CIMT and carotid plaque showed that aPL (aCL and/or LA) are independent risk factors for subclinical atherosclerosis (Ahmad et al., 2007). The multiethnic cohort study LUMINA which determined the baseline risk factors associated with the subsequent occurrence of vascular events (cardiovascular, cerebrovascular and peripheral vascular) confirmed aPL as independent predictors of these complications (OR = 4.7; 95%CI: 1.8-13.2) (Toloza et al., 2004). Similarly, study of longitudinal cohort of SLE patients also found aPL, and especially anti-beta2-glycoprotein I antibodies (aβ2-GPI) and aCL, baseline predictors of the first ever cardiovascular event (Gustafsson et al., 2009). Interestingly, an investigation performed in rheumatoid arthritis patients (premenopausal women, non-diabetic, non-hypertensive) disclosed advanced atherosclerosis in these patients shown as an increase of CIMT and plaque formation. Antiphospholipid antibodies (aCL and aβ2-GPI) were significantly more frequent in patients group supporting an idea that these antibodies represent an important risk factor for atherosclerosis in patients with rheumatoid arthritis (Pahor et al., 2006).

In accordance, our study on subclinical atherosclerosis in SLE patients which analyzed many serologic markers of the disease including aPL (aCL, LA, aβ2-GPI, anti-prothrombin antibodies (aPT) and aoxLDL) disclosed interesting association between CIMT and selected aPL. The presence of both isotypes of aCL IgG or IgM, LA and aPT IgA significantly increased the risk of thickening of intima-media and the relative risk was 4.4 (95%CI: 1.3-14.9), 4.0 (95%CI: 1.1-19.4) and 5.5 (95%CI: 1.1-30.2), respectively. We also confirmed the relationship between coexistence of APS and early atherosclerotic abnormalities in analyzed patients group. Additionally, the presence of aCL IgM significantly influenced carotid atherosclerotic plaque development (OR = 3.8; 95%CI: 1.1-13.1) (Fischer et al., 2007). Furthermore, our evaluation of risk factors for ischemic heart disease and myocardial infarction in SLE patients showed that these manifestations were more frequent in patients with coexistent APS (OR = 4.2 and 12.8, respectively). Ischemic heart disease was associated with aCL IgG (OR = 2.9) and myocardial infarction with aCL IgG and/or IgM (OR = 5.6) (Ostanek et al., 2006a). Furthermore, our next study on echocardiographic assessment of cardiovascular abnormalities documented a significant association between mitral valve involvement and aβ2-GPI IgA (OR = 13.63; 95%CI: 1.2-139.8) as well as aPT IgA (OR = 17.5; 95%CI: 1.3-231.0). Anticardiolipin antibodies IgG were significantly related to the increased amount of pericardial fluid (OR = 2.5; 95%CI: 1.1-6.1) (Ostanek et al., 2006b).

An investigation undertaken to examine the relationship of aPL with valvular, myocardial and arterial disease in SLE also documented significant correlation with mitral valve nodules and mitral regurgitation. Though, aPL were not related to myocardial hypertrophy, systolic dysfunction, coronary or carotid atherosclerosis and other analyzed vascular abnormalities (Farzaneh-Far et al., 2006).

Current studies also did not prove any association between aPL and atherosclerosis in SLE patients. Results from the Hopkins' Lupus Cohort regarding the relation of aPL (aCL, LA and aβ2-GPI) to thrombosis and non-thrombotic manifestations as well as atherosclerotic changes disclosed their significant relationship with venous and arterial thrombosis and selected cerebrovascular complications. Lupus anticoagulant was a sole antibody associated with myocardial infarction but there was no connection between aPL and CIMT, plaques and coronary calcification (Petri, 2010). In addition, the investigation focused on risk factors for coronary artery disease performed in SLE patients of the LASER study did not confirm any relation of aPL to cardiovascular risk (Haque et al., 2010).

3.2 Selected pathomechanisms in atherogenesis – The role of antiphospholipid antibodies

In regard to contrary reports from clinical studies there is large evidence that aPL may display proatherogenic effects which was disclosed by in vitro and in vivo studies.

Paraoxonase, an enzyme present in the arterial wall and in the HDL particle, inhibits LDL oxidation and is the major contributor to the antioxidant defense of plasma (Ames et al., 2009b). The paraoxonase gene is located at q21-q22 on the long arm of chromosome 7 (Durrington et al., 2001). It was shown in animal model that mice in which the paraoxonase gene was removed are devoid of protection against lipid peroxidation and HDL isolated from these mice were unable to prevent LDL oxidation in a co-cultured cell model of the artery wall (Jara et al., 2003). Furthermore, another experiment on non-lupus murine model investigated whether aCL could affect oxidant/antioxidant balance as an early biochemical step of APS. This study documented that aCL are associated with the decreased paraoxonase activity and reduced nitric oxide (sum of nitrite and nitrate) levels (Delgado Alves et al., 2005).

The study performed in SLE and PAPS patients paid attention to prevalence of anti-high-density lipoprotein antibodies (aHDL) and their relationship with aCL, aβ2-GPI and paraoxonase activity. Patients with SLE had decreased levels of HDL and its subfraction HDL_2 and HDL_3 and this lipoprotein or some of its components may represent target antigens for aHDL, which were significantly elevated in both analyzed patients groups. Moreover, there was strong inverse correlation between aHDL IgG and paraoxonase activity in SLE patients. In PAPS group, paraoxonase activity was inversely correlated with aCL IgG, aβ2-GPI IgG and IgM. However, on the basis on multiple regression model only aβ2-GPI IgG were found an independent predictor of decreased paraoxonase activity ($r= -0.483$, $p = 0.003$). The reported interactions may be relevant to the development of atherosclerosis in SLE and PAPS (Delgado Alves et al., 2002). Other observations also supported findings on the role of paraoxonase activity in SLE-related vascular abnormalities. The significantly decreased paraoxonase activity was found in SLE patients as compared to controls. Notably reduced paraoxonase activity was shown especially in lupus patients suffering from cardiovascular and cerebrovascular events (angina pectoris, myocardial infarction, transient ischemic attack, ischemic stroke) as compared to patients without such manifestations. Interestingly, also disturbed microcirculation was significantly associated with reduced paraoxonase activity in patients with Raynaud's phenomenon. These observations suggest that decreased paraoxonase activity in SLE patients may have pathogenic significance in accelerated atherosclerosis and its complications development (Kiss et al., 2007). More recent study evaluated vascular structure and function in women with aPL and assessed their relationship with paraoxonase activity. Patients with aPL in comparison with the controls had greater CIMT and arterial stiffness measured by pulse wave velocity, and lower flow-mediated dilatation pointing out an impaired endothelial function. Paraoxonase activity was lower in women with aPL than in controls and was inversely associated with CIMT and pulse wave velocity in these patients. Additionally, it was proved that HDL from women with aPL reduced nitric oxide bioavailability. That group was found to have an impaired anti-inflammatory and antioxidant properties (Charakida et al., 2009).

Some experimental studies clearly pointed out that aPL may enhance the development of atherosclerosis by oxidative modification of lipoproteins [LDL or Lp(a)] and by promoting the uptake of subendothelial lipoproteins by macrophage scavenger receptors causing an excessive intracellular accumulation of oxLDL and foam cell formation (Bassi et al., 2007). Oxidized LDL has chemotactic, proinflammatory and toxic properties, and promotes T-cell activation (Frostegård, 2005). The presence of oxLDL in atherosclerotic lesions in animal models and in humans has been shown (George et al., 2000). Enhanced oxidative stress and lipid peroxidation were also demonstrated in SLE patients (Frostegård, 2005).

A number of studies were addressing to the role of aoxLDL in atherosclerosis development in SLE patients. In our study we did not find any association between subclinical atherosclerotic lesions and these antibodies (Fischer et al., 2007). Other reports also provided discrepant results. The study of SLE patients in which aoxLDL and antibodies against oxidation epitopes in LDL were assessed showed aoxLDL more frequent in SLE patients with a history of cardiovascular disease in comparison to the controls (Svenungsson et al., 2001). It was also demonstrated that the titres of these IgG antibodies are high in SLE patients and that there is a good correlation between aoxLDL levels and the maximum intima-media thickness (Doria et al., 2003). High titres of aoxLDL IgG were also found in hypertensive SLE patients (Radulescu et al., 2004). On the other hand, the analysis of aoxLDL in SLE patients with and without APS, although, documented high frequency of aoxLDL in SLE patients with coexistent APS (not with PAPS) but did not find evidence suggesting that these antibodies may be associated with atherosclerosis. However, weak significant correlation between aoxLDL IgG and aCL IgG as well as aβ2-GPI IgG and association with a history of venous thrombosis were confirmed (Hayem et al., 2001).

Noteworthy, a number of early studies performed in the general population showed that aoxLDL are associated with myocardial infarction (Erkkilä et al., 2000) and, moreover, the effect was independent of LDL-cholesterol levels (Puurunen et al., 1994). Similarly, in patients with early-onset peripheral vascular disease the titres of aoxLDL were increased. There was also an interesting tendency for higher antibody levels in patients with more extensive atherosclerotic lesions (Bergmark et al., 1995). On the contrary, there are even reports on an inverse correlation between aoxLDL titre and CIMT (Fukumoto et al., 2000). More detailed analysis indicated that in humans aoxLDL are low at an early stage of cardiovascular disease development in nonautoimmune disease and in healthy individuals but they are increased at later stages and in more advanced disease (Frostegård, 2005).

Furthermore, these antibodies are heterogeneous in immunoglobulin class and in their epitope specificity and affinity. Thus, present opinion indicates that IgG aoxLDL antibodies seem to be pathogenic for subclinical atherosclerosis development in SLE patient (Bassi et al., 2007). While, IgM aoxLDL are thought to provide protection against proinflammatory oxidized moieties, which was shown in animal models (Matsuura et al., 2006a).

Crossreactivity between selected aPL and aoxLDL is an additional issue. Cardiolipin was found a component of LDL and the crossreactivity of aCL and aoxLDL has been documented (McMahon & Hahn, 2007). In addition, in vitro macrophage uptake of oxLDL has been significantly enhanced in the presence of beta2-glycoprotein I (β2-GPI) and aβ2-GPI IgG (Hasunuuma et al., 1997). The macrophage uptake of liposomes containing β2-GPI ligands also has been demonstrated indicating the possible proatherogenic role of aβ2-GPI IgG (Matsuura et al., 2005). The in vitro interaction between oxLDL and β2-GPI occurs quickly and evolve into stable covalent bonds making the complexes nondissociable. The similar mechanism has been postulated in vivo in the intima of arterial wall. Circulating oxLDL/β2-GPI complexes were demonstrated in SLE patients. In vitro investigations showed enhanced macrophage uptake of IgG immune complexes with oxLDL/β2-GPI. Measurement of oxLDL/β2-GPI complexes may represent a more physiological, clinically relevant, and accurate way of assessing oxidative stress and atherogenesis (Lopez et al., 2007).

The prolonged persistence of oxLDL/β2-GPI complexes can stimulate immune mechanisms and antibody production (aoxLDL/β2-GPI) that contribute to atherosclerosis (Lopez et al., 2007). The study performed in patients with selected systemic connective tissue diseases including SLE and APS showed aoxLDL/β2-GPI IgG significantly increased in SLE patients. Significantly higher levels of these antibodies were also confirmed in SLE patients with coexistence of APS with a positive predictive value for APS of 90%. Moreover, the predictive value for arterial thrombosis was 94%. It was considered that the presence of circulating oxLDL/β2-GPI complexes and IgG antibodies to these complexes indicates significant vascular injury and oxidative stress and proved an active role of autoimmune-mediated atherothrombosis (Matsuura et al., 2006b). Further studies disclosed contribution of these complexes and related antibodies to organ damage (especially renal involvement) and confirmed their association with thrombotic events in SLE patients (Bassi et al., 2009). Their relationship with both CIMT and reduced paraoxonase activity in PAPS patients has been also demonstrated (Ames et al., 2006).

Antiphospholipid antibodies may also have a direct effect on endothelium. Early in vitro studies documented that IgG from patients with high titre of aCL enhanced monocyte adhesion to human umbilical vein endothelial cells via mechanism dependent on β2-GPI (Simantov et al., 1995). Additionally, aβ2-GPI mediates binding of aCL to endothelial cells leading to their activation, and contributing to thrombosis and thrombocytopenia in patients in whom aCL were present (Le Tonquéze et al., 1995).

The other atherothrombotic mechanism has been also postulated based on decreased binding of annexin V to endothelial cells in the course of SLE. Among analyzed antibodies aCL IgG significantly influenced this decreased binding. Moreover, there was a positive association between annexin V binding and CIMT ($r = 0.73$, $p < 0.001$). Interestingly, immunochistochemical analysis revealed presence of annexin V in all human atherosclerotic plaques tested, especially at sites prone to rupture (Cederholm et al., 2005). The novel in vitro findings confirmed these observations showing reduced annexin A5 binding to endothelium by monoclonal aCL IgG via dose-dependent mechanism. Of note, preincubation of intravenous (IV) immunoglobulins at therapeutically relevant doses with aPL and monoclonal aCL restored annexin A5 binding to comparable levels when normal healthy serum was used. On the contrary, IV immunoglobulins per se reduced annexin A5 binding to endothelial cells when added to normal healthy serum suggesting that some antibodies in IV immunoglobulins may be involved in atherothrombosis and cardiovascular disease development during IV immunoglobulins treatment (Frostegård et al., 2010). The study conducted to investigate the association of plasma annexin V, anti-annexin V antibodies and aCL with acute myocardial infarction showed that patients suffering from acute myocardial infarction had significant low levels of annexin V and high levels of antibodies to this protein ($p = 0.002$ and $p = 0.004$, respectively). This combination indicated a hypercoagulable state in patients with acute myocardial infarction which was not related to traditional cardiovascular risk factors because plasma antibodies and annexin V levels were not correlated with hypertention, diabetes mellitus, hyperlipidemia, gender, age and smoking habits (Shojaie et al., 2009).

Antiphospholipid antibodies may act at various stages of atherogenesis process: activating endothelium, mediate adhesion of leukocytes and potentiating the uptake of oxLDL by scavenger receptor to generate foam cells. Crossreactivity of aPL to lipoprotein antigens may further facilitate atherogenesis (Narshi et al., 2011). However, SLE characteristics can mask the pathogenic role of some of autoantibodies in the development of atherosclerosis (Bassi et al., 2007). Therefore, the utility of aPL in related to SLE cardiovascular risk estimation in clinical practice remains controversial.

4. Atherosclerosis in primary antiphospholipid syndrome

Primary antiphospholipid syndrome is a systemic autoimmune disease characterized by the occurrence of arterial or venous thrombosis or pregnancy complications together with the persistence of aPL in the absence of other known autoimmune conditions (Miyakis et al., 2006).

Although, an accelerated atherosclerosis in APS coexistent with SLE is a well known clinical problem (Fischer, 2008; Belizna et al.; 2007; Roman et al., 2001). In patients with PAPS arterial ischemic events may occur even in the absence of evident atherosclerosis. Therefore, there is the risk of misdiagnosing young patients with potentially life-threatening symptoms including myocardial infarction (Gualtierotti et al., 2011). Furthermore, recent reports showed that a number of PAPS patients can develop Syndrome X defined as a condition with the presence of angina-like chest pain, positive response to stress testing and normal coronary angiograms often existing in the absence of traditional cardiovascular risk factors. It is suggested that microvascular abnormalities secondary to endothelial dysfunction may cause this complication development (Sangle et al., 2008).

Accordingly, there is accumulating evidence to confirm an impaired endothelial function in the course of PAPS. The study performed in 31 young patients with PAPS (mean age 35 years) documented a significant endothelial dysfunction in comparison with the controls. Moreover, patients with arterial involvement had importantly more prominent decrease of flow-mediated dilatation in comparison with patients with venous involvement. The presence of classic atherosclerotic risk factors did not differ between patients and the control group. Additionally, association between aCL IgG/IgM as well as variety of therapy and impaired endothelial function was not confirmed (Mercanoglu et al., 2004). Similarly, another study in which parameters of endothelial dysfunction were analyzed also proved endothelial dysfunction in 25 PAPS patients and, in addition, showed significant inverse correlation between endothelial dysfunction and selected markers of endothelial activation/damage (Štalc et al., 2006). In contrast, another group did not show in 20 PAPS patients neither impaired endothelial function, pathological values of plasma markers of endothelial or platelet activation nor progenitor and mature endothelial cells, suggesting that the alteration leading to thrombosis in PAPS concerns primarily the clotting system (Gresele et al., 2009). On the other hand, results showed in 44 PAPS patients in whom subclinical atherosclerosis was evaluated by endothelial function assessment and CIMT measurement clearly documented both abnormal values of CIMT and parameters of endothelial function. Moreover, there was negative linear correlation between flow-mediated vasodilation and CIMT. The von Willebrand factor level was also significantly higher in PAPS patients than in the control group, reflecting an endothelial injury. Similarly to other reports, significant difference regarding traditional cardiovascular risk factors between PAPS patients and the controls was not shown. Moreover, there was no correlation between impaired endothelial function and aPL serum levels. The authors pointed out that a relationship exists between the presence rather than the amount of aPL and subclinical atherosclerosis (Der et al., 2007). However, study performed in subjects with idiopathic aPL showed association between aCL IgG titre and CIMT. In addition, it confirmed aCL IgG as well as homocysteine and fibrinogen as independent predictors of CIMT indicating that measurement of homocysteine and fibrinogen may help to identify aPL patients who are more likely to develop atherosclerosis (Ames et al., 2002). More recent studies also confirmed a usefulness of CIMT measurement in a detection of early atherosclerotic changes and showed an association between CIMT and aPL in thrombotic PAPS patients (Ames et al., 2009a) as well as in patients with APS secondary to SLE (Belizna et al., 2008). Furthermore, a relationship between increased CIMT and stroke in the course of PAPS was reported (Medina et al., 2003).

A number of studies confirmed a clinical utility of other noninvasive imaging methods in atherosclerosis diagnosis in PAPS patients showing increased arterial stiffness (Belizna et al., 2008; Charakida et al., 2009) or abnormal ankle-brachial index (Barón et al., 2005).

Epidemilogical data from a multicenter, consecutive, prospective study on 1,000 APS patients disclosed at disease onset that some of the most common manifestations were cerebrovascular disorders (stroke - 13.1% and transient ischemic attack - 7.0%). Myocardial infarction was present in 2.8% of patients. Though, cumulative clinical features during the evolution of disease showed a higher prevalence of both neurologic manifestations (including stroke - 19.8% and transient ischemic attack - 11.1%) as well as selected cardiac complications - myocardial infarction (5.5%), angina (2.7%) and coronary bypass rethrombosis (1.1%) (Cervera et al., 2002). Myocardial infarction and stroke were also the most common causes of death in this cohort (18.9% and 13.2% respectively) (Cervera et al., 2009).

Accelerated atherosclerosis in the course of PAPS should be considered an example of atherothrombotic event caused by aPL playing both proatherogenic and prothrombotic role

(Der et al., 2007). Selected cardiovascular complications can exist without overt atherosclerosis (Gualtierotti et al., 2011). Therefore, early diagnosis of subclinical atherosclerotic changes with different imaging methods is extremely important.

5. Relationship between antiphospholipid antibodies and atherosclerosis in the general population

The new theories developed in the last century enabled the better understanding of atherosclerosis pathogenesis. The "response-to-injury" theory formulated by Ross and Glomset in 1973 showed endothelial damage to be a key initiator of atherosclerotic lesions. Further investigations disclosed that endothelial cells have the potential to play an active role both in the formation of lipid-laden foam cells and in the accumulation of necrotic tissue which are hallmarks of the atherosclerotic lesion (DiCorleto & Chisolm, 1986). The role of immunological and inflammatory factors in the pathogenesis of atherosclerotic lesions was confirmed in the 1990s (Ross, 1993). The interplay of inflammatory and immunological mediators including cytokines, chemokines, adhesion molecules, leukocytes, complement as well as antibodies, promotes damage of endothelium and progressive atherosclerotic plaque development (Hansson, 2001).

The potential role of aPL in atherosclerosis and atherosclerotic vascular events development in the general population has been extensively studied over the last few decades.

A case-control study, which included patients operated on for atherosclerotic peripheral vascular disease before 50 years of age, tested the hypothesis whether antibodies associated with an immune/inflammatory damage to the vascular wall were associated also with early atherosclerosis. Subjects were compared for the prevalence of aCL and anti-endothelial cell antibodies (AECA), classic risk actors for atherosclerosis and signs of inflammation. The presence of analyzed antibodies significantly differed between patients and controls ($p < 0.05$). The presence of aCL and AECA was confirmed in 14.5% and 12.9% patients, respectively. None of the patients with antibodies had clinical or laboratory features of systemic connective tissue disease. The patients had higher values of laboratory parameters suggesting inflammation. However, there was no correlation between the presence of antibodies and laboratory signs of inflammation. Interestingly, the occurrence of hyperlipidemia/dyslipidemia was lower in patients with aCL and/or AECA, as compared to patients without these antibodies suggesting that these antibodies have a role in vascular damage (Nityanand et al., 1995). These observations were confirmed by other investigators. The next study analyzed patients who had undergone elective supraiguinal (aortofemoral, femoral-femoral, iliac endarterectomy, or axillofemoral bypass grafting) or infrainguinal procedures for atherosclerotic occlusive disease. Patients were assessed for the presence of aPL- aCL IgG, IgM, IgA and LA and their association with the progression of the disease. There was statistically significant difference between aPL positive and negative patients in the progression of arterial occlusive disease in at least one artery during the 9 years follow-up (73% versus 37%, $p < 0.0001$). Furthermore, multivariate logistic regression analysis was used to test the effect of atherosclerotic risk factors on disease progression. Antiphospholipid antibodies status and traditional atherosclerotic risk factors, heart disease, chronic renal insufficiency, warfarin therapy and type of procedure were examined. Of note, only the presence or absence of aPL significantly contributed to progression in those patients who had undergone elective lower extremity revascularization for chronic ischemia (Lam et al., 2001). Interesting study was performed in 411 patients with atherosclerotic vascular disease who underwent at least one of the following events: unstable angina, myocardial infarction, angioplasty, coronary artery bypass surgery, claudication, transient ischemic attack and ischemic stroke. All subjects were tested for the presence of aCL IgG and IgM. It was shown on the basis of stepwise logistic regression analysis that for any atherosclerotic vascular disease event, significant independent, positive correlates included selected classic atherosclerotic factors (age, diabetes, male gender, hypertension and the family history of vascular atherosclerotic disease) and aCL IgM. Moreover, for those patients having a myocardial infarction, coronary bypass surgery and/or angioplasty, aCL IgM was a significant independent positive predictor of cardiovascular events. Additionally, aCL IgM was a positive significant independent risk factor for vascular events, including myocardial infarction, at ≤ 55 years of age. Levels of aCL IgG were positively associated with aCL IgM. The authors suggested that aCL IgG and IgM should be routinely measured as ancillary atherothrombotic risk factors in all patients with atherosclerotic vascular disease events, in patients at high risk of atherosclerotic vascular disease, and in patients where thrombosis is a major pathoetiology (Glueck et al., 1999). These results are consistent with the data from a prospective cohort study of the relation of aCL and risk of myocardial infarction and cardiac death performed in middle-aged men of Helsinki Heart Study. The levels of aCL IgG were significantly higher in subjects than controls ($p < 0.005$). Persons with the highest levels of aCL IgG were at 2-fold higher risk of myocardial infarction and the risk was independent of traditional risk factors for atherosclerosis (Vaarala et al., 1995). The clinical importance of high levels of aCL also documented study of patients with focal cerebral ischemia harboring aCL of at least 10 GPL units at the time of their index event. Patients were prospectively followed to estimate the effect of aCL titer on time to and risk of subsequent thrombo-occlusive events (stroke, transient ischemic attack, deep venous thrombosis, pulmonary embolism, myocardial infarction) and death. Patents with aCL titers > 40 GPL were younger, had more prior strokes, more frequent subsequent thrombo-occlusive events and death, and a shorter median time to event (Levine et al., 1997). The more recent study performed in 432 Taiwanese adults with cerebral ischemia disclosed an interesting impact of aCL IgG. Patients were classified into five subtypes according to the cause of cerebrovascular event: large-artery atherosclerotic disease, stroke of unknown etiology, small-artery occlusive disease, cardioembolism, and stroke of other known etiology. It was shown that aCL IgG selectively increases in patients with large-artery atherosclerosis and stroke of unknown etiology, reflecting selective activation of humoral immunity for aCL in the pathogenesis of cerebral ischemia (Chen et al., 2006). On the other hand, a multicenter cohort study performed in premenopausal women with a first myocardial infarction or ischemic stroke showed a significant relationship of LA to myocardial infarction (OR = 5.3) and ischemic stroke (OR = 43.1). Anti-beta2-glycoprotein I antibodies also were associated with an increased risk of ischemic stroke (OR = 2.3). However, neither aCL nor aPT affected the risk of those manifestations (Urbanus et al., 2009).

Finally, an inclusion of aPL to the estimation of risk of atherothrombotic vascular events development in the general population seems to be justified, especially in young patients without coexistent classic cardiovascular risk factors.

6. Selected non-criteria antiphospholipid antibodies and their relationship to atherosclerosis

Early studies performed in 1990s have already put attention to aPL directed against non-cardiolipin antigens in SLE. They documented significantly increased levels of selected aPL in lupus patients and described wide profile of potential antigens (Maneta-Peyret et al., 1991; Toschi et al. 1993).

Many studies on the clinical significance of aPT have been reported in APS patients (Galli & Barbui, 1999) and several pathogenic mechanisms providing to hypercoagulable state of APS via aPT were suggested (Atsumi & Koike, 2002). Interesting study performed in animal model provided the first direct evidence for thrombus induction by aPT. Mice were immunized with prothrombin, β2-GPI or β2-GPI followed by prothrombin. The presence of clinical manifestations of APS was analyzed. Thrombosis was studied in an ex-vivo model in which aorta was sutured for 1 minute and the presence or absence of visible thrombus was qualitatively evaluated. All prothrombin-immunized mice developed thrombus within the aorta confirming prothrombotic properties of aPT (Haj-Yahja et al., 2003). Moreover, the study performed in middle-aged men with dyslipidemia showed higher levels of aPT in patients who developed myocardial infarction or cardiac death than in controls. The relative risk of these complications was 2.5-fold higher (95%CI: 1.2-5.3) in patients with aPT (Vaarala et al., 1996). These data were supported by the investigation performed in young women with acute ischemic stroke. Anti-prothrombin antibodies were more frequent in patients with cerebrovascular manifestations in comparison with the healthy controls (OR = 182.0; 95%CI: 23.4-1416.6) and nonischemic neurological disorders patients (OR = 26.7; 95%CI: 5.7-123.7). In 43% of stroke patients aPT were the only antibodies detected (Cojocaru et al., 2008).

The clinical significance of these aPL was also intensively investigated in our studies. Our earlier reports demonstrated the usefulness of aPT in diagnosis of APS in SLE patients and the highest specificity showed aPT IgG (95.12%). Additionally, aPT IgG were significantly associated with selected central nervous system manifestations, and aPT IgM importantly influenced risk of development of cardiac complications and mononeuropathy. Interestingly, aPT IgA were significantly related to pleurisy and leucopenia, but they did not associate with the coexistence of APS (Ostanek et al., 2005). While, our study focused on atherosclerotic changes development in SLE patients disclosed a significant influence of aPT IgA and AECA on increase of CIMT (Fischer et al., 2007; Fischer et al., 2006). Moreover, this finding for aPT IgA was also confirmed by multivariate backward stepwise analysis (Fischer et al., 2007).

The analysis of other aPL in diagnosing APS and their role in main clinical complications related to APS showed that anti-phosphatidylserine antibodies (aPS) IgG and IgM are valuable diagnostic tool with a high significant predictive value for thrombotic events - arterial as well as venous (Lopez et al., 2004; Bertolaccini & Hughes, 2006; Szodoray et al, 2009). However, the case report of SLE patient with myocardial infarction and without associated traditional cardiovascular risk factors and classic aPL disclosed interesting relation to aPS IgA suggesting that complete evaluation for aPL should include testing for all three isotypes (Jansen et al., 1996). The data on an association between aPS and cerebrovascular disorders have been also frequently reported. The study which evaluated the relevance of different aPL in patients with cryptogenic stroke and with determined causes of stroke displayed a significant role of aPS IgG and, interestingly, aβ2-GPI IgA in stroke etiology (Kahles et al., 2005). Similarly, it was shown in 203 patients suffering from ischemic stroke that, in addition to classic aPL, also aPS IgG may be considered risk factors for stroke (Saidi et al., 2009). The analysis of 250 persons with cerebral infarction (lacunar, atherothrombotic and cardiogenic cerebral embolism) including SLE patients disclosed, moreover, that in aPS or anti-phosphatidylinositol (aPI) positive patients an increase of CIMT as well as presence of carotid plaques and carotid stenosis ≥ 50% were more frequent. Among 250 patients, 13.6% were positive either aPS or aPI and 6.8% were positive for both. The majority of patients with aPS and/or aPI were negative for classical aPL (aCL, aβ2-GPI, LA). On the other hand, 70.6% of these patients were positive for antinuclear antibodies. The authors pointed out that aPL are a risk factor for cerebral infarction especially in SLE patients and in younger population (Okuma et al., 2010). Moreover, a significant association between CIMT and the risk of ischemic stroke has been well documented (Chambless et al., 2000; Touboul et al., 2005).

There is also an increasing evidence of a relationship between the clinical manifestations of APS and antibodies directed against phosphatidylethanolamine (aPE) (Mcintyre & Wagenknecht, 2000). These antibodies were also often reported as the only aPL particularly in patients suffering from thrombotic disease (Bérard et al., 1996; Sanmarco et al., 2001). Furthermore, these antibodies, especially IgG isotype, may contribute to detect more patients with aPL-related clinical manifestations in SLE patients and their significant correlation with valvulopathies and livedo reticularis in patients with SLE was reported (Balada et al., 2001).

The study performed in 185 patients, including SLE patients, suffering from stroke showed aPE in 35% of patients. Furthermore, the presence of aPE was the most frequent finding in patients who were suspected to have an associated APS (Gonzales-Portillo et al., 2001). The next study on young non-SLE patients without obvious causes of arterial thromboembolism who underwent ischemic cerebrovascular incidences also demonstrated the presence of wide profile of non-cardiolipin aPL, including aPE. However, the frequency of aPE was lower - 10.4% (Toschi et al., 1998). In addition, the finding of aPE in the cerebral spinal fluid of patient with a documented ischemic stroke may suggest a possibility of an intrathecal production of aPL in the course of central nervous system disorders. However, this observation needs to be confirmed by further investigations (Sokol et al., 2000). A number of reports confirmed also an association between aPE and atherosclerosis. The analysis of the clinical features of 20 patients with aPE only, among whom 17 had symptoms potentially related to APS, showed significant relationship between aPE and arteriosclerosis with peripheral arteriopathy (Desauw et al., 2002).

Finally, the association between wide profile of aPL including aPS, aPI as well as anti-phosphatidic acid antibodies and cardiac impairment in lupus patients was reported indicating an adjunctive pathogenic role of aPL in these complications (Amoroso et al., 2006).

This short description emphasizes that rare non-criteria aPL are associated with selected vascular disorders in the course of SLE. The determination of these antibodies may provide an additional tool for APS diagnosis and appears to be of interest in patients negative for the serologic markers of APS but presenting a clinical picture highly suggestive of this syndrome.

7. Management and monitoring of atherosclerosis and cardiovascular risk factors in systemic lupus erythematosus patients

European League Against Rheumatism published in 2010 recommendations for monitoring SLE patients in clinical practice and in observational studies. It is proposed to assess cardiovascular risk factors at baseline and during follow-up at least once a year. Although data from the literature have clearly shown that traditional cardiovascular risk factors cannot fully explain the increased incidence of atherosclerosis and its complications in this patients population, an agreement exists on the need for monitoring conventional risk factors and treating modifiable risk factors. The evaluation of cardiovascular risk includes: assessment of smoking, vascular events (cerebral/cardiovascular), physical activity, oral contraceptive, hormonal therapies and family history of cardiovascular disease, blood cholesterol, glucose, blood pressure and body mass index (and/or waist circumference). More frequent assessment may be required in certain situations, for instance, in patients on glucocorticosteroids therapy (Mosca et al., 2010).

The guidelines for risk factors management developed to prevent cardiovascular disease in SLE patients contain indications regarding ideal targets values for risk factors and recommended therapy (Table 1.) (Wajed et al., 2004).

Risk factor	Ideal target values
Blood pressure	< 130 mmHg systolic and diastolic < 80 mmHg
LDL cholesterol	< 2.6 mmol/l
Diabetes mellitus	Fasting blood glucose < 7.0 mmol/l
	Random blood glucose < 11.0 mmol/l
Smoking	Stop smoking
Obesity	Body mass index < 25 kg/m^2

Table 1. Summary of ideal targets for risk factors in patients with systemic lupus erythematosus (Wajed et al., 2004)

Subjects with SLE tend to develop hypertension more often than general population. The drugs indicated as a first line treatment of hypertension in SLE patients are diuretics and ACE agents. Treatment with ACE is also recommended for heart failure, coronary heart disease, ventricular hypertrophy or renal failure. These agents are protective of brain stroke or microvascular injury in the course of diabetes mellitus (Table 2). Aspirin is an agent of proven value in primary and secondary coronary heart disease. It seems to be beneficial in terms of survival for SLE patients. However, its universal role for SLE treatment is not proven yet, its use is indicated in specific situations like in subjects with previous cardiovascular events, smokers, subjects positive for aPL (Table 2) (Wajed et al., 2004).

Glucocrticosteroids are commonly used in SLE patients and their relation to the risk of developing atherosclerotic lesions is now well established (Manzi et al., 1999; McDonald et al., 1992). On the other hand, antimalarial drugs have been shown to have a beneficial effect in SLE (Rahman et al., 1999; Molad et al., 2002). Additionally, in patients with APS anticoagulation therapy is used. The long-therm antithrombotic therapy provides protection against thrombotic events, but it does not have an antiatherogenic potential (Der et al., 2007).

Agent	Indication
Aspirin	Known vascular disease
	Systemic lupus erythematosus plus one other risk factor
	Anticardiolipin antibodies/lupus anticoagulant
ACE inhibitors	Prevalent cardiovascular disease including heart failure
	Left ventricular hypertrophy
	Diabetes mellitus
	Preferred second drug for hypertension

Table 2. Specific recommendation for aspirin and ACE inhibitors in patients with systemic lupus erythematosus (Wajed et al., 2004)

Moreover, the addition of aspirin also has no significant benefit, so aspirin therapy may not be necessary in this group (Wajed et al., 2004).

Keypoints of APS diagnosis and treatment in patients with acute coronary syndrome are summarized in table 3 (Gualtierotti et al., 2011).

Situations when the diagnosis of antiphospholipid syndrome should be taken into account in patients with acute coronary syndrome:
- in young patients (< 55 years in men and < 65 years in women)
- coronary arteries display normal angiography
- there are no other traditional cardiovascular risk factors
- there is no history of drug abuse
- there are no other causes of heart diseases (congenital abnormalities, etc.)
Treatment of acute coronary thrombosis is not different in aPL-positive and aPL-negative patients
Anticoagulation with a target INR > 3.0 has been suggested in APS patients with arterial thrombosis
The persistent medium-high aPL is a risk for arterial recurrences and anticoagulation should be continued
The elimination or reduction of other cardiovascular risk is mandatory
There are no data to recommend additional treatments (aspirin, hydroxychloroquine, or statins, etc.)

Table 3. Antiphospholipid syndrome diagnosis and therapy in patients with acute coronary syndrome (Gualtierotti et al., 2011)

In aPL related atherosclerosis treatment may be directed at managing the effects of aPL or at decreasing their titer. In this regard, statins may be potent drugs with positive effect on the immune system, vascular endothelium, paraoxonase activity and reduction of inflammation (Ames et al., 2009b). Furthermore, biological therapies may be helpful to prevent atherothrombotic events in APS/SLE patients (Der et al., 2004). However, anti-CD20 accomplished so far lowering of aPL titers in some PAPS patients but not others (Ames et al., 2009b).

8. Conclusions

Patients with SLE are at risk of accelerated and premature atherosclerosis and cardiac complications development. Sensitive noninvasive imaging techniques enable to evaluate atherosclerotic changes at every stage of their development and should be commonly used for diagnosis and progression monitoring. Traditional risk factors fail to fully account for cardiovascular risk in SLE patients. Therefore much attention has been put to investigate the role of selected immune mechanisms involved in atherosclerotic lesions pathogenesis. A heterogeneous group of antibodies in SLE may accelerate the inflammatory process of atherosclerosis. There is a growing body of evidence that aPL may display proatherogenic effect in several in vitro and in vivo studies. However, clinical studies provided discrepant reports on association between aPL and subclinical atherosclerosis as well as cardiovascular manifestations in patients with SLE and large prospective studies are needed to establish the role of these autoantibodies in identifying patients at risk. Furthermore, management of SLE-related atherosclerosis still remains an unsolved issue. The official recommendations and guidelines are focused on traditional modifiable risk factors and conventional anticoagulation therapy. The identification of autoantibody biomarkers may provide a useful tool to recognize patients with subclinical changes and avoid an irreversible cardiovascular damage and, on the other hand, may help to identify new therapeutic goals.

9. References

Ahmad, Y.; Shelmerdine, J.; Bodill, H.; Lunt, M. & Pattrick, MG.; The, LS.; Bernstein, LM.; Walker, MG.; Bruce, IN. (2007) Subclinical atherosclerosis in systemic lupus erythematosus (SLE): the relative contribution of classic risk factors and the lupus phenotype. *Rheumatology (Oxford)*, Vol.46, No.6, pp. 983-988.

Ames, PR.; Antinolfi, I.; Scenna, G.; Gaeta, G.; Margaglione, M. & Margarita, A. (2009a) Atherosclerosis in thrombotic primary antiphospholipid syndrome. *J Thromb Haemost*, Vol.7, No.4, pp. 537-542.

Ames, PRJ.; Delgado Alves, J.; Lopez, LR.; Gentile, F.; Margarita, A.; Pizzella, M.; Batuca, J.; Scenna, G.; Brancaccio, V. & Matsuura, E. (2006) Antibodies against β_2-glycoprotein I complexed with an oxidized lipoprotein relate to intima thickening of carotid arteries in primary antiphospholipid syndrome. *Clin Dev Immunol*, Vol.13, No.1, pp. 1-9.

Ames, PRJ.; Margarita, A.; Delgado Alves, J.; Tommasino, C.; Iannaccone, L. & Brancaccio, V. (2002) Anticardiolipin antibody titre and plasma homocysteine level independently predict intima media thickness of carotid arteries in subjects with idiopathic antiphospholipid antibodies. *Lupus*, Vol.11, No.4, pp. 208-214.

Ames, PRJ.; Margarita, A. & Delgado Alves, J. (2009b) Antiphospholipid antibodies and atherosclerosis: insights from systemic lupus erythematosus and primary antiphospholipid syndrome. *Clinic Rev Allergy Immunol*, Vol.37, No.1, pp. 29-35.

Amoros, A.; Cacciapaglia, F.; De Castro, S.; Battagliese, A.; Coppolino, G.; Galluzzo, S.; Vadacca, M. & Afeltra, A. (2006) The adjunctive role of antiphospholipid antibodies in systemic lupus erythematosus cardiac involvement. *Clin Exp Rheumatol*, Vol.24, No.3, pp. 287-294.

Atsumi, T. & Koike, T. (2002) Clinical relevance of antiprothrombin antibodies. *Autoimmun Rev*, Vol.1, No.1-2, pp. 49-53.

Balada, E.; Ordi-Ros, J.; Paredes, F.; Villarreal, J.; Mauri, M. & Virardell-Tarrés, M. (2001) Antiphosphatidylethanolamine antibodies contribute to the diagnosis of antiphospholipid syndrome in patients with systemic lupus erythematosus. *Scand J Rheumatol*, Vol.30, No.4, pp. 235-241.

Barón, MA.; Khamashta, MA.; Hughes, GRV. & D'Cruz, DP. (2005) Prevalence of an abnormal ankle-brachial index in patients with primary antiphospholipid syndrome: preliminary data. *Ann Rheum Dis*, Vol.64, No.1, pp. 144-146.

Bassi, N.; Ghirardello, A.; Iaccarino, L.; Zampieri, S.; Rampudda, ME.; Atzeni, F.; Sarzi-Puttini, P.; Shoenfeld, Y. & Doria, A. (2007) OxLDL/β_2GPI-anti-oxLDL/β_2GPI complex and atherosclerosis in SLE patients. *Autoimmun Rev*, Vol.7, No.1, pp. 52-58.

Bassi, N.; Zampieri, S.; Ghirardello, A.; Tonon, M.; Zen, M.; Beggio, S.; Matsuura, E. & Doria, A. (2009) oxLDL/β2-GPI complex and anti-oxLDL/β2-GPI in SLE: prevalence and correlates. *Autoimmunity*, Vol.42, No.4, pp. 289-291.

Belizna, CC.; Richard, V.; Primard, E.; Kerleau, JM.; Cailleux, N.; Louvel, JP.; Marie, I.; Hamidou, M.; Thuillez, C. & Lévescue, H. (2008) Early atheroma in primary and secondary antiphospholipid syndrome: an intrinsic finding. *Semin Arthritis Rheum*, Vol.37, No.6, pp. 373-380.

Belizna, CC.; Richard, V.; Thuillez, C. Lévescue, H. & Shoenfeld, Y. (2007) Insights into atherosclerosis therapy in antiphospholipid syndrome. *Autoimmun Rev*, Vol.7, No.1, pp. 46-51.

Bérard, M.; Chantome, R.; Marcelli, A. & Boffa, MC. (1996) Antiphosphatidylethanolamine antibodies as the only antiphospholipid antibodies. I. Association with thrombosis and vascular cutaneous diseases. *J Rheumatol*, Vol.23, No.8, pp. 1369-1374.

Bergmark, C.; Wu, R.; de Faire, U.; Levfert, AK. & Swedenborg, J.(1995) Patients with early-onset peripheral vascular disease have increased levels of autoantibodies against oxidized LDL. *Arterioscler Thromb Vasc Biol*, Vol.15, No.4, pp. 441-445.

Bertolaccini, ML. & Hughes, GR. (2006). Antiphospholipid antibody testing: which are most useful for diagnosis? *Rheum Dis Clin North Am*, Vol.32, No.3, pp. 455-463.

Bjarnegård, N.; Bengtsson, C.; Brodszki, J.; Sturfelt, G.; Nived, O. & Länne, E. (2006) Increase aortic pulse wave velocity in middle age women with systemic lupus erythematosus. *Lupus*, Vol.15, No.10, pp. 644-650.

Bombardier, C.; Gladman, DD.; Urowitz, MB.; Caron, D. & Chang, CH. (1992) Derivation of the SLEDAI. A disease activity index for lupus patients. The Committee on Prognosis Studies in SLE. *Arthritis Rheum*, Vol.35, pp. 630-640.

Borchers, AT.; Keen, CL.; Shoenfeld, Y. & Gershwin, ME. (2004) Surviving the butterfly and the wolf: mortality trends in systemic lupus erythematosus. *Autoimmun Rev*, Vol.3, No.6, pp. 423-453.

Boros, CA.; Bradley, TJ.; Cheung, MM.; Bargman, JM.; Russell, JM.; McCrindle, BW.; Adeli, K.; Hamilton, J. & Siverman, ED. (2011) Early determinants of atherosclerosis in paediatric systemic lupus erythematosus. *Clin Exp Rheumatol*, Vol.29, No.3, pp. 575-581.

Bruce, IN.; Gladman, DD. & Urowitz, MB. (2000). Premature atherosclerosis in systemic lupus erythematosus. *Rheum Dis Clin North Am*, Vol.26, No.2, pp. 257-278.

Bulkley, BH. & Roberts, WC. (1975). The heart in systemic lupus erythematosus and the changes induced in it by corticosteroid therapy. A study of 36 necropsy patients. *Am J Med*, Vol.58, No.2, pp. 243-264.

Cederholm, A.; Svenungsson, E.; Jensen-Urstad, K.; Trollmo, C.; Ulfgren, AK.; Swedenborg, J.; Fei, GZ. & Frostegård, J. (2005). Decreased binding of annexin V to endothelial cells: a potential mechanism in atherothrombosis of patients with systemic lupus erythematosus. *Arterioscler Thromb Vasc Biol*, Vol.25, No.1, pp. 198-203.

Celermajer, DS.; Sorensen, KE.; Gooch, VM.; Spiegelhalter, DJ.; Miller, OI.; Sullivan, ID.; Lloyd, JK. & Deanfield JE. (1992) Non-invasive detection of endothelial dysfunction in children and adults at risk of atherosclerosis. *Lancet*, Vol.340, No.8828, pp. 1111-1115.

Cervera, R.; Khamashta, MA.; Shoenfeld, Y.; Camps, MT.; Jacobsen, S.; Kiss, E.; Zeher, MM.; Tincani, A.; Kontopoulou-Griva, I.; Galeazzi, M.; Bellisai, F.; Meroni, PL.; Derksen, RH.; de Groot, PG.; Gromnica-Ihle, E.; Baleva, M.; Mosca, M.; Bombardieri, S.; Houssiau, F.; Gris, JC.; Quéré, I.; Hachulla, E.; Vasconcelos, C.; Roch, B.; Fernández-Nebro, A.; Piette, JC.; Espinosa, G.; Bucciarelli, S.; Pisoni, CN.; Bertolaccini, ML.; Boffa, MC. & Hughes, GR. Euro-Phospholipid Project Group (European Forum on Antiphospholipid Antibodies). (2009) Morbidity and mortality in the antiphospholipid syndrome during a 5-year period: a multicentre prospective study of 1000 patients. *Ann Rheum Dis*, Vol.68, No.9, pp. 1428-1432.

Cervera, R.; Piette, J-C.; Font, J.; Khamashta, MA.; Shoenfeld, Y.; Camps, MT.; Jacobsen, S.; Lakos, G.; Tincani, A.; Kontopoulou-Griva, I.; Galeazzi, M.; Meroni, PL.; Derksen, RH.; de Groot, PG.; Gromnica-Ihle, E.; Baleva, M.; Mosca, M.; Bombardieri, S.; Houssiau, F.; Gris, JC.; Quéré, I.; Hachulla, E.; Vasconcelos, C.; Roch, B.; Fernández-Nebro, A.; Boffa, MC.; Hughes, GR. & Ingelmo M; Euro-Phospholipid Project Group. (2002) Antiphospholipid syndrome: clinical and immunologic manifestations and patterns of disease expression in a cohort of 1000 patients. *Arthritis Rheum*, Vol.46, No.4, pp.1019-1027.

Chambless, LE.; Folsom, AR.; Clegg, LX.; Sharrett, AR.; Shahar, E.; Nieto, FJ.; Rosamond, WD. & Evans, G. (2000) Carotid wall thickness is predictive of incident clinical stroke. The Atherosclerosis Risk in Communities (ARIC) Study. *Am J Epidemiol*, Vol.151, No.5, pp. 478-487.

Charakida, M.; Besler, C.; Batuca, JR.; Sangle, S.; Marques, S.; Sousa, M.; Wang, G.; Tousoulis, D.; Delgado Alves, J.; Loukogeorgakis, SP.; Mackworth-Young, C.; D'Cruz, D.; Luscher, T.; Landmesser, U. & Deanfield, JE. (2009) Vascular abnormalities, paraoxonase activity, and dysfunctional HDL in primary antiphospholipid syndrome. *JAMA*, Vol.302, No.11, pp. 1210-1217.

Chen, WH.; Kao, YF.; Lan, MY.; Chang, YY.; Chen, SS. & Liu, JS. (2006) The increase of blood anticardiolipin antibody depends on the underlying etiology in cerebral ischemia. *Clin Appl Thromb Hemost*, Vol.12, No.1, pp. 69-76.

Cojocaru, IM.; Cojocaru, M.; Tănăsescu, R.; Burcin, C.; Mitu, AC.; Iliescu, I.; Dumitrescu, L.; Pavel, I. & Silosi, I. (2008) Detecting anti-prothrombin antibodies in young women with acute ischemic stroke. *Rom J Intern Med*, Vol.46, No.4, pp. 337-341.

Colombo, BM.; Murdaca, G.; Caiti, M.; Rodriguez, G.; Grassia, L.; Rossi, E.; Indiveri, F. & Puppo, F. (2007) Intima-media thickness a marker of accelerated atherosclerosis in woman with systemic lupus erythematosus. *Ann N Y Acad Sci*, Vol.1108, pp. 121-126.

Corretti, MC.; Anderson, TJ.; Benjamin, EJ.; Celermajer, D.; Charbonneau, F.; Creager, MA.; Deanfield, J.; Drexler, H.; Gerhard-Herman, M.; Herrington, D.; Vallance, P.; Vita, J.

& Vogel. R. International Brachial Artery Reactivity Task Force (2002) Guidelines for the ultrasound assessment of endothelial-dependent flow mediated vasodilatation of the brachial artery: a report of the International Brachial Artery Reactivity Task Force. *J Am Coll Cardiol*, Vol.39, No.2, pp. 257-265.

Delgado Alves, J.; Ames, PRJ.; Donohue, S.; Stanyer, L.; Nourooz-Zadeh, J.; Ravirajan, C. & Isenberg, DA. (2002) Antibodies to high-density lipoprotein and β_2-glycoprotein I are inversely correlated with paraoxonase activity in systemic lupus erythematosus and primary antiphospholipid syndrome. *Arthritis Rheum*, Vol.46, No.10, pp. 2686-2694.

Delgado Alves, J.; Mason, LJ.; Ames, PRJ.; Chen, PP.; Rauch, J.; Levine, JS.; Subang, R. & Isenberg, DA. (2005) Antiphospholipid antibodies are associated with enhanced oxidative stress, decreased plasma nitric oxide and paraoxonase activity in an experimental mouse model. *Rheumatology (Oxford)*, Vol.44, No.10, pp. 1238-1244.

Denarié, N.; Gariepy, J.; Chironi, G.; Massonneau, M.; Laskri, F.; Salomon, J.; Levenson, J. & Simon, A. (2000) Distribution of ultrasonographically–assessed dimensions of common carotid arteries in healthy adults of both sexes. *Atherosclerosis*, Vol.148, No.2, pp. 297-302.

Der, H.; Kerekes, G.; Veres, K.; Szodoray, P.; Toth, J.; Lakos, G.; Szegedi, G. & Soltesz, P. (2007) Impaired endothelial function and increased carotid intima-media thickness in association with elevated von Willebrand antigen level in primary antiphospholipid syndrome. *Lupus*, Vol.16, No.7, pp. 497-503.

Desauw, C.; Hachulla, E.; Boumbar, Y.; Bouroz-Joly, J.; Ponard, D.; Arvieux, J.; Dubucquoi, S.; Fauchais, AL.; Hatron, PY. & Devulder, B. (2002) (Antiphospholipid syndrome with only antiphosphatidylethanolamine antibodies: report of 20 cases). *Rev Med Interne*, Vol.23, No.4, pp. 357-63.

DiCorleto, PE & Chisolm, GM 3rd. (1986). Participation of the endothelium in the development of the atherosclerotic plaque. *Prog Lipid Res*, Vol.25, No.1-4, pp. 365-374.

Doria, A.; Sherer, Y.; Meroni, PL. & Shoenfeld, Y. (2005) Inflammation and accelerated atherosclerosis: Basic mechanisms. *Rheum Dis Clin North Am*, Vol.31, No.2, pp. 355-362.

Doria, A.; Shoenfeld, Y.; Wu, R.; Gambari, PF.; Puato, M.; Ghirardello, A.; Gilburd, B.; Corbanese, S.; Patnaik, M.; Zampieri, S.; Peter, JB.; Favaretto, E.; Iaccarino, L.; Sherer, Y.; Todesco, S. & Pauletto, P. (2003) Risk factors for subclinical atherosclerosis in prospective cohort of patients with systemic lupus erythematosus. *Ann Rheum Dis*, Vol.62, No.11, pp. 1071-1077.

Durrington, PN.; Mackness, B. & Mackness MI. (2001) Paraoxonase and atherosclerosis. *Arterioscler Thromb Vasc Biol*, Vol.21, No.4, pp. 473-480.

Ebrahim, S.; Papacosta, O.; Whincup, P.; Wannamethee, G.; Walker, M.; Nicolaides, AN.; Dhanjil, S.; Griffin, M.; Belcaro, G.; Rumley, A. & Lowe, GD. (1999) Carotid plaque, intima media thickness, cardiovascular risk factors, and prevalent cardiovascular disease in men and women. The British Regional Heart Study. *Stroke*, Vol.30, No.4, pp. 841-850.

El-Magadmi, M.; Bodill, H.; Ahmad, J.; Durrington, PN.; Mackness, M.; Walker, M.; Bernstein, RM. & Bruce, IN. (2004) Systemic lupus erythematosus: an independent risk factor for endothelial dysfunction in women. *Circulation*, Vol.110, No.4, pp. 399-404.

Erkkilä, AT.; Närvänen, O.; Seppo, L.; Uusitupa, MI. & Ylä-Herttuala, S. (2000) Autoantibodies against oxidized low-density lipoprotein and cardiolipin in patients with coronary heart disease. *Arterioscler Thromb Vasc Biol*, Vol.20, No.1, pp. 204-209.

Esdaile, JM.; Abrahamowicz, M.; Grodzicky, T.; Li, Y.; Panaritis, C.; du Berger, R.; Côte, R.; Grover, SA.; Fortin, PR.; Clarke, AE. & Senécal, JL. (2001) Traditional Framingham risk factors fail to fully account for accelerated atherosclerosis in systemic lupus erythematosus. *Arthritis Rheum*, Vol.44, No.10, pp. 2331-2337.

Farzaneh-Far, A.; Roman, MJ.; Lockshin, MD.; Devereux, RB.; Paget, SA.; Crow, MK.; Davis, A.; Sammaritano, L.; Levine, DM. & Salmon, JE. (2006) Relationship of antiphospholipid antibodies to cardiovascular manifestations of systemic lupus erythematosus. *Arthritis Rheum*, Vol.54, No.12, pp. 3918-3925.

Fischer, K. (2008) (Risk factors of thickened intima-media and atherosclerotic plaque development in carotid arteries in patients with systemic lupus erythematosus). *Ann Acad Med Stetin*, Vol.54, No.2, pp. 22-32.

Fischer, K. & Brzosko, M. (2009) Diagnosis of early atherosclerotic lesions, and selected atherosclerotic risk factors, in patients with systemic lupus erythematosus. *Pol Arch Med Wewn*, Vol.119, No.11, pp. 736-741.

Fischer, K.; Brzosko, M.; Walecka A.; Ostanek, L. & Sawicki, M. (2007) (Significance of antiphospholipid syndrome and antiphospholipid antibodies in patients with systemic lupus erythematosus in estimation of risk of subclinical atherosclerosis development). *Pol Arch Med Wewn*, Vol.117, Suppl 1, pp. 13-17.

Fischer, K.; Brzosko, M.; Walecka, A.; Ostanek, L. & Sawicki, M. (2006) (Antiendothelial cell antibodies as a risk factor of atherosclerosis in systemic lupus erythematosus). *Ann Acad Med Stetin*, Vol.52, Suppl 2, pp. 95-99.

Frostegård, J. (2005) SLE, atherosclerosis and cardiovascular disease. *J Intern Med*, Vol.257, No.6, pp. 485-495.

Frostegård, AG.; Su, J.; von Landenberg, P. & Frostegård, J. (2010) Effects of anti-cardiolipin antibodies and IVIg on annexin A5 binding to endothelial cells: implications for cardiovascular disease. *Scand J Rheumatol*, Vol.39, No.1, pp. 77-83.

Fukumoto, M.; Soji, T.; Emoto, M.; Kawagishi, T.; Okuno, Y. & Nishizawa, Y. (2001) Antibodies against oxidized LDL and carotid artery intima-media thickness in a healthy population. *Arterioscler Thromb Vasc Biol*, Vol.20, No.3, pp. 703-707.

Galli, M. & Barbui, T. (1999) Antiprothrombin antibodies: detection a clinical significance in the antiphospholipid syndrome. *Blood*, Vol.7, No.1, pp. 2149-2157.

George, J.; Afek, A.; Gilburd, B.; Harats, D. & Shoenfeld, Y. (2000) Autoimmunity in atherosclerosis: lessons from experimental models. *Lupus*, Vol.9, No.3, pp. 223-227.

Gladman, DD. & Urowitz, MB. (1987) Morbidity in systemic lupus erythematosus. *J Rheumatol Suppl*, Vol.14, Suppl 13, pp. 223-226.

Glueck, CJ.; Lang, JE.; Tracy, T.; Sieve-Smith, L. & Wang, P. (1999) Evidence that anticardiolipin antibodies are independent risk factors for atherosclerotic vascular disease. *Am J Cardiol*, Vol.83, No.10, pp. 1490-1494.

Gonzales-Portillo, F.; Mcityre, JA.; Wagenknecht, DR.; Williams, LS.; Bruno, A. & Biller, J. (2001) Spectrum of antiphospholipid antibodies (aPL) in patients with cerebrovascular disease. *J Stroke Cerebrovasc Dis*, Vol.10, No.5, pp. 222-226.

Gordon, PA.; George, J.; Kamashta, M.; Harats, D.; Hughes, G. & Shoenfeld, Y. (2001) Atherosclerosis and autoimmunity. *Lupus*, Vol.10, No.4, pp. 249-252.

Graham, I.; Atar, D.; Borch-Johnsen, K.; Boysen, G.; Burell, G.; Cifkova, R.; Dallongeville, J.; De Backer, G.; Ebrahim, S.; Gjelsvik, B.; Herrmann-Lingen, C.; Hoes, A.; Humphries, S.; Knapton, M.; Perk, J.; Priori, SG.; Pyorala, K.; Reiner, Z.; Ruilope, L.; Sans-Menendez, S.; Scholte op Reimer, W.; Weissberg, P.; Wood, D.; Yarnell, J.; Zamorano, JL.; Walma, E.; Fitzgerald, T.; Cooney, MT.; Dudina, A; European Society of Cardiology (ESC) Committee for Practice Guidelines (CPG). (2007) European guidelines on cardiovascular disease prevention in clinical practice: executive summary Fourth Joint Task Force of the European Society of Cardiology and Other Societies on Cardiovascular Disease Prevention in Clinical Practice (Constituted by representatives of nine societies and by invited experts). *Eur Heart J*, Vol.28, No.19, pp. 2375-2414.

Gresele, P.; Migliacci, R.; Vedovati, MC.; Ruffatti, A.; Becattini, C.; Facco, M.; Guglielmini, G.; Boscaro, E.; Mezzasoma, AM.; Momi, S. & Pengo. V. (2009) Patients with primary antiphospholipid antibody syndrome and without associated vascular risk factors present a normal endothelial function. *Thromb Res*, Vol.123, No.3, pp. 444-451.

Gualtierotti, R.; Biggioggero, M. & Meroni, PL. (2011) Cutting-edge in coronary disease and the primary antiphospholipid syndrome. *Clinic Rev Allergy Immunol*, DOI 10.1007/s12016-011-8268-9 [Epub ahead of print].

Gustafsson, J.; Gunnarsson, I.; Börjesson, O.; Pettersson, S.; Möller, S.; Fei, GZ.; Elvin, K.; Simard, JF.; Hansson, LO.; Lundberg, IE.; Larsson, A. & Svenungsson, E. (2009) Predictors of the first cardiovascular event in patients with systemic lupus erythematosus - a prospective cohort study. *Arthritis Res Ther*, Vol.11, R186, DOI: 10.1 186/ar2878.

Haj-Yahja, S.; Sherer, Y.; Blank, M.; Kaetsu, H.; Smolinsky, A. & Shoenfeld, Y. (2003) Anti-prothrombin antibodies cause thrombosis in a novel qualitative ex-vivo animal model. *Lupus*, Vol.12, No.5, pp. 364-369.

Hansson, GK. (2001) Immune mechanisms in atherosclerosis. *Arterioscler Thromb Vasc Biol*, Vol.21, No.12, pp. 1876-1890.

Haque, S.; Gordon, C.; Isenberg, D.; Rahman, A.; Lanyon, P.; Bell, A.; Emery, P.; McHugh, N.; Teh, LS.; Scott, DG.; Akil, M.; Naz, S.; Andrews, J.; Griffiths, B.; Harris, H.; Youssef, H.; McLaren, J.; Toescu, V.; Devakumar, V.; Teir, J. & Bruce, IN. (2010) Risk factors for coronary heart disease in systemic lupus erythematosus: the lupus and atherosclerosis evaluation of risk (LASER) study. *J Rheumatol*, Vol.37, No.2, pp. 322-329.

Hatsunuuma, Y.; Matsuura, E.; Makita, Z.; Katahira, T.; Nishi, S. & Koike, T. (1997) Involvement of beta 2-glycoprotein I and anticardiolipin antibodies in oxidatively modified low-density lipoprotein uptake by macrophages. *Clin Exp Immunol*, Vol.107, No.3, pp. 569-573.

Hayem, G.; Nicaise-Roland, P.; Palazzo, E. de Bandt, M.; Tubach, F.; Weber, M. & Meyer, O. (2001) Anti-oxidized low-density-lipoprotein (oxLDL) antibodies in systemic lupus erythematosus with and without antiphospholipid syndrome. *Lupus*, Vol.10, No.5, pp. 346-351.

Hirata, K.; Kadirvelu, A.; Kinjo, M.; Sciacca, R.; Sugioka, K.; Otsuka, R.; Choy, A.; Chow, SK.; Yoshiyama, M.; Yoshikawa, J.; Homma, S. & Lang, CC. (2007) Altered coronary vasomotor function in young patients with systemic lupus erythematosus. *Circulation*, Vol.56, No.6, pp. 1904-1909.

Jansen, NL.; Snell, JR. & Moy, JN. (1996) Myocardial infarction as the presenting manifestation of systemic lupus erythematosus with antiphosphatidylserine antibodies. *Ann Allergy Asthma Immunol*, Vol.76, No.3, pp. 266-268.

Jara, LJ.; Medina, G.; Vera-Lastra, O. & Shoenfeld, Y. (2003) Atherosclerosis and antiphospholipid syndrome. *Clin Rev Allergy Immunol*, Vol.25, No.1, pp. 79-88.

Jiménez, S.; Garcia-Criado, MA.; Tássies, D.; Reverter, JC.; Cervera, R.; Gilabert, MR.; Zambón, D.; Ros, E.; Bru, C. & Font, J. (2005) Preclinical vascular diseases in systemic lupus erythematosus and primary antiphospholipid syndrome. *Rheumatology (Oxford)*, Vol.44, No.6, pp. 756-761.

Kahles, T.; Humpich, M.; Steinmetz, H.; Sitzer, M. & Lindhoff-Last, E. (2005) Phosphatidylserine IgG and beta-2-glycoprotein I IgA antibodies may be a risk factor for ischaemic stroke. *Rheumatology*, Vol.44, No.9, pp. 1161-1165.

Kiss, E.; Seres, I.; Tarr, T.; Kocsis, Z.; Szegedi, G. & Paragh, G. (2007) Reduced paraoxonase1 activity is a risk factor for atherosclerosis in patients with systemic lupus erythematosus. *N Y Acad Sci*, Vol.1108, pp. 83-91.

Kiss, E.; Soltesz, P.; Der, H.; Kocsis, Z.; Tarr, T.; Bhattoa, H.; Shoenfeld, Y. & Szegedi, G. (2006) Reduced flow-mediated vasodilatation as a marker for cardiovascular complications in lupus patients. *J Autoimmun*, Vol.27, No.4, pp. 211-217.

Lam, EY.; Taylor, LM.; Landry, GJ.; Porter, JM. & Moneta, GL. (2001) Relationship between antiphospholipid antibodies and progression of lower extremity arterial occlusive disease after lower extremity bypass operations. *J Vasc Surg*, Vol.33, No.5, pp. 976-982.

Le Tonquéze, M.; Salozhin, K..; Dueymes, M.; Piette, JC.; Kovalev, V.; Shoenfeld, Y.; Nassonov, E. & Youinou, P. (1995) Role of β_2-glycoprotein I in the antiphospholipid antibody binding to endothelial cells. *Lupus*, Vol.4, No.3, pp. 179-186.

Lee, AB.; Godfrez, T.; Rowlez, KG.; Karschimkus, CS.; Dragicevic, G.; Romas, E.; Clemens, L.; Wilson, AM.; Nikpour, M.; Prior, DL.; Best, JD.; Jenkins, AJ. (2006) Traditional risk factors assessment does not capture the extent of cardiovascular risk in systemic lupus erythematosus. *Intern Med J*, Vol.36, No.4, pp. 237-243.

Levine, SR.; Salowich-Palm, L.; Sawaya, KL.; Perry, M.; Spencer, HJ.; Winkler, HJ.; Alam, Z. & Carey, JL. (1997) IgG anticardiolipin antibody titer > 40 GPL and the risk of subsequent thrombo-occlusive events and death. A prospective cohort study. *Stroke*, Vol.28, No.9, pp. 1660-1665.

Lopez, LR.; Buckner, TR.; Hurley, BL.; Kobayashi, K. & Matsuura, E. (2007) Determination of oxidized low-density lipoproteins (ox-LDL) versus ox-LDL/β_2GPI complexes for the assessment of autoimmune-mediated atherosclerosis. *N Y Acad Sci*, Vol.1109, pp. 303-310.

Lopez, L.; Dier, KJ.; Lopez, D.; Merrill, JT. & Fink, CA. (2004) Anti-β_2-Glycoprotein I and antiphosphatidylserine antibodies are predictors of arterial thrombosis in patients with antiphospholipid syndrome. *Am J Cli Pathol*, Vol.121, No.1, pp. 142-149.

Maneta-Peyet, L.; Previsani, C.; Sultan, Y.; Bezian, JH. & Cassagne, C. (1991) Autoantibodies against all the phospholipids: a comparative systematic study with systemic lupus erythematosus and healthy sera. *Eur J Clin Chem Clin Bioch*, Vol.29, No.1, pp. 39-43.

Manzi, S.; Meilahn, EN.; Rairie, JE.; Conte, CG.; Medsger, TA Jr.; Jansen-McWilliams, L.; D'Agostino, RB. & Kuller, LH. (1997) Age-specific incidence of myocardial infarction and angina in women with systemic lupus erythematosus: comparison with the Framingham study. *Am J Epidemiol*, Vol.145, No.5, pp. 408-415.

Manzi, S.; Selzer, F.; Sutton-Tyrrell, K.; Fitzgerald, SG.; Rairie, JE.; Tracy, RP. & Kuller, LH. (1999) Prevalence and risk factors of carotid plaque in women with systemic lupus erythematosus. *Arthritis Rheum*, Vol.42, No.1, pp. 51-60.

Matsuura, E.; Kobayashi, K.; Hurley, BL. & Lopez, LR. (2006b) Atherogenic oxidized low-density lipoprotein/β2-GP I (oxLDL/β2-GPI) complexes in patients with systemic lupus erythematosus and antiphospholipid syndrome. *Lupus*, Vol.15, No.7, pp. 478-483.

Matsuura, E.; Kobayashi, K.; Inoue, K.; Loez, LR. & Shoenfeld, Y. (2005) Oxidized LDL/β2-GPI I complexes: new aspects in atherosclerosis. *Lupus*, Vol.14, No.9, pp. 736-741.

Matsuura, E.; Kobayashi, K.; Tabuchi, M. & Lopez, LR. (2006a) Oxidative modification of low-density lipoprotein and immune regulation of atherosclerosis. *Prog Lipid Res*, Vol.45, No.6, pp. 466-486.

McDonald, J.; Stewart, J.; Urowitz, MB. & Gladman, DD. (1992) Peripheral vascular disease in patients with systemic lupus erythematosus. *Ann Rheum Dis*, Vol.51, No.1, pp. 56-60.

Mcintyre, JA. & Wagenknecht, DR. (2000) Anti-phosphatidylethanolamine (aPE) antibodies: the survey. J Autoimmun, Vol.15, No.2, pp. 185-193.

McMahon, M. & Hahn, BH. (2007) Atherosclerosis and systemic lupus erythematosus – mechanistic basis of the association. *Curr Opin Immunol*, Vol.19, No. 6, pp. 633-639.

Medina, G.; Casaos, D.; Jara, LJ.; Vera-Lastra, O.; Fuentes, M.; Barile, L. & Salas, M. (2003) Increased carotid intima-media thickness may be associated with stroke in primary antiphospholipid syndrome. *Ann Rheum Dis*, Vol.62, No.7, pp. 607-610.

Mercanoglu, F.; Erdogan, D.; Oflaz, H.; Kücükkaya, R.; Selcukbiricik, F.; Gül, A. & Inanc, M. (2004) Impaired brachial endothelial function in patients with primary anti-phospholipid syndrome. *J Clin Pract*, Vol.58, No.11, pp. 1003-1007.

Miyakis, S.; Lockshin, MD.; Atsumi, T.; Branch, DW.; Brey, RL.; Cervera, R.; Derksen, RH.; DE Groot, PG.; Koike, T.; Meroni, PL.; Reber, G.; Shoenfeld, Y.; Tincani, A.; Vlachoyiannopoulos, PG. & Krilis, SA. (2006) International consensus statement on an update of the classification criteria for definite antiphospholipid syndrome (APS). *J Thromb Haemost*, Vol.4, No.2, pp. 295-306.

Molad, Y.; Gorshtein, A.; Wysenbeek, AJ.; Guedj, D.; Majadla, R.; Weinberger, A. & Amit-Vazina, M. (2002) Protective effect of hydroxychloroquine in systemic lupus erythematosus. Prospective long term study of an Israeli cohort. *Lupus*, Vol.11, No.6, pp. 356-361.

Mosca, M.; Tani, C.; Aringer, M.; Bombardieri, S.; Boumpas, D.; Brey, R.; Cervera, R.; Doria, A.; Jayne, D.; Khamashta, MA.; Kuhn, A.; Gordon, C.; Petri, M.; Rekvig, OP.; Schneider, M.; Sherer, Y.; Shoenfeld, Y.; Smolen, JS.; Talarico, R.; Tincani, A.; van Vollenhoven, RF.; Ward, MM.; Werth, VP. & Carmona, L. (2010) European League Against Rheumatism recommendations for monitoring systemic lupus erythematosus patients in clinical practice and in observational studies. *Ann Rheum Dis*, Vol.69, No.7, pp. 1269-1274.

Muñoz, LE.; Lauber, K.; Schiller, M.; Manfredi, AA. & Herrmann, M. (2010) The role of defective clearance of apoptotic cells in systemic autoimmunity. *Nat Rev Rheumatol*, Vol.6, No.5, pp. 280-289.

Narshi, CB.; Giles, IP. & Rahman, A. (2011) The endothelium: an interface between autoimmunity and atherosclerosis in systemic lupus erythematosus. *Lupus*, Vol.20, No.1, pp. 5-13.

Nityanand, S.; Bergmark, C.; De Faire, U.; Swedenborg, J.; Holm, G. & Lefvert, AK. (1995) Antibodies against endothelial cells and cardiolipin in young patients with peripheral atherosclerotic disease. *J Int Med*, Vol.238, No.5, pp. 437-43.

O'Leary, DH.; Polak, JF.; Kronmai, FA.; Manolio, TA.; Burke, GL. & Wolfson, SK Jr. (1999) Carotid-artery intima and media thickness as a risk factor for myocardial infarction and stroke in older adults. *N Engl J Med*, Vol.340, No.1, pp. 14-22.

Okuma, H.; Kitagawa, Y. & Takagi, S. (2010) Investigation of antiphosphatidyl-serine antibody and antiphosphatidyl-inositol antibody in ischemic stroke patients. *Clin Dev Immunol*, Article ID 439230, 4 pp.

Ostanek, L.; Brzosko, M. & Fischer, K. (2005) (Usefulness of different antiphospholipid antibodies in the assessment of the secondary antiphospholipid syndrome in lupus erythematosus patients - review and own experiences). *Reumatologia*, Vol.43, No.6, pp. 354-357.

Ostanek, L.; Brzosko, M.; Fischer, K. & Płońska, E. (2006a) (Antiphospholipid syndrome and antiphospholipid antibodies as a risk factors of ischemic heart disease and myocardial infarction in patients with systemic lupus erythematosus). *Pol Arch Med Wewn*, Vol.115, No.5, pp. 407-413.

Ostanek, L.; Płońska, E.; Peregud-Pogorzelska, M.; Mokrzycki, K.; Brzosko, M.; Fischer, K. & Fliciński, J. (2006b) (Cardiovascular abnormalities in systemic lupus erythematosus patients in echocardiographic assessment). *Pol Merk Lek*, Vol.20, No.117, pp. 305-308.

Pahor, A.; Hojs, R.; Holc, I.; Ambrozic, A.; Cucnik, S.; Kveder, T. & Rozman, B. (2006) Antiphospholipid antibodies as a possible risk factor for atherosclerosis in patients with rheumatoid arthritis. *Immunobiology*, Vol.211, No.9, pp. 689-694.

Petri, M.; Perez-Gutthann, S.; Spence, D. & Hochberg, MC. (1992) Risk factors for coronary artery disease in patients with systemic lupus erythematosus. *Am J Med*, Vol.93, No.5, pp. 513-519.

Petri, M. (2010). Update on anti-phospholipid antibodies in SLE: the Hopkins' Lupus Cohort. *Lupus*, Vol.19, No.4, pp. 419-423.

Puurunen, M.; Mänttäri, M.; Manninen, V.; Tenkanen, L.; Alfthan, G.; Ehnholm, C.; Vaarala, O.; Aho, K. & Palosuo, T. (1994) Antibody against oxidized low-density lipoprotein predicting myocardial infarction. *Arch Intern Med*, Vol.154, No.28, pp. 2605-2609.

Radulescu, L.; Stancu, C. & Antohe, F. (2004) Antibodies against human oxidized low-density lipoprotein (LDL) as markers for human plasma modified lipoproteins. *Med Sci Monit*, Vol.10, No.7, pp. 207-214.

Rahman, P.; Gladman, DG.; Urowitz, MB.; Yuen, K.; Hallett, D. & Bruce, IN. (1999) The cholesterol lowering effect of antimalarial drugs is enhanced in patients with lupus taking corticosteroid drugs. *J Rheumatol*, Vol.26, No.2, pp. 325-330.

Roman, MJ.; Devereux, RB.; Schwartz, MD.; Lockshin, MD.; Paget, SA.; Davis, A.; Crow, MK.; Sammaritano, L.; Levine, DM.; Shankar, BA.; Moeller, E. & Salmon, JE. (2005) Arterial stiffness in chronic inflammatory diseases. *Hypertention*, Vol.46, No.1, pp. 194-199.

Roman, MJ.; Salmon, JE.; Sobel, R.; Lockshin, MD.; Sammaritano, L.; Schwartz, JE. & Devereux, RB. (2001) Prevalence and relation to risk factors of carotid atherosclerosis and left ventricular hypertrophy in systemic lupus erythematosus and antiphospholipid syndrome. *Am J Cardiol*, Vol.87, No.5, pp. 663-666.

Ross, R. (1993) The pathogenesis of atherosclerosis: a prospective for the 1990s. *Nature*, Vol.362, No.6423, pp. 801-809.

Ross, R. & Glomset, JA. (1973) Atherosclerosis and the arterial smooth muscle cell. *Science*, Vol.180, No.4093, pp. 1332-1339.

Saidi, S.; Mahjoub, T. & Almawi, WY. (2009) Lupus anticoagulants and anti-phospholipid antibodies as risk factors for a first episode of ischemic stroke. *J Thromb Haemost*, Vol.7, No.7, pp. 1075-1080.

Sangle, SR. & D'Cruz, DP. (2008) Syndrome X (angina pectoris with normal coronary arteries) and myocardial infarction in patients with antiphospholipid (Hughes) syndrome. *Lupus*, Vol.17, No.2, pp. 83-85.

Sanmarco, M.; Alessi, MC.; Harle, JR.; Sapin, C.; Aillaud, MF.; Gentile, S.; Juhan-Vague, I. & Weiller, PJ. (2001) Antibodies to phosphatidylethanolamine as the only antiphospholipid antibodies found in patients with unexplained thromboses. *Thromb Haemost*, Vol.85, No.5, pp. 800-805.

Schanberg, LE.; Sandborg, C.; Barnhart, HX.; Ardoin, SP.; Yow, E.; Evans, GW.; Mieszkalski, KL.; Ilowite, NT.; Eberhard, A.; Levy, DM.; Kimura, Y.; von Scheven, E.; Silverman, E.; Bowyer, SL.; Punaro, L.; Singer, NG.; Sherry, DD.; McCurdy, D.; Klein-Gitelman, M.; Wallace, C.; Silver, R.; Wagner-Weiner, L.; Higgins, GC.; Brunner, HI.; Jung, L.; Soep, JB. & Reed, A; Atherosclerosis Prevention in Pediatric Lupus Erythematosus Investigators. (2009) Premature atherosclerosis in pediatric systemic lupus erythematosus: risk factors for increased carotid intima-media thickness in the Atherosclerosis Prevention in Pediatric Lupus Erythematosus Cohort. *Arthritis Rheum*, Vol.60, No.5, pp. 1496-1507.

Selzer, F.; Sutton-Tyrrell, K.; Fitzgerald, S.; Tracy, R.; Kuller, L. & Manzi, S. (2001) Vascular stiffness in women with systemic lupus erythematosus. *Hypertention*, Vol.37, No.4, pp. 1075-1082.

Shoenfeld, Y.; Alarcon-Segovia, D.; Buskila, D.; Abu-Shakra, M.; Lorber, M.; Sherer, Y.; Berden, J.; Meroni, PL.; Valesini, G.; Koike, T. & Alarcon-Riquelme, ME. (1999) Frontiers of SLE: review of the 5th International Congress of Systemic Lupus Erythematosus, Cancun, Mexico, April 20 - 25, 1998. *Semin Arthritis Rheum*, Vol.29, No.2, pp. 112-130.

Shojaie, M.; Sotoodah, A.; Roozmeh, S.; Kholoosi, E. & Dana, S. (2009) Annexin V and anti-annexin V antibodies: two interesting aspects in acute myocardial infarction. *Thromb J*, Vol.7, pp.13.

Simantov, R.; LaSala, JM.; Lo, SK.; Gharavi, AE.; Sammaritano, LR.; Salmon, JE. & Silverstein, RL. (1995) Activation of cultured vascular endothelial cells by antiphospholipid antibodies. *J Clin Invest*, Vol.96, No.5, pp. 2211-2219.

Sokol, DK.; Mcintyre, JA.; Short, R.; Gutt, J.; Wagenknecht, DR.; Biller, J. & Garg, B. (2000) Henoch-Schönlein purpura and stroke: antiphosphatidylethanolamine antibody (aPE) in CSF and serum. *Neurology*, Vol.55, No.9, pp. 1379-1381.

Štalc, M.; Poredoš, P.; Peternel, P.; Tomsic, M.; Sebestjen, M. & Kveder, T. (2006) Endothelial function is impaired in patients with primary antiphospholipid syndrome. *Thromb Res*, Vol.118, No.4, pp. 455-461.

Sun, Y.; Lin, CH.; Lu, CJ.; Yip, PK. & Chen, RC. (2002) Carotid atherosclerosis, intima-media thickness and risk factors - an analysis of 1781 asymptomatic subjects in Taiwan. *Atherosclerosis*, Vol.164, No.1, pp. 89-94.

Svenungsson, E.; Jensen-Urstad, K.; Heimbürger, M.; Silveira, A.; Hamsten, A.; de Faire, U.; Witztum, JL. & Frostegård, J. (2001) Risk factors for cardiovascular disease in systemic lupus erythematosus. *Circulation*, Vol.104, No.16, pp. 1887-1893.

Szodoray, P.; Tarr, T; Tumpek, J.; Kappelmayer, J.; Lakos, G.; Poor, G.; Szegedi, G. & Kiss, E. (2009) Identification of rare anti-phospholipid/protein co-factor autoantibodies in patients with systemic lupus erythematosus. *Autoimmunity*, Vol.42, No.6, pp. 497-506.

Takashi, W.; Tsutomu, F. & Kentaro, F. (2002) Ultrasonic correlates of common carotid atherosclerosis in patients with coronary artery disease. *Angiology*, Vol.53, No.2, pp. 177-183.

Tanaka, H.; DeSouza, CA. & Seals, DR. (1998) Absence of age-related increase in central arterial stiffness in physically active women. *Arterioscl Thromb Vasc Biol*, Vol.18, No.1, pp. 127-132.

Theodoridou, A.; Bento, L.; D'Cruz, DP.; Khamashta, MA. & Hughes, GR. (2003) Prevalence and associations of an abnormal ankle-brachial index in systemic lupus erythematosus: a pilot study. *Ann Rheum Dis*, Vol.62, No.12, pp. 1199-1203.

Toloza, SM.; Uribe, AG.; McGwin Jr, G.; Alarcón, GS.; Fessler, BJ.; Bastian, HM.; Vilá, LM.; Wu, R.; Shoenfeld, Y.; Roseman, JM. & Reveille, JD; LUMINA Study Group. (2004) Systemic lupus erythematosus multiethnic US cohort (LUMINA): baseline predictors of vascular events. *Arthritis Rheum*, Vol.50, No.12, pp. 3947-3957.

Toschi, V.; Motta, A.; Castelli, C.; Gibelli, S.; Cimminiello, C.; Molaro, GL. & Gibelli, A. (1993) Prevalence and clinical significance of antiphospholipid antibodies to noncardiolipin antigens in systemic lupus erythematosus. *Haemostasis*, Vol.23, No.5, pp. 275-283.

Toschi, V.; Motta, A.; Castelli, C.; Paracchini, ML.; Zerbi, D. & Gibelli, A. (1998) High prevalence of antiphosphatidylinositol antibodies in young patients with cerebral ischemia of undetermined cause. *Stroke*, Vol.29, No.9, pp. 1759-1764.

Touboul, PJ.; Labreuche, J.; Vicaut, E. & Amarenco, P; GENIC Investigators. (2005) Carotid intima-media thickness, plaques, and Framingham risk score as independent determinants of stroke risk. *Stroke*, Vol.36, No.8, pp. 1741-1745.

Urbanus, RT; Siegerink, B.; Roest, M.; Rosendaal, FR.; de Groot, PG. & Algra, A. (2009) Antiphospholipid antibodies and risk of myocardial infarction and ischemic stroke in young women in the RATIO study: a case-control study. *Lancet Neurol*, Vol.8, No.11, pp. 998-1005.

Urowitz, MB.; Bookman, AAM.; Koehler, BE.; Gordon, DA.; Smythe, HA. & Ogryzlo, MA. (1976) The bimodal mortality pattern of systemic lupus erythematosus. *Am J Med*, Vol.60, No.2, pp. 221-225.

Urowitz, MB.; Ibanez, D. & Gladman, DD. (2007) Atherosclerotic vascular events in a single large lupus cohort: prevalence and risk factors. *J Rheumatol*, Vol.34, No.1, pp. 70-75.

Vaarala, O.; Mänttäri, M.; Manninen, V.; Tenkanen, L.; Puurunen, M.; Aho, K. & Palosuo, T. (1995) Anti-cardiolipin antibodies and risk of myocardial infarction in a prospective cohort of middle-aged men. *Circulation*, Vol.91, No.1, pp. 23-27.

Vaarala, O.; Puurunen, M.; Mänttäri, M.; Manninen, V.; Aho, K. & Palosuo, T. (1996) Antibodies to prothrombin imply a risk of myocardial infarction in middle-aged men. *Thromb Haemost*, Vol.75, No.3, pp. 456-459.

Wajed, J.; Ahmad, Y.; Durrindton, PN. & Bruce, IN. (2004) Prevention of cardiovascular disease in systemic lupus erythematosus—proposed guidelines for risk factor management. *Rheumatology (Oxford)*, Vol.43, No.1, pp. 7-12.

Walecka, A.; Sawicki, M.; Brzosko, M.; Ostanek, L.; Fischer, K. & Kordowski J. (2004) Value of high resistance index - HRI calculated from Doppler spectrum of popliteal arteries in patients with systemic lupus erythematosus (SLE). *Med Sci Monit*, Vol.10, Suppl 3, pp. 58-62.

Wright, SA.; O'Prey, FM.; Rea, DJ.; Plumb, RD.; Gamble, AJ.; Leahey, WJ.; Devine, AB.; McGivern, RC.; Johnston, DG.; Finch, MB.; Bell, AL. & McVeigh, GE. (2006) Microcirculatory hemodynamics and endothelial dysfunction in systemic lupus erythematosus. *Arterioscler Thromb Vasc Biol*, Vol.26, No.10, pp. 2281-2287.

7

The Kidney in Antiphospholipid Syndrome

Alexandru Caraba[1], Viorica Crişan[1], Andreea Munteanu[1], Corina Şerban[1], Diana Nicoară[2] and Ioan Romoşan[1]
[1]*University of Medicine and Pharmacy „Victor Babeş", Timişoara*
[2]*Selfmed Clinique, Timişoara*
Romania

1. Introduction

Graham Hughes described in 1983 a syndrome, characterized by recurrent arterial and venous thrombosis, pregnancy morbidity, thrombocytopenia, and the presence of antiphospholipid antibodies (aPL), which was named *antiphospholipid syndrome* [Hughes, 1983]. Many other features of this syndrome were identified during the time. In present, antiphospholipid syndrome is considered a systemic form of autoantibody-induced thrombophilia, which involves many organs [Wilson et al., 1999].

Antiphospholipid antibodies (aPL) are: lupus anticoagulant (LA), anticardiolipin antibodies (aCL), and anti-β_2-glycoprotein I antibodies [Cervera et al., 2002]. Classification criteria for the antiphospholipid syndrome had been updated by Miyakis et al. in 2006 [Miyakis et al., 2006].

Antiphospholipid syndrome was first described in patients with systemic lupus erythematosus. Now, it is known that this syndrome may be associated with another disorder (autoimmune diseases, malignancies, infections or drugs), or, may be appear alone, named as primary antiphospholipid syndrome [Sinico et al., 2010].

This disorder may involve any organ in the body, due to vascular thrombosis. The kidney involvement represents one of the most important features of this syndrome. Renal manifestations reflect the extension of thrombotic process in the kidney vascular bed: main renal arteries, intrarenal arteries and arterioles, glomerular capillaries, renal veins [Tektonidou et al., 2000; Vlachoyiannopoulos et al., 2001]. Besides the thrombotic lesions, glomerulonephritis were described in patients with primary antiphospholipid syndrome, too [Nochy et al., 2002; Fakhouri et al., 2003; Sinico et al., 2010].

Renal involvement appears in 2.7% of patients with antiphospholipid syndrome [Cervera et al., 2002], but the real incidence is greater. The explanations of this underestimated incidence are represented by the fact that renal biopsy is a high-risk procedure in patients treated with anticoagulants, and, on the other hand, renal manifestations of antiphospholipid syndrome are frequently attributed to other conditions, as essential hypertension, or, lupus nephritis [Tektonidou, 2009]. In catastrophic antiphospholipid syndrome, kidney involvement was reported in 78% of cases [Uthman, Khamashta, 2006]. Renal manifestations associated with antiphospholipid syndrome are summarized in table 1 [Uthman, Khamashta, 2006].

Renal manifestation	Main clinical and laboratory findings
Renal artery lesions	• hypertension • decreased glomerular filtration rate
Hypertension	• hypertension • decreased glomerular filtration rate
Antiphospholipid syndrome nephropathy	• hypertension • proteinuria • hematuria • decreased glomerular filtration rate
Renal vein thrombosis	• proteinuria (even nephrotic syndrome) • hematuria
End stage renal disease/renal transplant	• decreased glomerular filtration rate • vascular thrombosis of renal allograft

Table 1. Renal manifestations in antiphospholipid syndrome

2. Renal artery lesions

Renal artery lesions are represented by stenosis or occlusion. Renal artery stenosis, thrombosis and renal infarction were described by many authors [Asherson et al., 1991; Ames et al., 1992; Mandreoli et al., 1992; Godfrey et al., 2000]. The first case of renal artery involvement in antiphospholipid syndrome was reported by Ostuni et al. [Ostuni et al., 1990]. They described the appearance of renal artery thrombosis and hypertension in a young female patient with high titers of aCL and a false positive venereal disease research laboratory test. Then, Asherson et al. reported the case of young man with primary antiphospholipid syndrome, who suddenly developed severe hypertension due to right renal artery stenosis [Asherson et al., 1991]. Another patient described by Ames and collaborators presented hypertension and oliguria, bilateral renal artery occlusions on renal arteriography and high titers of circulating aPL [Ames et al., 1992]. Sangle et al., using magnetic resonance angiography, identified that 26% of the aPL-positive patients with severe, poorly controlled arterial hypertension had renal artery stenosis, compared with 8% in young aPL-negative hypertensive patients [Sangle et al., 2003]. The renal artery stenosis in aPL-positive patients has two patterns. In the first, most common, the stenosis is smooth, well-delineated, often non-critical, localized distal to the renal artery ostium. Another pattern, less common, is localized proximally, occasionally involving the aorta [Uthman, Khamashta, 2006; Tektonidou, 2009]. The common features of renal artery stenosis are represented by: renovascular hypertension and decrease of glomerular filtration rate [Mandreoli, Zuccheli, 1993]. Reno-vascular hypertension in patients with antiphospholipid syndrome and inadequate anticoagulation has a progressive evolution, leading to the renal impairment function [Sangle et al., 2005]. Based on the thrombotic basis of these renal lesions, Sangle et al. recommended that all the hypertensive patients with aPL-related renal artery stenosis need to be treated with anticoagulant drugs, irrespective of the presence of previous thrombotic events [Sangle et al., 2005]. Renal artery thrombosis determines the occurrence of severe hypertension or a worsening of a previously arterial hypertension. In some cases, these patients present pain in lumbar area, hematuria, or decreased of renal function. This renal artery disorder is caused by in situ thrombosis or embolism from heart valve. Other factors involved in the appearance of thrombosis are represented by increased levels of endothelin and accelerated atherosclerosis. The complete occlusion of renal arteries leads to renal infarcts. They may be symptomatic (uni-, bilateral lumbar pain, hypertension, hematuria, oliguria if the lesions are bilateral), or may have a subclinical evolution. In the latter case, the old infarcts may be discovered by imagistic methods [Sonpal et al., 1993].

Imagistic methods such as renal ultrasonography (including main renal artery Doppler ultrasonography), computed tomography, renal scintigraphy, renal angiography, and gadolinium enhanced magnetic resonance angiography contribute to the diagnosis and severity assessment of the renal arteries lesions [Mandreoli, Zuccheli, 1993; Sangle et al., 2003].

The treatment consists in antihypertensive, anticoagulants and antiplatelets drugs. Because the high values of blood pressure have a negative impact on renal function, it is reasonable to diminish these values, without worsening the renal function [Asherson et al., 1991; Godfrey T et al., 2000; Tektonidou, 2009]. Although the renal arteries stenoses are often non-critical, it is recommendable to avoid the use of angiotensin-converting enzyme inhibitors and angiotensin receptor blockers in hypertension therapy of these patients [D'Cruz, 2009]. But other authors reported a good control of high blood pressure with angiotensin-converting enzyme inhibitors, angiotensin receptor blockers and calcium channel blockers, without worsening the renal function [Godfrey et al., 2000]. Poststenotic reduction of renal perfusion pressure stimulates the appearance of high levels of angiotensin II, resulting vasoconstriction of the efferent arteriole, which preserves the glomerular capillary filtration pressure. Angiotensin-converting enzyme inhibitors and angiotensin receptor blockers inhibit this compensatory mechanism, and results a reduction of glomerular filtration rate. But the reduction of the glomerular filtration rate is not specific to angiotensin-converting enzyme inhibitors or angiotensin receptor blockers. The reduction of high blood pressure may impair the autoregulation of intrarenal circulation, and then the renal function declines, irrespective of antihypertensive agents. That is why is very important to closely check the renal function after the initiation of antihypertensive therapy [Mimran, 1992]. Remondino et al. demonstrated that the oral anticoagulation may contribute to the recanalization after bilateral renal artery thrombosis with the subsequent normalizing the high blood pressure [Remondino et al., 2000]. The beneficial role of oral anticoagulant therapy (INR of 3.0 to 4.5) in control of arterial hypertension and improve of the renal function was demonstrated by Sangle et al. A value of INR < 3.0 is associated with poorly controlled blood pressure, and deterioration of glomerular filtration rate [Sangle et al., 2005]. Other therapeutic methods are: thrombolysis, transluminal balloon angioplasty with or without stenting, surgical interventions [Rysana et al., 1998; Sangle et al., 2005; Tektonidou, 2009].

3. Arterial hypertension

Hypertension is common in patients with antiphospholipid syndrome. Hughes described in 1983 the features of arterial hypertension in these patients. He sustained that hypertension in patients with antiphospholipid syndrome often fluctuates, apparently correlating with the severity of the livedo, inferring the relationship between thrombotic renal lesions and high blood pressure [Hughes, 1984].

The etiology of hypertension in antiphospholipid syndrome is represented by the stenosis or occlusion of renal artery, or, by the intrarenal vascular lesions. Cacoub et al. studied the kidney lesions in a group of 5 patients with antiphospholipid syndrome and malignant hypertension, in the absence of lupus nephritis. These lesions were represented by ischemic glomeruli without proliferation, focal intimal fibrosis, and thrombosis [Cacoub et al., 1992]. Another study performed by Kincaid-Smith et al., revealed fibrin thrombi in glomeruli and in intrarenal arterioles [Kincaid-Smith et al., 1988]. Nochy et al. reported the presence of high blood pressure in 93% of the 16 patients with primary antiphospholipid syndrome. In some cases, hypertension represented the unique sign of renal involvement in this syndrome. In this study, the authors revealed that the causes of hypertension are represented by intrarenal vascular lesions: arteriosclerosis, fibrous intimal hyperplasia, arterial and arteriolar fibrous, fibrocellular occlusions and thrombotic microangiopathy [Nochy et al., 1999]. In 25 patients with severe essential hypertension, Rollino et al. identified aPL in 8% of them, a frequency higher than in control population [Rollino et al., 2004]. High levels of anti-β_2-glycoprotein I antibodies were identified by Frostegard et al. in 73 borderline hypertensive patients [Frostegard et al., 1998].

Hypertensive aPL-positive patients had to be extensively investigated: glomerular rate filtration, urinary sediment, proteinuria, renal ultrasonography (including Doppler of renal arteries, veins, and intrarenal vessels) (fig. 1), renal angiography [Tektonidou, 2009].

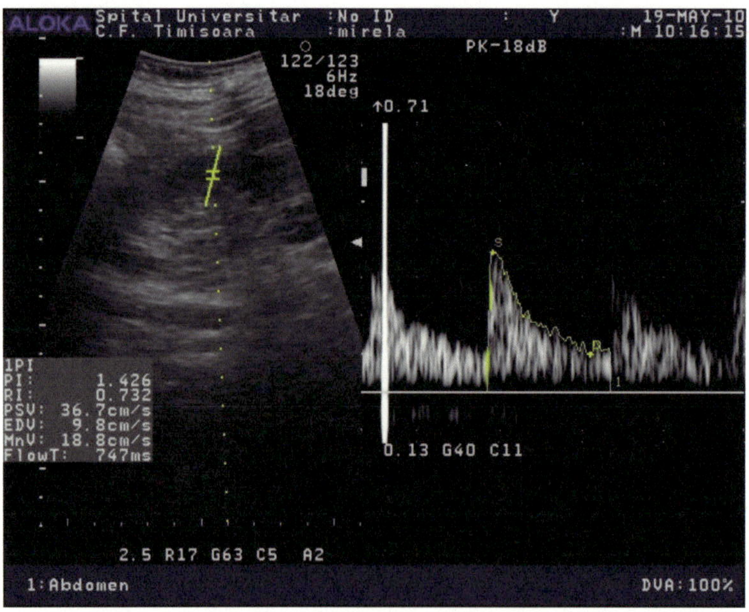

Fig. 1. Increased resistive index (RI) of interlobar renal arteries in hypertensive patient with antiphospholipid syndrome

The objective of the treatment is to obtain reduced blood pressure values in order to preserve the renal function. It is achieved by an association between antihypertensive drugs and anticoagulants [Nochy et al., 2002; Tektonidou, 2009, Sinico et al., 2010].

4. Antiphospholipid syndrome nephropathy

The intrarenal vascular lesions associated with antiphospholipid syndrome define antiphospholipid syndrome nephropathy. These lesions are represented by: thrombotic microangiopathy, arteriosclerosis, fibrous intimal hyperplasia of arterioles and interlobular arteries, organized thrombi in arteries and arterioles with or without recanalization, fibrous arterial and arteriolar occlusions, focal cortical atrophy [Nochy et al., 1999]. Nochy et al. and Tektonidou et al. revealed that the characteristic features of antiphospholipid syndrome nephropathy are: arterial hypertension, acute or chronic renal failure, proteinuria and microscopic hematuria [Nochy et al., 1999; Tektonidou et al., 2008; Tektonidou, 2009].

Systemic hypertension was identified in 93% of studied patients by Nochy et al. The severity of hypertension varied from mild to severe, even malignant. Malignant hypertension was described in only one patient, who developed acute renal failure associated with microangiopathic hemolytic anemia, requiring dialysis and progressing to end stage renal disease [Nochy et al., 1999]. It is considered that hypertension represents the most common feature of antiphospholipid syndrome nephropathy. The intrarenal vascular lesions generate systemic hypertension, which may worsen these lesions. Appearance of hypertension in a patient diagnosed with primary antiphospholipid syndrome may reveal the development of nephropathy associated with this disorder. Therefore, the patient with antiphospholipid syndrome who develops hypertension must be extensively investigated, including renal biopsy, irrespective of the presence of proteinuria, hematuria or decreased glomerular rate filtration [Nochy et al., 1999; Tektonidou, 2009; Sinico et al., 2010].

In his study, Nochy identified renal insufficiency in 87% of patients. It was mild in the most patients (mean value of serum creatinine 1.64 mg/dl), being associated with proteinuria and hematuria. End stage renal disease appeared only in one patient [Nochy et al., 1999]. Usually, proteinuria is mild (< 1 g/24 hours). In 25% of patients, it becomes in nephrotic range. Renal lesions in antiphospholipid syndrome nephropathy were described by many authors [Nochy et al., 1999; Griffiths et al., 2000; Tektonidou, 2009, Gigante et al., 2009].

Thrombotic microangiopathy represents the most characteristic lesion in this nephropathy [Amigo et al., 1992; Griffiths et al., 2000]. It is defined by the presence of fibrin thrombi in glomerular capillaries and in intrarenal vessels, without inflammatory cells or immune deposits. The most frequently affected vessels are: preglomerular arterioles, small interlobular arteries, glomerular capillaries. Complete noninflammatory vascular occlusions by intraluminally, subendothelial, and medial accumulation of fragmented erythrocytes, leucocytes and eosinophilic fibrinoid material may be observed. Old lesions are associated with recanalization thrombi. Immunofluorescence shows that the fibrin is the main constituent of these thrombi. Vasculitis was absent in many performed studies [Nochy et al., 1999; Gigante et al., 2009]. Arteriosclerosis lesions consist of fibrous intimal thickening and reduction of arcuate and interlobular arteries lumen. Arteriolar hyalinosis and arteriolosclerosis are identified, too [Gigante et al., 2009]. Fibrous intimal hyperplasia is characterized by intense myofibroblastic intimal cellular proliferation, which determines thickening of intima and tortuosity of interlobular arteries and their branches. The intima seems to be much more cellular than it observed in aging arteriosclerosis. Media may be atrophic and fibrous, or hypertrophic (hypertrophic myocites). Reduced lumen is caused by fibrous thickening of intima or recanalization after thrombosis. The organized thrombi may be seen. Small interstitial arteries present fibrocellular and fibrous occlusions [Nochy et al., 1999; Gigante et al., 2009]. Focal cortical atrophy is placed in the superficial zones of the subcapsular cortex, near the renal capsule, which presents a contour depression. It is identified a sharp border between focal cortical atrophy and the normal kidney cortex. This lesion is considered to be very specific for the nephropathy associated with antiphospholipid syndrome. In the regions of focal cortical atrophy, some histological characteristics were described. Glomeruli present two patterns, which may be seen in the same biopsy. Some of them are small and sclerotic, but others are voluminous and pseudocystic. Dense interstitial fibrosis, tubular atrophy, thyroidization and fibrous intimal hyperplasia of the vessels are other histological features. The arterioles are occluded by fibrin thrombi or by fibrous tissue [Gigante et al., 2009]. The main histological features of glomeruli, tubules, interstitium, and intrarenal vessels are presented in table 2.

Glomeruli	*Light microscopy* • enlarged • normal glomerular cellularity • increased number of capillary loops • diffusely thickened of capillary walls • double contours of glomerular basement membrane (the outer contour is wrinkled with redundant folds) • cellular interposition between the glomerular basement membrane and endothelial cells • central mesangiolysis *Immunofluorescence* • negative *Electron microscopy* • lucent flocculent material between the endothelial cells and glomerular basement membrane
Tubules	• atrophied • thyroidization
Interstitium	• fibrosis
Intrarenal vessels	*Grade 1* • endothelial swelling • mild fibrous arterial intimal thickening and/or • mild patchy arteriolar hyalinosis *Grade 2* • moderate fibrous arterial intimal thickening or • moderate arteriolar hyalinosis *Grade 3* • severe occlusive intimal thickening • thrombosis

Table 2. The main histological features in antiphospholipid syndrome nephropathy

Griffiths et al. and D'Cruz et al. showed that the redundant, wrinkled segments of glomerular basement membrane and duplicate straighter thin membrane represents pathognomonic findings of antiphospholipid syndrome nephropathy [Griffiths et al., 2000; D'Cruz, 2009]. The reports of Asherson, Bucciarelli et al., and Erkan et al. demonstrated that the kidney is one of the most frequently affected organs in catastrophic antiphospholipid syndrome [Asherson, 1992; Erkan et al., 2003; Bucciarelli et al., 2006]. Because of this form of antiphospholipid syndrome is very rare (less than 1% of antiphospholipid syndrome cases), there are few data about renal histological characteristics. Some cases of catastrophic antiphospholipid syndrome with renal involvement, in which renal biopsies were performed, showed fibrin thrombi in arteries and glomerular capillaries. Chronic vascular lesions were only rare identified [Tektonidou et al., 2008; Tektonidou, 2009]. The efficacy of anticoagulants in the treatment of antiphospholipid syndrome nephropathy wasn't evaluated. Based on the intrarenal thrombotic lesions which characterized this nephropathy, oral anticoagulation seems to be an acceptable therapy, even the long-term effects on renal function are not known, yet [Sinico et al., 2010]. Korkmaz et al. reported that proteinuria was reduced and renal function improved after a combined treatment with immunosuppressive, anticoagulants, calcium channel blockers and angiotensin-converting enzyme inhibitors [Korkmaz et al., 2003].

5. Renal vein thrombosis

Asherson et al. described for the first time renal vein thrombosis in two patients with proliferative lupus nephritis and positive LA [Asherson et al., 1993]. D'Cruz suggested that the aPL had an important role in the development of renal vein thrombosis [D'Cruz, 2005].

This lesion is more frequently among the patients with antiphospholipid syndrome and systemic lupus erythematosus than in patients without lupus. Nephrotic syndrome is the main clinical manifestation. Because of this situation, it is indicated that any patient with antiphospholipid syndrome who develops sudden nephrotic range proteinuria should be evaluated by imagistic methods the renal veins (fig. 2).

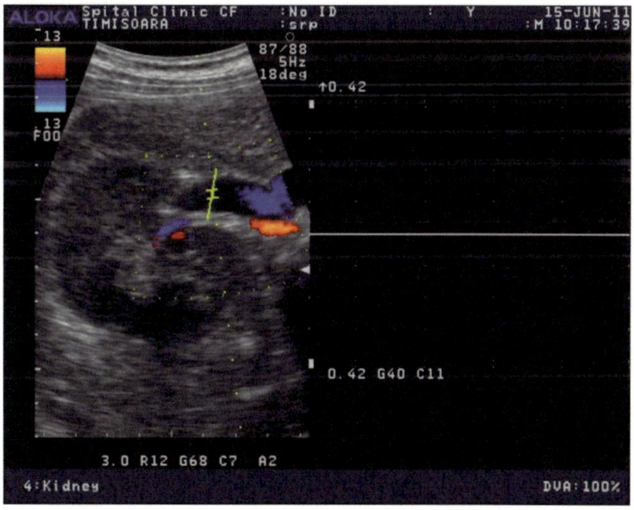

Fig. 2. Renal vein thrombosis (Duplex ultrasonography of the right renal vein)

Renal failure is a consequence of bilateral vein thrombosis. Anticoagulation represents the therapeutic key of this renal complication in antiphospholipid syndrome [Nochy et al., 2002; Tektonidou, 2009].

6. End-stage renal disease/renal transplantation

In patients undergoing hemodialysis for end-stage renal disease, it was reported a high prevalence of aPL. In a group of 97 patients with end-stage renal disease treated by hemodialysis, Brunet et al. identified LA in 16.5% of them, and aCL in 15.5% [Brunet et al., 1995]. No relations between aPL and sex, age, duration of dialysis, hepatitis viruses B, C were identified [Tektonidou, 2009]. Some studies established a relationship between aPL and vascular access thrombosis, especially in patients with LA [Lesar et al., 1999; Haviv, 2000]. Among the patients with renal transplant, it was identified a high incidence of aPL [Tektonidou, 2009]. The risk for vascular thrombosis and renal graft failure was increased in these patients [Andrassy et al., 2004]. Ducloux et al. identified aPL in 28% of transplant recipients; among them, 18% developed thrombotic complications [Ducloux et al., 1999]. The risk of thrombotic complications was greater in aPL-positive patients with systemic lupus erythematosus [Moroni et al., 2005]. The role of anticoagulant therapy in aPL-positive renal transplanted patients remains controversial, and prospective studies are necessary in order to establish the best modality for prevention of thrombotic complications [Tektonidou, 2009].

7. Antiphospholipid antibodies and systemic lupus erythematosus

Antiphospholipid antibodies are identified in approximately 30-40% of patients with systemic lupus erythematosus (SLE) [Tektonidou, 2009], but antiphospholipid syndrome appeared in 30% of cases [Tektonidou et al., 2004]. Hypertension from mild to malignant, hematuria, proteinuria from mild to nephrotic range, acute or chronic renal failure are the main clinical and laboratory findings in patients with SLE and aPL [Kleinknecht et al., 1989]. But all these findings may be the consequence of antiphospholipid syndrome nephropathy without any lesion of lupus nephropathy, or lupus nephropathy alone, or lupus nephropathy associated with antiphospholipid nephropathy. In these conditions, renal biopsy is a mandatory procedure for all the patients with SLE and aPL, who develop renal disease. This procedure provides useful data for prognosis, guiding the therapy [Asherson, Klumb, 2008; Gigante et al., 2009].

The most common renal lesion in patients with SLE and aPL is thrombotic microangiopathy. These patients present mainly arterial hypertension. Acute thrombotic lesions have a progressive evolution to chronic proliferative, obstructive, and fibrotic forms (focal cortical atrophy, fibrous intimal hyperplasia of arterioles, arteriolar occlusions, and sclerotic lesions). Chronic lesions are correlated with raised levels of serum creatinine. The patients who present hypertension and raised levels of serum creatinine at the time of kidney biopsy have an accelerated evolution to end stage renal disease [Tektonidou et al., 2004].

Antiphospholipid syndrome may occur in any class of lupus nephropathy. The studies didn't demonstrate a correlation between the class of lupus nephropathy and the presence of antiphospholipid syndrome. It was no correlation between antiphospholipid syndrome and activity or chronicity index scores, or between aPL titers and anti-DNAds antibodies or serum complement levels [Fofi et al., 2001; Hill, Nochy, 2007].

In patients with any class of lupus nephropathy and aCL, renal biopsies showed a greater degree of sclerosis, crescent formation and glomerular necrosis. Moss and Isenberg demonstrated that in classes III and IV of lupus nephropathy the presence of aPL is associated with thrombosis of glomerular capillaries, which may evolve to glomerular sclerosis [Moss, Isenberg, 2001]. Moroni et al. identified a strong association between aPL and class V of lupus nephropathy [Moroni et al., 2004].

Positivity for antinucleosome antibodies at the time of antiphospholipid syndrome diagnosis may predict the subsequent development of SLE [Hill, Nochy, 2007]. Andreoli et al. reported a high frequency of antinucleosome antibodies in patients with antiphospholipid syndrome. Some of these patients developed SLE during the period of follow-up [Andreoli et al., 2008]. Antiphospholipid syndrome patients with membranous nephropathy or proliferative glomerulonephritis represent a group with high risk for developing SLE. Thus, the antiphospholipid syndrome patients with antinucleosome antibodies, membranous nephropathy or proliferative glomerulonephritis need a careful monitoring in order to detect the appearance of SLE [Hill, Nochy, 2007; Andreoli et al., 2008]. On the other hand, Loizou et al. demonstrated that in patients with SLE, the association between aCL, high titers of anti-DNAds and anti-C_{1q} antibodies is very specific for renal involvement [Loizou et al., 2000].These patients benefit by the association between anticoagulants, steroid and immunosuppressive therapy. Immunoadsorption treatment was used in order to reduce the antibodies levels [Hauser et al., 2005].

8. Glomerulonephritis and antiphospholipid syndrome

Beside the renal lesions which define the antiphospholipid syndrome nephropathy, in patients with primary antiphospholipid syndrome, kidney biopsies revealed glomerular lesions. Fakhouri et al. identified glomerular lesions in 9 from 29 patients with antiphospholipid syndrome. They were represented by: membranous glomerulonephritis (three cases), pauci-immune crescentic glomerulonephritis (one case), glomerulonephritis with C_3 mesangial deposits (two cases), minimal change disease/focal segmental glomerulosclerosis (three cases). The patients from this study presented proteinuria, even in nephrotic range, hematuria, decreased of renal function. They were treated with antihypertensive (six cases), anticoagulants (five cases), steroids (four cases), and antiplatelets drugs (three cases). At last follow-up, renal function was stabilized in seven of these patients [Fakhouri et al., 2003].

Membranous nephropathy was the most described glomerulonephritis among the patients with antiphospholipid syndrome [Dorel et al., 2000; Fakhouri et al., 2003].

Crescentic glomerulonephritis may be present in patients with primary antiphospholipid syndrome. Cisternas et al. and Dede et al. reported two cases of crescentic glomerulonephritis who developed in patients with primary antiphospholipid syndrome [Cisternas et al., 2000, Dede et al., 2008]. Cisternas et al. showed an association between catastrophic antiphospholipid syndrome and crescentic glomerulonephritis with renal failure [Cisternas et al., 2000]. Dede et al. described the case of a young female with pauci-immune glomerulonephritis, p-ANCA positive that had a favourable evolution under the therapy consisted of steroids and cyclophosphamide. After 3 months of follow-up, the patient was in clinical and laboratory remission [Dede et al., 2008].

Abdalla et al. reported a case of membrano-proliferative glomerulonephritis with no evidence of thrombotic microangiopathy or systemic lupus erythematosus. The authors sustained the role of immune deposits in pathogenesis of proliferative glomerulonephritis associated with primary antiphospholipid syndrome [Abdalla et al., 2006].

Another type of glomerular lesion was identified by Bhowmik et al. They described a case of focal segmental glomerulosclerosis who had a favourable course under the treatment with aspirin, heparin (during pregnancy), then angiotensin-converting enzyme inhibitors, angiotensin receptor blockers and steroids [Bhowmik et al., 2005].

The therapy of glomerulonephritis associated with antiphospholipid syndrome is based on steroids, immunosuppressive drugs, angiotensin-converting enzyme inhibitors, angiotensin receptor blockers, aspirin or anticoagulants [Dorel et al., 2000; Fakhouri et al., 2003; Bhowmik et al., 2005; Abdalla et al., 2006; Dede et al., 2008].

9. References

Abdalla, A.H., Kfoury, H.K., Al-Suleiman, M, Al-Khader AA. (2006). Proliferative glomerulonephritis and primary antiphospholipid syndrome. *Saudi Medical Journal,* Vol. 27, No. 7, (July, 2006), pp. 1063-1065.

Ames, P.R.; Cianciaruso, B.; Bellizzi, V.; Balletta, M.; Lubrano, E.; Scarpa, R.; Brancaccio, V. (1992). Bilateral renal artery occlusion in a patient with primary antiphospholipid antibody syndrome: thrombosis, vasculitis or both? *The journal of rheumatology*, vol. 19, Nr.11, (November, 1992), pp. 1802-1806.

Amigo, M.C.; Garcia-Torres, R.; Robles, M.; Bochiccio, T.; Reyes, P.A. (1992). Renal involvement in primary antiphospholipid syndrome, *The journal of rheumatology,* Vol. 19, (August, 1992), pp. 1181-1185.

Andrassy, J.; Zeier, M.; Andrassy, K. (2004). Do we need screening for thrombophilia prior to kidney transplantation? *Nephrology, Dialysis, Transplantation,* Vol. 19 (suppl. 4), (July, 2004), pp. 64-68.

Andreoli L, Pregnolato F, Burlingame RW, Allegri F, Rizzini S, Fanelli V, et al. (2008). Antinucleosome antibodies in primary antiphospholipid syndrome: A hint at systemic autoimmunity. *Journal of Autoimmunity,* Vol. 30, pp. 51-57.

Asherson, R.A. (1992). The catastrophic antiphospholipid syndrome. *The journal of rheumatology*, Vol. 19, No.4, (April, 1992), pp. 508-512.

Asherson RA, Klumb EM. (2008). Antiphospholipid syndrome nephropathy in different scenarios. *The Journal of Rheumatology,* Vol. 35, pp. 1909-1911.

Asherson, R.A.; Noble, G.E. Hughes, G.R. (1991). Hypertension, renal artery stenosis and the primary antiphospholipid syndrome. *The journal of rheumatology,* Vol. 18, No.9, (September, 1991), pp. 1413-1415.

Bhowmik D, Dadhwal V, Dinda AK, Handa R, Dash SC. (2005). Steroid-responsive focal segmental glomerulosclerosis in primary antiphospholipid syndrome with successful pregnancy outcome. *Nephrology, Dialysis, Transplant,* Vol. 20, pp. 1726-1728.

Brunet, P.; Aillaud, M.F.; San Marco, M.; et al. (1995). Antiphospholipid in hemodialysis patients: relationship between lupus anticoagulant and thrombosis. *Kidney International,* Vol. 48, No.3, (September, 1995), pp. 794-800.

Bucciarelli, S.; Espinosa, G.; Cervera, R. et al. (2006). European Forum on Antiphospholipid Antibodies. Mortality in the catastrophic antiphospholipid syndrome: causes of death and prognostic factors in a series of 250 patients. *Arthritis and rheumatism,* Vol. 54, (August, 2006), pp. 2568-2576.

Cacoub, P.; Piette, J.C., Beaufils H et al. (1992). Malignant hypertension in the antiphospholipid syndrome (APS) without lupus nephritis, *Arthritis and rheumatism,* Vol. 35, pp. S360.

Cervera, R.; Piette, J.C.; Font, J.; Shoenfeld, Y.; Camps, M.T.; Jacobsen, S. et al. (2002). Euro-Phospholipid Project Group: Antiphospholipid syndrome: clinical and immunological manifestations and pattern of disease expression in a cohort of 1000 patients. *Arthritis and rheumatism,* Vol. 46, No.4, (April, 2002), pp. 1019-1027.

Cisternas M, Gutierrez MA, Rosenberg H, Jara A, Jacobelli S. (2000). Catastrophic antiphospholipid syndrome associated with crescentic glomerulonephritis: a clinicopathologic case. *Clinical and Experimental Rheumatology,* Vol. 18, No.2, pp. 252-254.

D'Cruz D. (2009). Renal manifestations of the antiphospholipid syndrome. *Current Rheumatology Reports,* Vol. 11, pp. 52-60.

Dede F, Simsek Y, Odabas AR, Ayli D, Kayatas M. (2008). Pauci-immune glomerulonephritis associated with primary antiphospholipid syndrome. *Rheumatology International,* Vol. 28, No.5, pp. 499-501.

Dorel M, Daniel L, Liprandi A. (2000). Idiopathic membranous glomerulonephritis associated with primary antiphospholipid syndrome. *Nephron,* Vol. 86, pp. 366-367.

Ducloux, D.; Pellet, E.; Fournier, V.; Rebibou, J.M.; Bresson-Vautrin, C.; Racadot, E.; et al. (1999), Prevalence and clinical significance of antiphospholipid antibodies in renal transplant recipients. *Transplantation,* Vol. 67, No.1, (January, 1999), pp. 90-93.

Erkan, D.; Cervera, R.; Asherson, R.A. (2003). Catastrophic antiphospholipid syndrome: where we stand. *Arthritis and rheumatism,* Vol. 48, No.12, (December, 2003), pp. 3320-3327.

Fakhouri, F.; Noël, L.H.; Zuber, J.; Beaufils, H.; Martinez, F.; Lebon, P.; Papo, T.; et al. (2003). The expanding spectrum of renal diseases associated with antiphospholipid syndrome. *American Journal of Kidney Disease,* Vol. 41, No.6, (June, 2003), pp. 1205-1211.

Fofi C, Cuadrado MJ, Godfrey T, Abbs I, Khamashta MA, Hughes GR. (2001). Lack of association between antiphospholipid antibody and WHO classification in lupus nephritis. *Clinical and Experimental Rheumatology,* Vol. 19, pp. 75-77.

Frostegard, J.; Wli, R.; Gillis-Haegerstrand, C.; Lemne, C.; de Faire, U. (1998). Antibodies to endothelial cells in borderline hypertension. *Circulation,* Vol. 98, No.11, (September, 1998), pp. 1092-1098.

Gigante, A.; Gasperini, M.L.; Cianci, R.; Barbano, B.; Giannakakis, K.; Di Donato, D.; Fuiano G, Amoroso, A. (2009). Antiphospholipid antibodies and renal involvement. *American Journal of Nephrology,* Vol. 30, No.5, (August, 2009), pp. 405-412.

Godfrey T, Khamashta MA, Hughes GR. (2000). Antiphospholipid syndrome and renal artery stenosis. *QJM: An International Journal of Medicine,* Vol. 93, No.2, (February, 2000), pp. 127-129.

Griffiths, M.H.; Papadaki, L.; Neild, G.H. (2000). The renal pathology of primary antiphospholipid syndrome: a distinctive form of endothelial injury. *QJM: Monthly Journal of the Association of Physicians,* Vol. 93, pp. 457-467.

Hauser AC, Hauser L, Pabinger-Fasching I, Quehenberger P, Derfler K, Horl WH. (2005). The course of anticardiolipin antibody levels under immunoadsorption therapy. *American Journal of Kidney Disease,* Vol. 46, No.3, (September, 2005), pp. 446-454.

Haviv,Y.S. (2000). Association of anticardiolipin antibodies with vascular access occlusion in hemodialysis patients: cause or effect. *Nephron,* Vol. 86, (December, 2000), pp. 447-454.

Hill GS, Nochy D. (2007). Antiphospholipid syndrome in systemic lupus erythematosus. *Journal of the American Society of Nephrology,* Vol. 18, pp. 2461-2464.

Hughes G. (1984). Connective tissue diseases and the skin. The 1983 Posser-White Oration. *Clinical and Experimental Dermatology,* Vol. 9, No.6, (November, 1984), pp. 535-544.

Hughes GRV. (1983), Thrombosis, abortion, cerebral disease, and the lupus anticoagulant. *British Medical Journal* (Clin Res Ed), Vol. 287, pp. 1088-1089.

Kincaid-Smith, P.; Fairley KF, Kloss M. (1988). Lupus anticoagulant associated with renal thrombotic microangiopathy and pregnancy-related renal failure. *QJM: An International Journal of Medicine,* Vol. 68, No. 258, (October, 1988), pp. 795-815.

Kleinknecht D, Bobrie G, Meyer O, Noel LH, Callard P, Ramdane M. (1989). Recurrent thrombosis and renal vascular disease in patients with a lupus anticoagulant. *Nephrology, Dialysis, Transplantation,* Vol. 4, pp. 854-858.

Korkmaz C, Kabukcuoglu S, Isiksoy S, Yalcin AU. (2003). Renal involvement in primary antiphospholipid syndrome and its response to immunosuppressive therapy. *Lupus,* Vol. 12, No.10, pp. 760-765.

Lesar CJ, Merrick HW, Smith MR. (1999). Thrombotic complications resulting from hypercoagulable states in chronic hemodialysis vascular access. *Journal of the American College of Surgeons,* Vol. 189, No.1, (July, 1999), pp. 73-79.

Loizou S, Samarkos M, Norsworthy PJ, Cazabon JK, Walport MJ, Davies KA. (2000). Significance of anticardiolipin and anti-β_2-glycoprotein I antibodies in lupus nephritis. *Rheumatology,* Vol. 39, pp. 962-968.

Mandreoli, M.; Zuccala, A.; Zucchelli, P. (1992). Fibromuscular dysplasia of the renal arteries associated with antiphospholipid autoantibodies: two case reports. *American Journal of Kidney Disease,* Vol. 20, pp. 500-503.

Mandreoli, M.; Zucchelli, P. (1993). Renal vascular disease in patients with primary antiphospholipid antibodies. *Nephrology, Dialysis, Transplantation,* Vol. 8, No.11, pp. 1277-1280.

Mimran A. (1992). Renal effects of antihypertensive agents in parenchymal disease and renovascular hypertension. *Journal of the Cardiovascular Pharmacology,* Vol. 19 (Suppl. 6): 45.

Miyakis, S.; Lockshin, M.D.; Atsumi, T.; Branch, D.W.; Brey, R.L.; Cervera, R. et al. (2006). International consensus statement on an update of the classification criteria for definite antiphospholipid syndrome (APS). *Journal of Thrombosis and Hemostasis,* Vol. 4, No. 2, (February, 2006), 295-306.

Moroni, G.; Tantardini, F.; Galleli, B.; Quaglini, S.; Banfi, G; Poli F et al. (2005). The long-term prognosis of renal transplantation in patients with lupus nephritis. *American Journal of Kidney Disease,* Vol. 45, No.5, (May, 2005), pp. 901-911.

Moroni G, Ventura D, Riva P, Panzeri P, Quaglini S, Banfi G, et al. (2004). Antiphospholipid antibodies are associated with an increased risk for chronic renal insufficiency in patients with lupus nephropathy. *American Journal of Kidney Disease,* Vol. 43, pp. 28-36.

Moss KE, Isenberg DA. (2001). Comparison of renal disease severity and outcome in patients with primary antiphospholipid syndrome, antiphospholipid syndrome secondary to systemic lupus erythematosus (SLE) and SLE alone. *Rheumatology* (Oxford), Vol.40, pp. 863-867.

Nochy, D.; Daugas, E.; Droz, D.; Beaufils, H.; Grünfeld, J.P.; Piette, J.C. et al. (1999). The intrarenal vascular lesions associated with primary antiphospholipid syndrome. *Journal of the American Society of Nephrology,* Vol. 10, No. 3, (March, 1999), pp. 507-18.

Nochy, D.; Daugas, E.; Hill, G.; Grünfeld JP. (2002). Antiphospholipid syndrome nephropathy. *Journal of Nephrology,* Vol. 15, No.4, (July-August, 2002), pp. 446-461.

Ostuni PA, Lazzarin P, Pengo V et al. (1990). Renal artery thrombosis and hypertension in a 13 year old girl with antiphospholipid syndrome. *Annals of Rheumatic Diseases,* Vol. 49, No.3, (March, 1990), pp. 184-187.

Piette, J.C.; Cacoub, P.; Wechsler, B. (1994), Renal manifestations of the antiphospholipid syndrome. *Seminars in Arthritis and Rheumatism,* Vol. 23, No.6, (June, 1994), pp. 357-366.

Remondino, G.I.; Mysler, E.; Pissano, M.N et al. (2000). A reversible bilateral renal artery stenosis in association with antiphospholipid syndrome. *Lupus,* Vol.9, No.1, pp. 65-67.

Rollino, C.; Boero, R.; Elia, F.; Montaruli, B.; Massara, C.; Beltrame, G et al. (2004). Antiphospholipid antibodies and hypertension. *Lupus,* Vol. 13, No.10, pp. 769-772.

Rysana R, Zabka J, Peregin JH, Tesar V, Merta M, Rychlik I. (1998). Acute renal failure due to bilateral renal artery thrombosis associated with primary antiphospholipid syndrome. *Nephrology, Dialysis, Transplantation,* Vol. 13, No.10, (October, 1998), pp. 2645-2647.

Sangle, S.R.; D'Cruz, D.P.; Abbs, I.C.; Khamashta, M.A.; Hughes, G.R. (2005). Renal artery stenosis in hypertensive patients with antiphospholipid (Hughes) syndrome: outcome following anticoagulation. *Rheumatology* (Oxford), Vol. 44, No.3, (March, 2005), pp. 372-377.

Sangle, S.R., D'Cruz, D.P.; Jan, W.; Karim, M.Y.; Khamashta, M.A.; Abbs, I.C.; Hughes, G.R. (2003). Renal artery stenosis in the antiphospholipid (Hughes) syndrome and hypertension. *Annals of the Rheumatic Disease,* Vol. 62, No.10, (October, 2003), pp. 999-1002.

Sinico, R.A.; Cavazzana, I.; Nuzzo, M.; Vianelli, M.; Napodano, P.; Scaini, P.; Ticani, A. (2010). Renal involvement in primary antiphospholipid syndrome: retrospective analysis of 160 patients. *Clinical Journal of the American Society of Nephrology,* Vol. 5, No.7, (July, 2010), pp. 1211-1217.

Sonpal, G.M.; Sharma, A.; Miller, A. (1993). Primary antiphospholipid antibody syndrome, renal infarction and hypertension. *The Journal of Rheumatology,* Vol. 20, No.7, (July, 1993), pp. 1221-1223.

Tektonidou, M.G. (2009). Renal involvement in the antiphospholipid syndrome (APS)-APS nephropathy. *Clinical Reviews in Allergy and Immunology,* Vol. 36, No.2-3, (June, 2009), pp. 131-140.

Tektonidou, M.G.; Ioannidis, J.P.A.; Boki, K.A.; Vlachoyiannopoulos, P.G.; Moutsopoulos, H.M. (2000). Prognostic factors and clustering of serious clinical outcomes in antiphospholipid syndrome. *QJM: An International Journal of Medicine,* Vol. 93, Vol.8, (August, 2000), pp. 523-530.

Tektonidou MG, Sotsiou F, Moutsopoulos HM. (2008). Antiphospholipid syndrome (APS) nephropathy in catastrophic, primary and systemic lupus erythematosus-related APS. *The Journal of Rheumatology,* Vol. 35, No.10, (October, 2008), pp. 1883-1988.

Tektonidou MG, Sotsiou F, Nakopoulou L, Vlachoyiannopoulos PG, Moutsopoulos HM. (2004). Antiphospholipid syndrome nephropathy in patients with systemic lupus erythematosus and antiphospholipid antibodies. Arthritis and Rheumatism, Vol. 50, No. 8, pp. 2569-2579.

Uthman, I.; Khamashta, M. (2006). Antiphospholipid syndrome and the kidney. *Seminars in Arthritis and Rheumatism,* Vol. 35, No.6, (June, 2006), pp. 360-367.

Vlachoyiannopoulos, P.G.; Kanellopoulos, P.; Gektonidou, M.; Moutsopoulos, H.M. (2001). Renal involvement in antiphospholipid syndrome. *Nephrology, Dialysis, Transplantation,* Vol. 16 (suppl. 6), pp. 60-62.

Wilson, W.A.; Gharavi, A.E.; Koike, T. et al. (1999). International consensus statement on preliminary classification criteria for definite antiphospholipid syndrome: report of an international workshop. *Arthritis and rheumatism,* Vol. 42, No.7, (July, 1999), pp. 1309-1311.

8

The Management of Antiphospholipid Antibodies Affected Pregnancy

Kenji Tanimura, Yashuhiko Ebina,
Yoko Maesawa, Ryoichi Hazama and Hideto Yamada*
Department of Obstetrics and Gynecology,
Kobe University Graduate School of Medicine, Kobe
Japan

1. Introduction

Antiphospholipid antibody (aPL) is a heterogeneous group of autoantibodies directed against phospholipids-binding proteins. Antiphospholipid syndrome (APS) is defined by two major components: 1) presence of at least one type of aPLs, 2) the occurrence of at least one clinical feature from a list of potential disease manifestations, the most common of which are categorized as venous or arterial thromboses, and pregnancy complications. The pregnancy complications include recurrent spontaneous abortion (RSA), unexplained fetal death, severe pre-eclampsia, fetal growth restriction (FGR), and premature delivery. International consensus conferences have proposed and revised classification criteria for definite APS. Two types of aPLs were originally included in the laboratory criteria: IgG and IgM anticardiolipin antibody (aCL); and lupus anticoagulant (LA) (1). After that, IgG and IgM anti-β2 glycoprotein-I antibody (aβ2GPI) were included as laboratory criteria (2). However, scant evidence exists in regard to a relationship between the aPL profile and serious adverse pregnancy outcome.

With the widespread use of tests to detect aPLs, obstetricians often encounter pregnant or non-pregnant women who have positive aPL tests. Currently, a variety of aPLs in the human blood can be measured by laboratory systems, each of which requires evaluation in regard to whether an association with pregnancy complications exists. This review focused on risks of pregnancy complications and therapeutic modality in women with aPLs.

2. Antiphospholipid antibody and pregnancy complications

The detrimental effects of aPLs are attributed to pathological mechanisms including thrombotic changes, suppression of hCG release (3), induction of complement activation and placental injury (4), and a direct effect on trophoblast cell growth and differentiation (5). Live-birth rates in women with aPLs (range 62–84%) are found to be lower than those in women without aPLs (range 90–98%) (6-9).

---

* Corresponding Author

Many studies indicated that aPLs cause thromboembolism and mid-trimester fetal death; and probably RSA. However, the association between aPLs and risks of pregnancy-induced hypertension (PIH), pre-eclampsia, FGR, or premature delivery (PD) still remains controversial. In retrospective case-control studies, it was found that women with a history of severe pre-eclampsia or hemolysis-elevated liver enzymes-low platelets (HELLP) syndrome frequently tested positive for LA and aCL (10,11). However, prospective studies assessing associations between aPLs and PIH, pre-eclampsia or other pregnancy complications found conflicting results. Studies conducted in the 1990s noted that pre-eclampsia was associated with the presence of LA (6), aCL (6, 9), β_2–glycoprotein I dependent aCL (aCLβ_2GPI) (12) and aβ_2GPI (13). Similarly, fetal loss and FGR were associated with the presence of aCL (9, 12). Later prospective studies, however, denied the association between pre-eclampsia and the presence of LA (14), aCL (14-16) or aβ_2GPI (16). PIH (17) and HELLP syndrome (16) were not associated with the presence of aCL or aβ_2GPI.

Our group have assessed whether aPLs measurements during early pregnancy are useful for predicting pregnancy complications (18). The aPLs including LA, IgG, IgM, IgA aCL, IgG, IgM phosphatidylserine dependent antiprothrombin antibody (aPS/PT), and IgG kininogen dependent antiphosphatidylethanolamine antibody (aPE) were measured during the first trimester in a consecutive series of 1,155 women. We for the first time determined predictive risks of pregnancy complications, being adjusted with the life style-related confounding factors such as maternal age, parity, BMI, smoking and drinking. IgG aCL was asssociated with PIH; IgG aPE with PIH, severe PIH and PD; LA with PD and low birth weight (Table 1). Additionally, we found that multi-positive or double-positive aPLs (LA and aCL), were risk factor for severe PIH, PD and low birth weight. This is the first evidence in regard to the association between the multi/double-positive aPLs and severe PIH. Recent studies have also suggested that the multi-positive test is associated with a more severe course of APS disease, increasing significantly the rate of thrombosis (16, 19-21). Pregnant women with multi / double-positive aPLs should be more carefully managed during pregnancy.

The abovementioned study for the first time demonstrated IgG aPE was associated with PIH (18). aPE was frequently detected in patients with unexplained recurrent early fetal loss, mid-to-late fetal loss, unexplained thrombosis, systemic lupus erythematosus, heart valvulopathies and livedo reticularis (22-26). Sugi *et al.* measured the kininogen dependent aPE that probably binds to kininogen as a cofactor (27). The kallikrein-kinin system is involved in the blood pressure control and angiogenesis. Tissue kallikrein cleaves low-molecular-weight kininogen substrate to produce the vasodilator Lys-bradykinin, whereas plasma kallikrein forms bradykinin (BK) from high-molecular-weight kininogen (HMWK). Kininogen-deficient rats are susceptible to the development of salt-induced hypertension (28), and the *in vivo* angiogenesis is suppressed (29). The proangiogenic effect of BK and HMWK has been demonstrated in both *in vitro* and *in vivo* studies (30). Therefore, we assume that aPE pathophysiologically causes impairment of fetoplacental angiogenesis and vessel development, which subsequently may predispose women to PIH. Alternatively, disruption of kininogen cascade in the kallikrein-kinin system may reduce vasodilator production and cause a hypertensive disorder. A recent multicenter study demonstrated that aPE, but not LA or aCL, was closely associated with thrombosis with the highest odds ratio (31). The thrombotic insult may be causally associated with PIH.

Pregnancy complication	Antiphospholipid antibody	Odds ratio	95% CI
PIH	IgG aCL	11.4	2.7-48
	IgG aPE	8.3	2.4-29
Severe PIH	IgG aPE	20.4	4.5-91
	Multi-positive	143	9.8-1000
	Double-positive (LA and aCL)	250	11.1-1000
Premature delivery (<37 weeks)	LA	11.0	2.8-44
	Multi-positive	11.6	1.5-91
	Double-positive (LA and aCL)	22.2	1.9-250
Premature delivery (<34 weeks)	IgG aPE	12.7	3.1-50.0
Low birth weight	LA	8.0	2.1-31
	Double-positive (LA and aCL)	13.7	1.2-167

PIH, pregnancy induced hypertension; aCL, anticardiolipin antibody; aPE, kininogen dependent antiphosphatidylethanolamine antibody; LA, lupus anticoagulant;

Table 1. Antiphospholipid antibodies as risk factors for pregnancy complications determined by multivariate analysis

Subsequently, whether IgG, IgM aβ2GPI was associated with the development of PIH or pre-eclampsia, we evaluated in the case-control study in cohort (32). The case group comprises 36 patients who developed PIH during their pregnancies. Normal ranges of IgG (<2.2 Unit/ml) and IgM (<6.0 Unit/ml) aβ2GPI values with cut-off values of 99th percentile have been established using non-pregnant 132 healthy controls. The cut-off values of IgG (normal <1.0 Unit/ml) and IgM (normal <1.2 Unit/ml) aβ2GPI were established from the most appropriate values dividing pregnant subjects in this study. It was found that titers of IgG aβ2GPI ≥1.0 Unit/ml represent a risk factor for severe PIH (P=0.023, OR 5.7 95%CI 1.4-23). In addition, titers of IgM aβ2GPI ≥1.2 Unit/ml were found to be a risk factor for PIH (P=0.001, OR 8.8 95%CI 1.6-47.5). These results support the utility of aβ2GPI determination as one of the laboratory criteria for APS classification.

There is a large body of evidence for an involvement of aβ2GPI in hypercoagulation status and thrombosis. (33-38). A multivariate analysis in a multicenter study has demonstrated that aβ2GPI and aPE, but not LA or aCL, were significantly associated with thrombosis (31). aβ2GPI induce the activation of endothelial cells, resulting in a proinflammatory state which favours the prothrombotic diathesis (39). Recently, a study has demonstrated β2GPI naturally inhibits von Willebrand factor (VWF)-dependent platelet adhesion and aggregation. aβ2GPI of APS patients neutralized the β2GPI-VWF interactions, contributing to hypercoagulation status in these patients (40). It is likely that the thrombotic insult of aβ2GPI to placental angiogenesis or circulation is causally associated with PIH. Additionally, β2GPI binds to trophoblast cells (41). The antibody binding to β2GPI downregulates trophoblast chorionic gonadotropin synthesis and secretion (42). Such a direct effect to trophoblast cells may contribute to inhibition of trophoblast invasiveness and defective placentation (41), causing PIH.

3. Antiphospholipid antibody and recurrent spontaneous abortion

The mechanism of fetal loss is believed to be due to binding of aPLs to trophoblast cells, resulting in defective placentation.(43) Thromboembolic events in the uteroplacental circulation have also been proposed as a contributing mechanism(44). Jane *et al.* shown that complement activation plays an essential and causative role in pregnancy loss, and that blocking activation of the complement cascade rescues pregnancies using a mouse model of APS induced by passive transfer of human aPL (45).

It remained uncertain whether any combination of aPL screening in women with RSA is clinically valid. Our group determined the prevalence of a variety of aPLs, with and without a combination of measurements, present in 114 women who had a history of two or more spontaneous abortions (Table 2). aPLs measured included LA, aCLß2GPI, aCL, aPS/PT and aPE. The most frequent type of aPL was IgG aPE (20.2%), followed by IgG aCL and then IgG aCLß2GPI. The standard combinations of aPL measurements upon RSA screening may be LA plus IgG, IgM aCLß2GPI, and LA plus IgG, IgM aCL. Using these standard combinations as definition, 2.6% and 4.4% of women with RSA could be diagnosed as having aPL. When IgA aCLß2GPI, IgA aCL and IgG, IgM aPS/PT were combined with the standard aPL measurements for RSA screening, positive frequencies of aPL reached 7.0%. If IgG, IgM aPE were additionally included, positive frequencies of aPL increased remarkably to 26.3% among women with RSA.

Antiphospholipid antibody	Prevalence (%)	Mid-trimester (≥14 weeks) fetal losses	
		Yes (n = 15)	No (n = 99)
LA	1.8	13.3[a]	0[a]
IgG/IgM/IgA aCLβ2GPI	2.6/0.9/1.8	13.3[b]/6.7/13.3[c]	1.0[b]/0/0[c]
IgG/IgM/IgA aCL	4.4/0.9/4.4	20.0[d]/6.7/13.3	2.0[d]/0/3.0
IgG/IgM aPS/PT	1.8/0	13.3[e]/0	0[e]/0
IgG/IgM aPE	20.2/2.6	6.7/0	22.2/3.0
Combined measurements			
LA or aCLβ2GPI	2.6	13.3[f]	1.0[f]
LA or aCL	4.4	20.0[g]	2.0[g]
LA, aCLβ2GPI, aCL or aPS/PT	7.0	20.0	5.1
All aPLs measurement	26.3	20.0	27.3

aCL, anticardiolipin antibody; aCLβ2GPI, anticardiolipin β2-glyciprotein I antibody; aPS/PT, antiphosphatidylserine prothombin antibody; aPE, antiphosphatidylethanolamine antibody; LA, lupus anticoagulant. [a,b,c,d,e,f,g] $P<.05$

Table 2. Prevalence of antiphospholipid antibodies in women with recurrent spontaneous abortion

The prevalence of each aPL and the combinations of aPLs was compared between women with RSA who had experienced at least one mid-trimester fetal loss and those who did not. As a result, RSA women with mid-trimester fetal losses yielded a significantly higher prevalence of LA, IgG, IgA aCLß2GPI, IgG aCL, and IgG aPS/PT, but not aPE, as compared with women with early RSA. Thus, it was confirmed that mid-trimester fetal losses were associated with the presence of LA, aCLß2GPI, aCL, and aPS/PT in women with RSA (Table 2). The information provided here constituted a beneficial reference for clinical practice in the area of infertility.

4. Management and therapy for women with antiphospholipid antibody

The management of pregnancy in women with APS has been a subject of much debate, antiplatelet and anticoagulation therapies are usually recommended. A randomized controlled study demonstrated high live birth rate (71%) with low dose aspirin (LDA) plus unfractionated heparin (UFH) as compared with 42% with LDA alone in APS women (46). The LDA plus UFH had fewer maternal adverse effects, and was found to be superior to LDA plus steroids (47). American College of Chest Physicians guidelines recommend LDA in combination with prophylactic or intermediate-dose of UFH, or prophylactic dose of low molecular weight heparin (LMWH) for RSA women with aPL during their pregnancy (48).

Figure 1 shows an algorithm used in the Kobe University Hospital for the management and treatment of pregnant women with positive test of aPLs (LA, aCL, aβ2GPI, or aCLβ2GPI). Treatment modalities are classified by a history or presence of thromboembolism (TE) and pregnancy complications. In women with aPL and no history, LDA is used until 28 weeks of gestation (GW). If women have a history of RSA in the first trimester, LDA is used until 28 GW, plus use of prophylactic dose of UFH (5,000~10,000 U per day) until 15 GW is considered. In women with a history of IUFD, FGR and severe PIH, we recommend use of LDA until 28 GW plus UFH (10,000~12,000U per day) until 28-36GW. The timing of UFH completion can be determined due to a history of previous obstetric complications. In women with a history of TE event, warfarin should be substituted at 5 GW for LDA until 28 GW plus therapeutic dose of UFH, and UFH (continuous infusion or subcutaneous injection to maintain the aPTT within the therapeutic aPTT ranges) is continued throughout their pregnancies. During pregnancy fetal growth and well-being are monitored by ultrasonography including pulse doppler and cardiotocogram; and maternal D-dimer is measured regularly. If women have elevated D-dimer (especially >10.0 μg/ml), increases of UFH dose and ultrasound examination for deep venous thrombosis may be considered. If women yield multi-positive tests or a high titer of aPL, more intensive treatment should be considered (Figure 1).

5. Intravenous immunoglobulin infusion for aspirin-heparin resistant antiphospholipid syndrome

We often encountered APS women who underwent LDA plus heparin and failed to have a healthy infant. Such cases can be designated as aspirin-heparin resistant APS (AHRAPS) (49). In AHRAPS, intravenous immunoglobulin (IVIg) therapy may be effective. Carreras et al. (50) first reported successful IVIg therapy in a pregnant woman with LA and a history of 9 RSA. A randomized controlled trial comparing LDA plus heparin plus IVIg with LDA

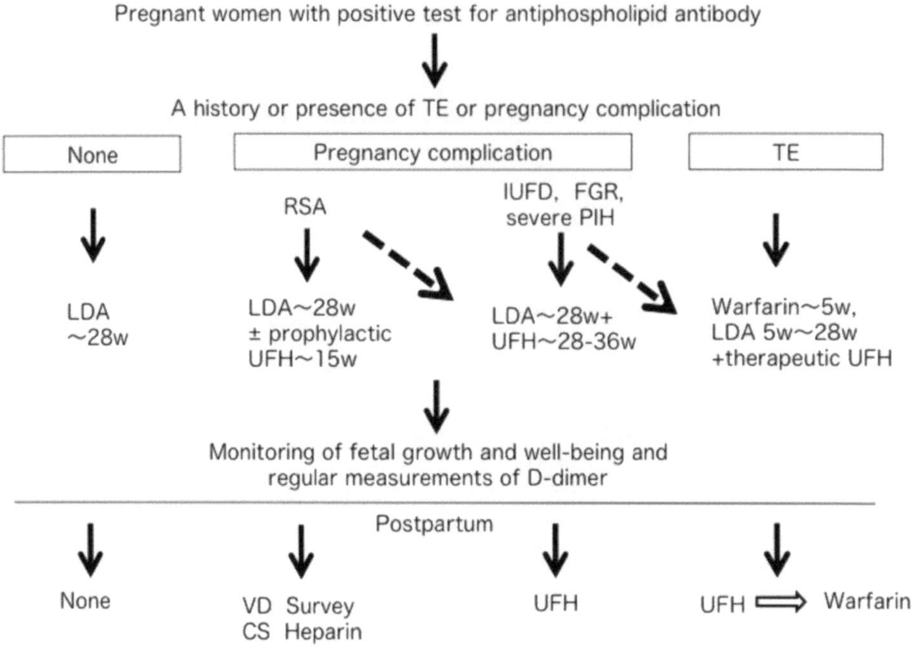

Antiphospholipid antibodies include lupus anticoagulant, anticardiolipin antibody, anti-β2 glycoprotein-I antibody, and β_2-glycoprotein I dependent anticardiolipin antibody. If women yield multi-positive tests or a high titer of antiphospholipid antibody, more intensive treatment should be considered as presented by dotted arrows.
TE, thromboembolism; RSA, recurrent spontaneous abortion; IUFD, intrauterine fetal death; FGR, fetal growth restriction; PIH, pregnancy-induced hypertension; LDA, low dose aspirin; UFH, unfractionated heparin; VD, vaginal delivery; CS, cesarean section

Fig. 1. Management strategy for pregnant women with positive test for antiphospholipid antibody

plus heparin therapies in 16 APS patients failed to show differences in the efficacy (51). Triolo et al. (52) reported that LDA plus low molecular weight heparin had a higher birth rate (84%) than that of IVIg alone (57%) in RSA women with aCLβ2GPI. But later, they also reported successful IVIg therapy in 8 of 10 APS women previously unresponsive to LDA plus heparin (53). There were several case reports of successful pregnancy outcome in APS patients with RSA (54-57). Therefore, a certain subgroup of APS women such as AHRAPS must have the possible advantage of IVIg therapy. The inhibitory effect of IVIg on aPLs, especially aCL, and LAC has been reported by several authors (58-61).

The optimal dosage of IVIg in APS women during pregnancy was not determined and still to be debated. Yamada et al., first performed a high dose IVIg therapy (20 g/day, 5 consecutive days, total 100 g) in early pregnancies of women with unexplained severe RSA, demonstrating a high live birth rate (62-64). Carreras et al. (50) performed IVIg therapy (400 mg/kg · day, 5 consecutive days at 17 GW; and 2 days at 22, 27 GW) in APS women. Others reported monthly 1g/kg IVIg therapies (53).

The mechanisms of IVIg efficacy for pregnant women with APS have not been fully assessed. Possible mechanisms to explain its broad activity comprised the following;

1) provision of anti-idiotypic antibodies and the function as immunomodulator; 2) interference with the complement activation and the cytokine network; 3) modulation of the expression and function of Fc receptors; and 4) differentiation and effector functions of T and B cells (65,66). As for the anti-idiotypic antibody function, inhibitory effects of IVIg on aCL and LA were reported (59,60,67). Caccavo et al. (67) demonstrated that aCL binding to cardiolipin was suppressed by $F(ab')_2$ fragments derived from IVIg in a dose-dependent manner. Galli et al. (59) also demonstrated dose-dependent suppression of LA activity in patients, using either IVIg or $F(ab)_2$ fragments. IVIg may induce long-term decrease in autoantibody production by acquiring the inactivation of idiotype-bearing B cell clones (68).

6. Acknowledgments

This work was supported in part by Grants-in-Aid from the Ministry of Health, Labor and Welfare of Japan (grant number; H23-Jisedai-Ippan-001), the Ministry of Education, Science, Sports and Culture of Japan (grant number; 23592403), and Japan Association of Obstetricians and Gynecologists (grant number; H22-Ogyah-Kenkin).

7. References

[1] Wilson WA, Gharavi AE, Koike T, Lockshin MD., Branch DW, Piette JC, Brey R, Sherer Y, Levy Y, Derksen R, Harris EN, Hughes GR, Triplett DA, Khamashta MA. 1999. International consensus statement on preliminary classification criteria for definite antiphospholipid syndrome: report of an international workshop. Arthritis Rheum. 42, 1309-1311.

[2] Miyakis S, Lockshin MD, Atsumi T, Branch DW, Brey RL, Cervera R., Derksen RH, DE Groot PG, Koike T, Meroni PL, Reber G, Shoenfeld Y, Tincani A, Vlachoyiannopoulos PG, Krilis SA. 2006. International consensus statement on an update of the classification criteria for definite antiphospholipid syndrome (APS). J Thromb Haemost. 4, 295-306.

[3] Di Simone N, De Carolis S, Lanzone A, Ronsisvalle E, Giannice R, Caruso A. 1995. In vitro effect of antiphospholipid antibody-containing sera on basal and gonadotrophin releasing hormonedependent human chorionic gonadotrophin release by cultured trophoblast cells. Placenta.16,75–83.

[4] Holers VM, Girardi G, Mo L, Guthridge JM, Molina H, Pierangeli SS, Espinola R, Xiaowei LE, Mao D, Vialpando CG, Salmon JE. 2002.Complement C3 activation is required for antiphospholipid antibody-induced fetal loss. J Exp Med. 195, 211–20.

[5] Chamley LW, Duncalf AM, Mitchell MD, Johnson PM. 1998. Action of anticardiolipin and antibodies to beta2-glycoprotein-I on trophoblast proliferation as a mechanism for fetal death. Lancet. 35, 1037–8.

[6] Pattison NS, Chamley LW, McKay EJ, Liggins GC, Butler WS. 1993. Antiphospholipid antibodies in pregnancy: prevalence and clinical associations. Br J Obstet Gynaecol. 100, 909–13.

[7] Lynch A, Marlar R, Murphy J, Davila G, Santos M, Rutledge J. 1994. Antiphospholipid antibodies in predicting adverse pregnancy outcome: a prospective study. Ann Intern Med. 120, 470–5.

[8] Lockwood CJ, Romero R, Feinberg RF, Clyne LP, Coster B, Hobbins JC. 1989. The prevalence and biologic significance of lupus anticoagulant and anticardiolipin antibodies in a general obstetric population. Am J Obstet Gynecol. 161, 369–73.
[9] Yasuda M, Takakuwa K, Tokunaga A, Tanaka K. 1995. Prospective studies of the association between anticardiolipin antibody and outcome of pregnancy. Obstet Gynecol. 86, 555–9.
[10] van Pampus MG, Dekker GA, Wolf H, Huijgens PC, Koopman MM, von Blomberg BM, Buller HR. 1999. High prevalence of hemostatic abnormalities in women with a history of severe preeclampsia. Am J Obstet Gynecol. 180, 1146-1150.
[11] von Tempelhoff GF, Heilmann L, Spanuth E, Kunzmann E, Hommel G. 2000. Incidence of the factor V Leiden-mutation, coagulation inhibitor deficiency, and elevated antiphospholipid-antibodies in patients with preeclampsia or HELLP-syndrome. Hemolysis, elevated liver-enzymes, low platelets. Thromb Res. 100, 363-365.
[12] Katano K, Aoki K, Sasa H, Ogasawara M, Matsuura E, Yagami Y. 1996. Beta 2-Glycoprotein I-dependent anticardiolipin antibodies as a predictor of adverse pregnancy outcomes in healthy pregnant women. Hum Reprod. 11, 509-512.
[13] Faden D, Tincani A, Tanzi P, Spatola L, Lojacono A, Tarantini M, Balestrieri G. 1997. Anti-beta 2 glycoprotein I antibodies in a general obstetric population: preliminary results on the prevalence and correlation with pregnancy outcome. Anti-beta2 glycoprotein I antibodies are associated with some obstetrical complications, mainly preeclampsia-eclampsia. Eur J Obstet Gynecol Reprod Biol. 73, 37-42.
[14] Dreyfus M, Hedelin G, Kutnahorsky R, Lehmann M, Viville B, Langer B, Fleury A, M'Barek M, Treisser A, Wiesel ML, Pasquali JL. 2001. Antiphospholipid antibodies and preeclampsia: a case-control study. Obstet Gynecol. 97, 29-34.
[15] Branch DW, Porter TF, Rittenhouse L, Caritis S, Sibai B, Hogg B, Lindheimer MD, Klebanoff, M, MacPherson C, VanDorsten JP, Landon M, Paul R, Miodovnik M, Meis P, Thurnau G. 2001. National Institute of Child Health and Human Development Maternal-Fetal Medicine Units Network. Antiphospholipid antibodies in women at risk for preeclampsia. Am J Obstet Gynecol. 184, 825-834.
[16] Lee RM, Brown MA, Branch DW, Ward K, Silver RM. 2003. Anticardiolipin and anti-beta2-glycoprotein-I antibodies in preeclampsia. Obstet Gynecol. 102, 294-300.
[17] Lynch A, Byers T, Emlen W, Rynes D, Shetterly SM., Hamman RF.1999. Association of antibodies to beta2-glycoprotein 1 with pregnancy loss and pregnancy-induced hypertension: a prospective study in low-risk pregnancy. Obstet Gynecol. 93, 193-198.
[18] Yamada H, Atsumi T, Kobayashi G, Ota C, Kato E, Tsuruga N, Ohta K, Yasuda S, Koike T, Minakami H. 2009. Antiphosholipid antibodies increase the risk of pregnancy-induced hypertension and adverse pregnancy outcomes. J Reproduct Immunol. 79,188-195.
[19] Detkova D, Gil-Aguado A, Lavilla P, Cuesta MV, Fontan G, Pascual-Salcedo D. 1999. Do antibodies to beta2-glycoprotein 1 contribute to the better characterization of the antiphospholipid syndrome? Lupus. 8, 430-438.
[20] Obermoser G, Bitterlich W, Kunz F, Sepp NT. 2003. Thromboembolic risk in patients with high titre anticardiolipin and multiple antiphospholipid antibodies. Thromb Haemost. 90, 108-115.

[21] Obermoser G, Bitterlich W, Kunz F, Sepp NT. 2004. Clinical significance of anticardiolipin and anti-beta2-glycoprotein I antibodies. Int. Arch. Allergy Immunol. 135, 148-153.

[22] Gris JC, Quere I, Sanmarco M, Boutiere B, Mercier E, Amiral J, Hubert AM, Ripart-Neveu S, Hoffet M, Tailland ML, Rousseau O., Monpeyroux F, Dauzat M., Sampol J, Daures JP, Berlan J, Marès P. 2000. Antiphospholipid and antiprotein syndromes in non-thrombotic, non-autoimmune women with unexplained recurrent primary early foetal loss. The Nimes Obstetricians and Haematologists Study-NOHA. Thromb Haemost. 84, 228–236.

[23] Sanmarco M, Alessi MC, Harle JR, Sapin C, Aillaud MF., Gentile S, Juhan-Vague I, Weiller PJ. 2001. Antibodies to phosphatidylethanolamine as the only antiphospholipid antibodies found in patients with unexplained thromboses. Thromb Haemost. 85, 800–805.

[24] Balada E, Ordi-Ros J, Paredes F, Villarreal J, Mauri M, Vilardell-Tarres M. 2001. Antiphosphatidylethanolamine antibodies contribute to the diagnosis of antiphospholipid syndrome in patients with systemic lupus erythematosus. Scand J Rheumatol. 30, 235-241.

[25] Yamada H, Atsumi T, Kato E, Shimada S, Morikawa M, Minakami H. 2003. Prevalence of diverse antiphospholipid antibodies in women with recurrent spontaneous abortion. Fertil Steril. 80, 1276-1278.

[26] Sugi T, Matsubayashi H, Inomo A, Dan L, Makino T. 2004. Antiphosphatidylethanolamine antibodies in recurrent early pregnancy loss and mid-to-late pregnancy loss. J Obstet Gynaecol Res. 30, 326–332.

[27] Sugi T, Katsunuma J, Izumi S, McIntyre JA, Makino T. 1999. Prevalence and heterogeneity of antiphosphatidylethanolamine antibodies in patients with recurrent early pregnancy losses. Fertil Steril. 71, 1060-1065.

[28] Majima M, Mizogami S, Kuribayashi Y, Katori M, Oh-ishi S. 1994. Hypertension induced by a nonpressor dose of angiotensin II in kininogen-deficient rats. Hypertension. 24, 111-119.

[29] Hayashi I, Amano H, Yoshida S, Kamata K, Kamata M, Inukai M, Fujita T, Kumagai Y, Furudate S, Majima M. 2002. Suppressed angiogenesis in kininogen-deficiencies. Lab Invest. 82, 871-880.

[30] Guo YL, Colman RW. 2005. Two faces of high-molecular-weight kininogen (HK) in angiogenesis: bradykinin turns it on and cleaved HK (HKa) turns it off. J Thromb Haemost. 3, 670-676.

[31] Sanmarco M, Gayet S, Alessi MC, Audrain M, de Maistre E, Gris JC, de Groot PG, Hachulla E, Harlé JR, Sié P, Boffa MC. 2007. Antiphosphatidylethanolamine antibodies are associated with an increased odds ratio for thrombosis. Thromb Haemost. 97. 949-954.

[32] Yamada H, Atsumi T, Olga A, Koike T, Furuta I, Ohta K, Kobayashi G. 2010. Anti-β2 glycoprotein-I antibody increases the risk of pregnancy-induced hypertension: a case-controlled study. J Reproduct Immunol. 84, 95-99.

[33] Martinuzzo, M.E, Forastiero, R.R. Carreras, L.O, 1995. Anti beta 2 glycoprotein I antibodies: detection and association with thrombosis. Br J Haematol. 89, 397-402.

[34] Amengual O, Atsumi T, Khamashta M, Koike T, Hughes GRV. 1996. Specificity of ELISA for antibody to beta2-glycoprotein I in patients with antiphospholipid syndrome. Br J Rheumatol. 35, 1239-1243.

[35] Zanon E, Prandoni P, Vianello F, Saggiorato G, Carraro G, Bagatella P, Girolami A. 1999. Anti-beta2-glycoprotein I antibodies in patients with acute venous thromboembolism: prevalence and association with recurrent thromboembolism. Thromb Res. 96, 269-274.

[36] Zoghlami-Rintelen C, Vormittag R, Sailer T, Lehr S, Quehenberger P, Rumpold H, Male C, Pabinger I. 2005. The presence of IgG antibodies against beta2-glycoprotein I predicts the risk of thrombosis in patients with the lupus anticoagulant. J Thromb Haemost. 3, 1160-1165.

[37] Pengo V, Biasiolo A, Pegoraro C, Cucchini U, Noventa F, Iliceto S. 2005. Antibody profiles for the diagnosis of antiphospholipid syndrome. Thromb Haemost. 93, 1147-1152.

[38] de Laat B, Derksen RH, Urbanus RT, de Groot PG. 2004. IgG antibodies that recognize epitope Gly40-Arg43 in domain I of beta 2-glycoprotein I cause LAC, and their presence correlates strongly with thrombosis. Blood. 105, 1540-1545.

[39] D'Ippolito S, Di Simone N, Di Nicuolo F, Castellani R, Caruso A. 2007. Antiphospholipid antibodies: effects on trophoblast and endothelial cells. Am J Reprod Immunol. 58, 150-158.

[40] Hulstein JJ, Lenting PJ, de Laat B, Derksen RH, Fijnheer R, de Groot PG. 2007. beta2-Glycoprotein I inhibits von Willebrand factor dependent platelet adhesion and aggregation. Blood. 110, 1483-1491.

[41] Di Simone N, Meroni PL, D'Asta M, Di Nicuolo F, D'Alessio MC, Caruso A. 2007. Pathogenic role of anti-beta2-glycoprotein I antibodies on human placenta: functional effects related to implantation and roles of heparin. Hum Reprod Update. 13, 189-196.

[42] Di Simone N, Raschi E, Testoni C, Castellani R, D'Asta M, Shi T, Krilis SA, Caruso A, Meroni PL. 2005. Pathogenic role of anti-beta 2-glycoprotein I antibodies in antiphospholipid associated fetal loss: characterisation of beta 2-glycoprotein I binding to trophoblast cells and functional effects of anti-beta 2-glycoprotein I antibodies in vitro. Ann Rheum Dis. 64, 462-467.

[43] Di Simone N, Luigi MP, Marco D, Fiorella DN, Silvia D, Clara DM, Alessandro C. 2007.. Pregnancies complicated with antiphospholipid syndrome: the pathogenic mechanism of antiphospholipid antibodies: a review of the literature. Ann N Y Acad Sci. 1108:505-514.

[44] Greer IA 2003. Thrombophilia: implications for pregnancy outcome. Thromb Res. 109, 73-81.

[45] Jane E. Salmon, G. 2008. Antiphosholipid antibodies and pregnancy loss: a disorder of inflammation. J Reprod Immunol; 77(1), 51-56

[46] Rai R, Cohen H, Dave M, Regan L. 1997. Randomised controlled trial of aspirin and aspirin plus heparin in pregnant women with recurrent miscarriage associated with phospholipid antibodies (or antiphospholipid antibodies). BMJ. 314, 253–7.

[47] Cowchock FS, Reece EA, Balaban D, Branch DW, Plouffe L. 1992. Repeated fetal losses associated with antiphospholipid antibodies: a collaborative randomized trial

comparing prednisone with low-dose heparin treatment. Am J Obstet Gynecol. 166, 1318–23.

[48] Bates SM, Greer IA, Pabinger I, Sofaer S, Hirsh J. 2008. Venous thromboembolism, thrombophilia, antithrombotic therapy, and pregnancy: American College of Chest Physicians Evidence-Based Clinical Practice Guidelines (8th Edition). Chest. 133, 844S-886S.

[49] Shimada S, Yamada H, Atsumi T, Yamada T, Sakuragi N, Minakami H, 2010. Intravenous immunoglobulin therapy for aspirin-heparinoid-resistant antiphospholipid syndrome. Reprod Med Biol. 9, 217-221.

[50] Carreras LD, Perez GN, Vega HR, Casavilla F. 1988. Lupus anticoagulant and recurrent fetal loss:successful treatment with gammaglobulin. Lancet. 2, 393-394.

[51] Branch DW, Peaceman AM, Druzin M, Silver RK, El-Sayed Y, Silver RM, Esplin MS, Spinnato J, Harger J. 2000. A multicenter, placebo-controlled pilot study of intravenous immune globulin treatment of antiphospholipid syndrome during pregnancy. The Pregnancy Loss Study Group. Am J Obstet Gynecol. 182, 122-127.

[52] Triolo G, Ferrante A, Ciccia F, Accardo-Palumbo A, Perino A, Castelli A, Giarratano A, Licata G. 2003. Randomized study of subcutaneous low molecular weight heparin plus aspirin versus intravenous immunoglobulin in the treatment of recurrent fetal loss associated with antiphospholipid antibodies. Arthritis Rheum. 48, 728-731.

[53] Triolo G, Ferrante A, Accardo-Palumbo A, Ciccia F, Cadelo M, Castelli A, Perino A, Licata G. 2004. IVIG in APS pregnancy. Lupus. 13, 731-735.

[54] Parke A, Maier D, Wilson D, Andreoli J, Ballow M. 1989. Intravenous gammaglobulin, antiphospholipid antibodies and pregnancy. Ann Intern Med. 110, 495-6.

[55] Scott JR, Branch DW, Kochenour NK, Ward K. 1989. Intravenous immunoglobulin treatment of pregnant patients with recurrent pregnancy loss caused by aniphospholipid antibodies and Rh immunization. Am J Obstet Gynecol. 159, 1055-6.

[56] Wapner RJ, Cowchock FS, Shapiro SS, 1989. Successful treatment in two women with antiphospholipid antibodies and refractory pregnancy losses with intravenous gammaglobulin infusions. Am J Obstet Gynecol. 616, 1271-2.

[57] Ron-el R, Vinder A, Golan A, Herman A, Raziel A, Caspi E, Sidi Y. 1993. The use of intravenous gammaglobulin, heparin and aspirin in the maintenance of pregnancy of freeze thawed embryo in a patient with lupus-type anticoagulant. Eur J Obstet Gynecol Reprod Biol. 52, 131-3.

[58] Caccavo D, Vaccaro F, Ferri GM, Amoroso A, Bonomo L. 1994. Anti-idiotypes against antiphospholipid antibodies are present in normal polyspecific immunoglobulins for therapeutic use. J Autoimmun. 7, 537-48.

[59] Galli M, Cortelazzo S, Barbui T. 1991. *In vivo* efficacy of intravenous gammaglobulins in patients with lupus anticoagulant is not mediated by anti-idiotypic mechanism. Am J Hematol. 30, 184-8.

[60] Said PB, Martinuzzo ME, Carreras LO. 1992. Neutralization of lupus anticoagulant activity by human immunoglobulin '*in vitro*'. Nouv Rev Fr Hematol. 34, 37-42.

[61] Matsuda J, Gohchi K, Kawasugi K., Tsukamoto M, Saitoh N, Kinoshita T. 1993. *In vitro* lupus anticoagulant neutralizing activity of intravenous immunoglobulin. Thromb Res. 70, 109-10 (letter).

[62] Yamada H, Kishida T, Kobayashi N, Kato EH, Hoshi N, Fujimoto S. 1998. Massive immunoglobulin treatment in women with four or more recurrent spontaneous primary abortions of unexplained aetiology. Hum Reprod. 13, 2620-2623.

[63] Morikawa M, Yamada H, Kato EH, Shimada S, Kishi T, Yamada T, Kobashi G, Fujimoto S. 2001. Massive intravenous immunoglobulin treatment in women with four or more recurrent spontaneous abortions of unexplained etiology: down-regulation of NK cell activity and subsets. Am J Reprod Immunol. 46, 399-404.

[64] Yamada H , Morikawa M, Furuta I, Kato E, Shimada S, Iwabuchi K, Minakami H. 2003. Intravenous immunoglobulin treatment in women with recurrent abortions: increased cytokine levels and reduced Th1/Th2 lymphocyte ratio in peripheral blood. Am J Reprod Immunol. 49, 84-89.

[65] Kazatchkine MD, Kaveri SV. 2001. Immunomodulation of autoimmune and inflammatory diseases with intravenous immune globulin. N Engl J Med. 345, 747-755.

[66] Bayary J, Dasgupta S, Misra N, Ephrem A, Van Huyen JP, Delignat S, Hassan G, Caligiuri G, Nicoletti A, Lacroix-Desmazes S, Kazatchkine MD, Kaveri S. 2006. Intravenous immunoglobulin in autoimmune disorders: an insight into the immunoregulatory mechanisms. Int Immunopharmacol. 6, 528-534.

[67] Caccavo D, Vaccaro F, Ferri GM, Amoroso A, Bonomo L. 1994. Anti-idiotypes against antiphospholipid antibodies are present in normal polyspecific immunoglobulins for therapeutic use. J Autoimmun. 7, 537-548.

[68] Sherer Y, Levy Y, Shoenfeld Y. 2000. Intravenous immunoglobulin therapy of antiphospholipid syndrome. Rheumatology. 39, 421-426.

9

Antiphospholipid Autoantibodies in Women with Recurrent Gestational Failures – Controversies in Management

Áurea García Segovia[1], Margarita Rodríguez-Mahou[2], Pedro Caballero[1] and Silvia Sánchez-Ramón[3,*]
[1]*Clínica Tambre, Madrid, Spain*
[2]*Laboratory of Autoimmunity*
[3]*Clinical Immunology Unit,*
Department of Immunology,
Hospital General Universitario
Gregorio Marañón, Madrid
Spain

1. Introduction

Antiphospholipid syndrome (APS) is the most common acquired thrombophilia in pregnant women. This syndrome is characterized by vascular thrombosis and/or pregnancy morbidity in association with the presence of circulating antiphospholipid antibodies (aPL). The APS may occur alone (primary APS), or in association with an underlying autoimmune connective tissue disorder (secondary APS).(1)(2) The APS diagnosis requires at least one of the clinical criteria and one of the laboratory criteria described in Table 1.

APS has been largely related to recurrent miscarriages (RM) and several pregnancy complications as pre-eclampsia, but their association with implantation failure (IF) after *in vitro* fertilization (IVF) is still a matter of debate. IF, defined as a failure in conceive after IVF treatment, is considered a cause of recurrent gestational failure (RGF), a current concept that includes both RM and IF. There is no consensus about the number of IVF failures cycles or the number of embryos transferred needed for the diagnostics of IF, but the majority of the clinicians consider 3 fresh IVF attempts' failures for the diagnosis.(3)

Assisted Reproduction Techniques (ART) development has tremendously increased the pregnancy rates (around 50%) by improvements in culture conditions, embryo selection and technical advances, but implantation is consider to be an important limiting factor in this field. Numerous anatomical, endocrine, immunological, thrombophilic and genetic alterations have been described as risk factors in IF. (4)

---

* Corresponding Author

Clinical criteria	
Vascular thrombosis	≥1 clinical episodes of arterial, venous, or small vessel thrombosis, in any tissue being confirmed by appropriate imaging studies or histopathology without evidence of inflammation in the vessel.
Pregnancy morbidity	≥1 unexplained deaths of a morphologically normal foetus at or beyond the 10th week of gestation, with normal foetal morphology documented.
	≥1 premature births of a morphologically normal neonate before the 34th week of gestation due to eclampsia and severe preeclampsia, or to recognized features of placental insufficiency.
	≥3 unexplained consecutive spontaneous abortions before the 10th week of gestation, with maternal anatomic or hormonal abnormalities, and paternal and maternal chromosomal causes excluded.
Laboratory criteria	
Lupus anticoagulant	Present in plasma, on ≥2 occasions at least 12 weeks apart, detected according to the guidelines of the International Society on Thrombosis and Haemostasis (Scientific Subcommittee on LAs/phospholipid-dependent antibodies)
Anticardiolipin antibody of IgG and/or IgM isotype	Present in serum or plasma at medium or high titre (>40 GPL or MPL, or >99th percentile), on >2 occasions, at least 12 weeks apart, measured by a standardized enzyme-linked immunosorbent assay (ELISA)
Anti-β2GPI antibody of IgG and/or IgM isotype	Present in serum or plasma (titre >99th percentile), ≥2 occasions, at least 12 weeks apart, measured by a standardized ELISA, according to recommended procedures

Table 1. Clinical and Laboratory criteria for the diagnosis of the APS. Adapted from Miyakis, S. *et al.* (2006). Abbreviations: β2GPI, β2 glycoprotein I; ELISA, enzyme-linked immunosorbent assay; GPL, IgG phospholipid units; GPM, IgM phospholipid units.

2. Implantation process

Embryo implantation and successful establishment of pregnancy require delicate interactions between the blastocyst and the maternal uterine cells. From the embryo phase, the trophectoderm and the throphoblast establish contact with the specialized maternal tissue, the uterine endometrium. Classically, implantation process has been divided into three phases: apposition, adhesion and invasion of a developmentally competent embryo in the receptive endometrium. Implantation begins with attachment of the blastocyst trophoblast (derived from the trophectoderm) at the embryonic pole through the outer epithelial uterine lining (day 6 from the fertilization). The site of implantation is marked on the surface by a coagulation plug left where the blastocyst has entered the uterine wall (day 12 from the fertilization). This phenomenon triggers changes in both the trophoblast and the connective tissue (stroma) beneath the uterine epithelium. Some trophoblast cells fuse to make a syncytium called the syncytiotrophoblast that releases proteolytic enzymes that allow passage of the blastocyst into the endometrial wall first, then into the stroma (carrying the whole conceptus with it).

During this migration, the trophoblast cells destroy the wall of the maternal uterine spiral arteries, converting them from muscular vessels into flaccid sinusoidal sacs. This vascular transformation is important to ensure an adequate blood supply to the feto-placental unit and the beginning of the histiotrophic nutrition. [5]

A change in endometrial gene expression is necessary to allow the embryo implantation. In fact, already in the late luteal phase, physiological changes occur in the endometrium to allow blastocyst implantation. Uterine cells changes their phenotype during the menstrual cycle and these critical events during this so called "window of implantation or receptivity" results in the presence of the embryo, in a decidual reaction, leading to programs of gene expression particular to pregnancy. Failure to properly begin these critical events results in early implantation failure.

3. Disorders of implantation

Adequate implantation is a limiting factor in human reproduction. The study of the possible causes responsible of this failure is technically difficult in the daily clinical routine. As previously described, implantation is the result of the remarkable synchronization between the development of the embryo and the differentiation of the endometrium.

Uterine pathologies like adhesions, septa, intrauterine polyps, hydrosalpinx, endometriosis and other disorders might impair implantation. Several studies suggest that reparatory surgery improves the conception rate. However, there is still an ongoing debate on the benefits of surgery in infertile patients. [6-10]

During the last few years several authors have reported different gene networks important for the endometrium receptivity that controls the expression of key transcription factors (e.g. HOXA10, STAT3, p53) [11-15], growth factors and cytokines [e.g. HB-EGF, leukaemia-inhibiting factor (LIF), prokineticin 1] [16-18](and cell adhesion molecules and their ligands (e.g. avb3 integrin, trophinin, L-selectin ligand) [19-21], all of which are essential for coordinated cross-talk with the implanting embryo. [22] Altmae *et al.* demonstrated that women with IF show a somewhat different endometrial gene profile during the window of implantation, [23] which is thought to contribute to the lower implantation rates seen in these patients. In particular, investigations focusing on endometrium of IF patients showed changes in known implantation markers, such as integrins, as well as leukaemia inhibitory factor (LIF) and interleukin-1 (IL-1). [24]

Natural killer (NK) cells have been recently identified among the relevant immunological factors for reproductive success [25]. Of note, uterine natural killer (NK) cells ($CD56^{bright}CD16^{-}$) represent the dominant type of immune cells in the decidua (around 70% of feto-maternal interface lymphocytes), and it has been suggested that they contribute to the normal trophoblast invasion control and angiogenesis process. An increased number and cytotoxic activity of blood NK cells ($CD56^{dim}CD16^{+}$) and their presence in the endometrium of pregnant women has been related to pregnancy loss. Circulating NK cell expansion has been also associated to the presence of antiphospholipid antibodies in women with RM and has been ascribed to antiphospholipid-mediated specific reactions [26].

4. Thrombophilias and IF

Acquired and inherited thrombophilias are associated with adverse pregnancy outcome. Thrombophilias has been largely related to RM and several pregnancy complications as pre-eclampsia, late foetal dead, foetal grow restriction and placenta abruption.

With respect to recurrent IF, although the medical literature is not as substantive as that of the recurrent pregnancy loss field, the data again suggest that thrombophilia is associated with repeated IF. Several authors have reported a significantly higher prevalence of thrombophilias in women with four or more failed IVF cycles when compared with spontaneous conceptions.[27-30] Due to the limitations on the knowledge of the implantation process, the mechanisms underlying these associations still remain unclear. Thrombophilias would affect on the ability of the endometrium to develop adequately, communicate effectively with the embryo, or potentially disrupt the early interactions with the maternal circulation.

The inherited thrombophilic conditions can be classified into five broad groups. Each inherited thrombophilia has variable frequency depending on race and ethnicity. In Caucasians, the most common are showed in Table 2. [31,32]

Trombophilia	Incident VTE (%)	Recurrent VTE (%)	Normal population
Factor V Leiden	20	40–50	3–7
Prothrombin G20210A mutation	3–8	15–20	1–3
Antithrombin deficiency	1–2	2–5	0.02–0.04
Protein C deficiency	2–5	5–10	0.2–0.5
Protein S deficiency	1–3	5–10	0.1–1

Table 2. Prevalence of genetic defects among Caucasians

APS has been largely related to recurrent miscarriages (RM) and several pregnancy complications such as pre-eclampsia, prematurity, abruption placentae and the HELLP syndrome (haemolysis, elevated liver enzymes, low platelets count), and others. It is considered the most frequently acquired risk factor for thrombophilia and the main risk of pregnancy loss. However, their association with IF after IVF is still a matter of debate. [33,34] *In vitro* and *in vivo* mice models have demonstrated that antiphospholipid antibodies (aPL) are able to increase thrombus formation in venous and arteries. [35,36]

Antiphospholipid syndrome antibodies (aPL), anticardiolipin (aCL), anti-β2 glycoprotein I (β2GPI) and lupus anticoagulant (LA), are believed to have a pathogenic role. Several authors have reported changes in endothelial adhesion molecules expression as well as in nitric oxide and tissue factor expression in the presence of aPL. These changes could induce coagulation cascade activation but the cells and the exact mechanism involved in clot formation still remains to be elucidated.

β2GPI-dependent aPL is considered the antibody subpopulation responsible for the thrombotic manifestations of APS. The expression of β2GPI on trophoblast cell membranes explains the placental tropism of anti-β2GPI antibodies and the possible role of these antibodies in pregnancy loss. Placental thrombosis, acute inflammation and complement activation have been described as possible responsible of foetal loss in APS patients.

In vitro studies showed that aPL might induce a procoagulant status at the placental level through several mechanisms including the ability of the aPL antibodies (specifically, anti-β2GPI antibodies) to disrupt the anticoagulant annexin A5 shield on trophoblast but histopathological studies have not demonstrated thrombosis findings in most APS women placentas. (37)

An adequate balance between pro-inflammatory and anti-inflammatory arms of the immune response is necessary for a successful pregnancy outcome (38). Complement activation could be involved in APS foetal loss pathogenesis because of the demonstration that the protective effect of heparin in the mouse model is linked to the anticomplement, rather than to the anticoagulant, activity. (39)

We still do not know the precise mechanisms responsible of the high diversity of clinical manifestations in APS patients. Several authors have reported studies *in vitro* and *in vivo* trying to explain pregnancy loss and vascular implications of the syndrome, but in IF cases the potential pathogenic mechanisms are less known. β2GPI-dependent antibodies bind to human trophoblast and could affect several cell functions needed for the correct embryo implantation like proliferation and syncytium formation. These antibodies could decrease production of human chorionic gonadotrophin and others important factors for the invasion of the trophoblast. (40) In addition, expression of important factors for the implantation in the endometrium has been found in reduced quantities in women with aPL. Also, it has been shown that β2GPI-dependent aPL are able to react with human stromal decidual cells *in vitro*, inducing a proinflammatory phenotype. (41,42)

A wide range of different antigenic specificities has been described in APS (Table 3), and could be determined when the clinical suspicion of obstetrical APS is strong and the classical anticardiolipin antibodies (aCL), anti- β2GPI and LA are all negative.

5. Prevalence of antiphospholipid antibodies in recurrent gestational failure

We consecutively studied 157 women that fulfilled diagnosis of RPL, of age range from 28 to 41 (mean age, 36.86±3.93), from whom 60 presented with RM with a mean of 3.28±1.14 prior miscarriages; and 97 presented with IF, with a mean of 4.75±2.17 prior failed IVF. In the group of RM, 13.62% showed positive antiphospholipid antibodies (mostly low titre anti-β2GPI or/and aCL); only a 4.60% showed moderate to high titres of antiphospholipid antibodies and therefore fulfilled criteria of APS. In the group of IF, 18.80% of patients showed positive antiphospholipid antibodies (all of them low titre anti-β2GPI or/and aCL). A 97% of patients with antiphospholipid antibodies in our series had also expanded circulating NK cells (above 12%). The allele frequency prevalence of the mutations in the genes of factor V Leiden, the prothrombin G20210A, and the methylenetetrahydrofolate reductase (MTHFR C677T) in the general population in the European population represent approximately a 2.5%, 2.2%, and 35.3%, respectively. (43) We systematically studied all three mutations in our cohort of patients with RPL. We observed that in the group of RM, the

Reagin
Anionic phospholipids
Cardiolipin
Phosphatidylserine
Phosphatidic acid
Phosfatidilinositol
Neutral phospholipids
Phosfatidilcoline
Dipolar phospholipids
Phosphatidyletanolamine
Phospholipid-linking proteins
β-2-glicoprotein I
Prothrombin
Annexin V
Protein C
Protein S
High and low molecular weight kininogens
Other

Table 3. Different specificities of antiphospholipid antibodies

10.8% was homozygous for MTHFR mutation and the 64.9% were carriers. In the group of IF, the 8.3% was homozygous for MTHFR mutation and the 55.6% were carriers. The frequencies of carriers of mutations of factor V Leiden were 3.12% in RM and 6.25% in IF, respectively; the frequencies of carriers of mutations of prothrombin were 3.12% in RM and 0% in IF, respectively. No homozygous for both factors were observed in our series of patients.

6. Clues in management of thrombophilia in recurrent pregnancy loss

In addition to the risk of embryo and foetal losses, there is a low but actual risk of maternal morbidity due to coagulation disorders. The risk of pulmonary embolism and/or deep vein thrombosis increases during pregnancy and puerperium, and is further enhanced by the presence of acquired or inherited thrombophilias. (1) This thromboembolic complications remain as a main cause of maternal death during pregnancy, and its incidence is increasing. For the presence of antiphospholipid antibodies, the risk of pregnancy-related severe maternal thrombosis has been estimated by an odds ratio of 15.8 (95%CI 10.9-22.8). (44)

Based on meta-analyses of randomized controlled studies, observational studies and clinical reports, the American College of Physicians has made the following recommendations: (45,46)

1. For women with aPL and recurrent pregnancy loss, and no history of venous or arterial thrombosis, a prophylactic dose of unfractionated heparin combined with low-dose aspirin antepartum is recommended (Grade 1B). This combination has been shown to be effective in reducing miscarriage rates in women with aPL and prior recurrent foetal loss. This treatment regimen is significantly more effective that others, such as corticosteroids either alone or with aspirin, and IV gammaglobulin. Two recent pilot

studies suggest that the combination of low molecular weight heparin (LMWH) and aspirin might be equivalent to unfractionated heparin and aspirin in preventing recurrent pregnancy loss. (47,48) Our protocol is based in the modified protocol proposed by Ray with combined low-dose aspirin and low-molecular weight heparin. (49)

2. For women at high risk for pre-eclampsia, low-dose aspirin throughout pregnancy is recommended (Grade 1B). Treatment seems to be more effective if started early in pregnancy and at appropriate dose (75–100 mg once daily). An effect of anticoagulant therapy on the risk of preeclampsia is biologically plausible. However, the results of previous small sized studies are still controversial, and the presence of thrombophilia has not been considered in randomized trials on prevention. (1)
3. For women with thrombophilia and previous late foetal loss, placental abruption and/or foetal growth retardation, the available data do not suffice to form the basis of a recommendable prophylactic protocol.

From a clinical perspective, there is still controversial the decision of the adequate thromboprophylaxis protocol for preventing IF and RM in several thrombophilic alterations, such as factor V Leiden and/or prothrombin mutations' carriers in otherwise asymptomatic women. In particular, MTHFR mutation has been shown to lack clinical significance alone. However, an argument to justify prophylaxis could be made that the recurrence risk of women with prior foetal loss, abruption, severe IUGR, or severe preeclampsia is high enough (5–30%). Although there are no randomized clinical trials to support such an approach, observational studies of low-dose aspirin, and LMWH have reported improvement in birth weight compared with untreated pregnancies. Such patients should be offered postpartum anticoagulation prophylaxis if they have an affected first-degree relative or thrombotic risk (e.g., caesarean delivery) (50) Finally, although low corticosteroid doses (<20 mg/day) are occasionally used, particularly in women unresponsive to the standard combination therapy (low-dose aspirin and heparin), there is no evidence to support the routine use of corticosteroids. (2)

7. Conclusions

Multiple acquired and genetic thrombophilic conditions may interact or act in addition as causes of recurrent pregnancy loss. Antiphospholipid antibodies are a heterogeneous group of autoantibodies with varying affinity for different phospholipids and protein-phospholipid complexes with direct pathogenic role resulting in lower blood flow and/or thrombosis at the maternal-foetal interface and final embryo/foetus loss, among other potential maternal complications. Our results in a cohort of patients with recurrent pregnancy loss suggest that aPL may have a similar role in IF patients as in RM patients. Quantification of these thrombosis risk factors in women with RPL will contribute to a better understanding of the interaction of genetic and acquired risk factors, and to better adjust in a more personalized approach the best management for a successful gestation.

8. Acknowledgments

We are grateful to all patients and healthy controls that participated in this study.

This work was supported by a grant from the Spanish Ministry of Health, Social Policy and Equality (EC10-026) and from the Fundación Tambre, Spain.

9. References

[1] Benedetto C, Marozio L, Tavella AM, Salton L, Grivon S, Di Giampaolo F.Ann. 2010. Coagulation disorders in pregnancy: acquired and inherited thrombophilias . N Y Acad Sci.;1205:106-17

[2] Meroni PL, Borghi MO, Raschi E, Tedesco F.2011. Pathogenesis of antiphospholipid syndrome: understanding the antibodies. Nat Rev Rheumatol.;7(6):330-9.

[3] Tan, B.K., Vandekerckhove, P., Kennedy, R., Keay, S.D., 2005. Investigation and current management of recurrent IVF treatment failure in the UK.

[4] Jauniaux E, Farquharson RG, Christiansen OB, Exalto N.2006. Evidence-based guidelines for the investigation and medical treatment of recurrent miscarriage. Hum Reprod;21:2216–22

[5] Daniel D. Carson. 1999. Embryo Implantation: Molecular, Cellular and Clinical Aspects.

[6] Bosteels, J., Weyers, S., Puttemans, P., Panayotidis, C., Van Herendael, B., Gomel, V., Mol, B.W., Mathieu, C., D'Hooghe, T., 2010. The effectiveness of hysteroscopy in improving pregnancy rates in subfertile women without other gynaecological symptoms: a systematic review. Hum.Reprod. Update 16, 1–11.

[7] Mollo, A., De Franciscis, P., Colacurci, N., Cobellis, L., Perino, A., Venezia, R., Alviggi, C., De Placido, G., 2009. Hysteroscopic resection of the septum improves the pregnancy rate of women with unexplained infertility: a prospective controlled trial. Fertil. Steril. 91, 2628–2631

[8] Perez-Medina, T., Bajo-Arenas, J., Salazar, F., Redondo, T., Sanfrutos, L., Alvarez, P., Engels, V., 2005. Endometrial polyps and their implication in the pregnancy rates of patients undergoing intrauterine insemination: a prospective, randomized study. Hum. Reprod. 20, 1632–1635.

[9] Strandell, A., Lindhard, A., Waldenstrom, U., Thorburn, J., Janson, P.O., Hamberger, L., 1999. Hydrosalpinx and IVF outcome: a prospective, randomized multicentre trial in Scandinavia on salpingectomy prior to IVF. Hum. Reprod. 14, 2762–2769.

[10] Barri, P.N., Coroleu, B., Tur, R., Barri-Soldevila, P.N., Rodriguez, I., 2010. Endometriosis-associated infertility: surgery and IVF, a comprehensive therapeutic approach. Reprod. Biomed. Online 21, 179–185

[11] Catalano RD, Johnson MH, Campbell EA, Charnock-Jones DS, Smith SK,Sharkey AM. Inhibition of Stat3 activation in the endometrium preventsimplantation: a nonsteroidal approach to contraception. Proc Natl AcadSci USA 2005;102:8585–8590.

[12] Nakamura H, Kimura T, Koyama S, Ogita K, Tsutsui T, Shimoya K, Taniguchi T, Koyama M, Kaneda Y, Murata Y. Mouse model of human infertility: transient and local inhibition of endometrial STAT-3 activation results in implantation failure. FEBS Lett 2006; 580:2717–2722.

[13] Hu W, Feng Z, Teresky AK, Levine AJ. p53 regulates maternal reproduction through LIF. Nature 2007;450:721–724.

[14] Vitiello D, Kodaman PH, Taylor HS. HOX genes in implantation. Semin Reprod Med 2007;25:431–436.

[15] Lynch VJ, Tanzer A, Wang Y, Leung FC, Gellersen B, Emera D, Wagner GP. Adaptive changes in the transcription factor HoxA-11 are essential for the evolution of pregnancy in mammals. Proc Natl Acad Sci USA 2008;105:14928–14933.

[16] Stewart CL, Kaspar P, Brunet LJ, Bhatt H, Gadi I, Kontgen F, Abbondanzo SJ. Blastocyst implantation depends on maternal expression of leukaemia inhibitory factor. Nature 1992;359: 76–79.

[17] Evans J, Catalano RD, Brown P, Sherwin R, Critchley HO, Fazleabas AT, Jabbour HN. Prokineticin 1 mediates fetal-maternal dialogue regulating endometrial leukemia inhibitory factor. FASEB J 2009; 23:2165–2175.
[18] Lim HJ, Dey SK. HB-EGF: a unique mediator of embryo–uterine interactions during implantation. Exp Cell Res 2009;315:619–626.
[19] Aoki R, Fukuda MN. Recent molecular approaches to elucidate the mechanism of embryo implantation: trophinin, bystin, and tastin asmolecules involved in the initial attachment of blastocysts to the uterus in humans. Semin Reprod Med 2000;18:265–271.
[20] Genbacev OD, Prakobphol A, Foulk RA, Krtolica AR, Ilic D, Singer MS, Yang ZQ, Kiessling LL, Rosen SD, Fisher SJ. Trophoblast L-selectin-mediated adhesion at the maternal–fetal interface. Science 2003;299:405–408.
[21] Donaghay M, Lessey BA. Uterine receptivity: alterations associated with benign gynecological disease. Semin Reprod Med 2007;25:461–475.
[22] Brosens JJ, Hodgetts A, Feroze-Zaidi F, Sherwin JR, Fusi L, Salker MS, Higham J, Rose GL, Kajihara T, Young SL, Lessey BA, Henriet P, Langford PR, Fazleabas AT.2010. Proteomic analysis of endometrium from fertile and infertile patients suggests a role for apolipoprotein A-I in embryo implantation failure and endometriosis. Mol Hum Reprod. Apr;16(4):273-85
[23] Altmae, S., Martinez-Conejero, J.A., Salumets, A., Simon, C., Horcajadas, J.A.,Stavreus-Evers, A., 2010. Endometrial gene expression analysis at the time of embryo implantation in women with unexplained infertility. Mol. Hum. Reprod. 16, 178-187, gap102 [PII].
[24] Toth B, Würfel W, Germeyer A, Hirv K, Makrigiannakis A, Strowitzki T.2011.Disorders of implantation - are there diagnostic and therapeutic options?. J Reprod Immunol.90(1):117-23.
[25] Cianchetta-Sívori M, Moraru M, García-Segovia A, Sánchez-Ramón S. Pregnancy as an immune phenomenon. Rev Iberoam Fert 2011, in press.
[26] Oliver-Minarro D., Gil J., Aguaron A., Rodriguez-Mahou M., Fernandez-Cruz E., Sánchez-Ramón S. 2009. NK cell expansion in obstetrical antiphospholipid syndrome: guilty by association? Eur J Obstet Gynecol Reprod Biol. 145(2):227.
[27] Azem F, Many A, Yovel I, Amit A, Lessing JB, Kupferminc MJ.2004. Increased rates of thrombophilia in women with repeated IVF failures. Hum Reprod 19: 368–70.
[28] Coulam CB, Jeyendran RS, Fishel LA, Roussev R.2006. Multiple thrombophilic gene mutations are risk factors for implantation failure. Reprod BioMed Online; 12:322–7.
[29] Qublan HS, Eid SS, Ababneh HA, Amarin ZO, Smadi AZ, Al-Khafaji FF, et al.2006. Acquired and inherited thrombophilia: implication in recurrent IVF and embryo transfer failure. Hum Reprod ;21:2694–8.
[30] Bellver J, Soares SR, Alvarez C, Munoz E, Ramirez A, Rubio C, et al.2008.The role of thrombophilia and thyroid autoimmunity in unexplained infertility, implantation failure and recurrent spontaneous abortion. Hum Reprod :23(2):278–84.
[31] Khan S, Dickerman JD. 2006. Hereditary thrombophilia. Thromb J. 12;4:15
[32] Crowther, M.A. & J.G. Kelton. 2003. Congenital thrombophilic states associated with venous thrombosis: a qualitative overview and proposed classification system. Ann. Intern. Med. 138: 128–134.
[33] Levine, J.S., D.W. Branch & J. Rauch. 2002. The antiphospholipid syndrome. N. Engl. J. Med. 346: 752–763.
[34] Vinatier,D., P. Dufour, M.Cosson & J.L.Houpeau. 2001. Antiphospholipid syndrome and recurrentmiscarriages. Eur. J. Obstet. Gynaecol. Reprod. Biol. 96: 37–50

[35] Jankowski, M. et al. 2003. Thrombogenicity of β2-glycoprotein I-dependent antiphospholipid antibodies in a photochemically induced thrombosis model in the hamster. Blood 101, 157-162 .
[36] Ramesh, S. et al.2011. Antiphospholipid antibodies promote leukocyte-endothelial cell adhesion and thrombosis in mice by antagonizing eNOS via β2GPI and apoER2. J. Clin. Invest. 121, 120-131.
[37] Park, A. L. in Hughes' Syndrome (ed. Khamashta, M. A.) Ch. 28 Placental pathology in antiphospholipid syndrome, 362-374 (Springer-Verlag, London, 2006).
[38] Chaouat, G. 2007. The Th1/Th2 paradigm: still important in pregnancy? Semin. Immunopathol. 29, 95-113.
[39] Girardi, G., Redecha, P. & Salmon, J. E. 2004. Heparin prevents antiphospholipid antibody-induced foetal loss by inhibiting complement activation. Nat. Med. 10, 1222-1226.
[40] Meroni, P. L. et al. 2010. Anti-phospholipid antibody mediated foetal loss: still an open question from a pathogenic point of view. Lupus 19, 453-456.
[41] Francis, J. et al. 2006. Impaired expression of endometrial differentiation markers and complement regulatory proteins in patients with recurrent pregnancy loss associated with antiphospholipid syndrome. Mol. Hum. Reprod. 12, 435-442.
[42] Borghi, M. O. et al. 2009. Antiphospholipid antibodies reactivity with human decidual cells: an additional mechanism of pregnancy complications in APS and a potential target for innovative therapeutic intervention [abstract OP-0119]. Ann. Rheum. Dis. 68 (Suppl. 3), 109.
[43] Antoniadi T, Hatzis T, Kroupis C, Economou-Petersen E, Petersen MB. 1999. Prevalence of factor V Leiden, prothrombin G20210A, and MTHFR C677T mutations in a Greek population of blood donors. Am J Hematol. 61(4):265-7
[44] James, A.H., M.G. Jamison, L.R. Brancazio, et al. 2006. Venous thromboembolism during pregnancy and the postpar- tum: incidence, risk factors, and mortality. Am. J. Obstet. Gynecol. 194: 1311-1315
[45] Guyatt, G., D. Gutterman, M.H. Baumann, et al. 2006. Grading strength of recommendations and quality of evidence in clinical guidelines: report from an American College of Phisicians Task Force. Chest 129: 174-181.
[46] American College of Obstetricians and Gynecologists. 2001.Thromboembolism in pregnancy. ACOG Practice Bulletin No. 19. Int. J. Gynaecol. Obstet. 75: 203-212.
[47] Noble, L.S., W.H. Kutteh, N. Lashey, et al. 2005. Antiphospholipid antibodies associated with recurrent pregnancy loss: prospective, multicenter, controlled pilot study comparing treatment with low molecular-weight heparin versus unfractionated heparin. Fertil. Steril. 83: 684-690.
[48] Stephenson, M.D., P.J. Ballem, P. Tsang, et al. 2004. Treatment of antiphospholipid antibodies syndrome (APS) in pregnancy: a randomized pilot trial comparing low molecular-weight heparin to unfractionated heparin. J Obstet Gynaecol. Can. 26: 729-734.
[49] Rai, R., Regan, L., 2006. Recurrent miscarriage. Lancet 368, 601- 611.
[50] Lockwood CJ. Inherited thrombophilias in pregnant patients: detection and treatment paradigm. Obstet Gynecol 2002;99:333-41.

10

Antiphospholipid Syndrome in Pregnancy

Kjell Haram[1], Eva-Marie Jacobsen[2,3] and Per Morten Sandset[2,3]
[1]*Department of Obstetrics and Gynaecology, Haukeland University Hospital, Bergen*
[2]*Department of Haematology, Oslo University Hospital Rikshospitalet, Oslo*
[3]*Institute of Clinical Medicine, University of Oslo, Oslo*
Norway

1. Introduction

The antiphospholipid syndrome (APS) is a multisystemic disease, characterized by venous or arterial thromboses, or certain obstetric complications, and the presence of antiphospholipid antibodies (APAs)(1-4). APAs are a heterogeneous group of autoantibodies that bind to negatively charged phospholipids, phospholipid-binding protein, or a combination of the two. Lupus anticoagulant (LA), anticardiolipin antibodies (aCL) and anti-beta 2 glycoprotein 1 (anti-β2GP1) antibodies are the main antibodies in this syndrome(1;2;5). APS occurs in isolation as a primary APS in more than 50% of the cases, but can be associated with other autoimmune diseases, most often with systemic lupus erythemathosus (SLE). Twenty to 35% of women with SLE develop APS(6). APS occurs for the most part in young women of fertile age(7). It occurs rarely in children, and only 12% of all APS occur after 50 years of age(8).

2. Antiphospholipid antibodies in pregnancy

Antiphospholipid antibodies in pregnancy are associated with recurrent miscarriage, intrauterine growth restriction (IUGR), preeclampsia, placental abruption, premature delivery or fetal death in addition to arterial or venous thrombosis(9;10). Thus, the woman may experience both early and late fetal loss. Vascular thrombosis can occur in any organ or tissue(2). Deep vein thrombosis in the legs is most frequent, but the renal vein, the pulmonary vein, the inferior vena cava and the hepatic and portal vein may also be affected. The most common site of arterial thrombosis is the cerebral circulation, but occlusion of coronary and retinal arteries has also been reported(3;11;12). APA, particularly LA, is an independent risk factor for first and possibly recurrent ischemic stroke in young adults(13). Cerebral ischemic events can occur in any vascular territory(14). Cerebral angiography typically demonstrates intracranial branch or trunk occlusion or is normal in about one third of patients so studied(15). In addition, leg ulcer, chorea, and migraine have been associated with APAs(3). A wide range of abdominal manifestations have been reported in APA-positive patients. Hepatic involvement is most numerous, thereafter thrombotic events in branches of the intestinal vasculature(16).

3. Diagnosis of APS in non-pregnant and pregnant women

According to the last updated consensus the diagnosis of obstetric APS needs to be based on: 1) one or more unexplained deaths of normal fetuses at or beyond the 10th week of gestation, or 2) one or more premature births before the 34th week of gestation because of eclampsia, severe preeclampsia, or placental insufficiency, or 3) three or more unexplained consecutive spontaneous abortions before the 10th gestational week[7]. Pregnant women with such complications should have laboratory testing.

The diagnosis of APS must be based both on clinical criteria and persistent positivity for APA[2;7]. Laboratory testing for APA is used to confirm or refute the diagnosis[2]. Thrombosis must be confirmed by strict objective criteria (angiography, venography, Doppler ultrasound examination or CT)[7]. CT is considered to be first-line investigation of suspected thrombosis in patients with abdominal symptoms. CT features of mesenteric ischemia are thickening of both small and large bowel walls with prominence of the supplying mesenteric vessels[17]. For histopathological confirmation thrombosis should be present without evidence of inflammation in the vessel wall[7]. Cerebral thrombosis can be diagnosed by cerebral angiography, transcranial Doppler technique, or magnetic resonance imaging (MRI)[13;18]. In some cases, MRI has revealed small foci of high signal in subcortical white matter scattered throughout the brain[13;19].

4. Venous thromboembolism

Pregnancy is a risk factor for venous thromboembolism (VTE). From two to ten-fold increase of VTE compared with the risk for non-pregnant women has been reported(20;21).The risk of thrombosis in the lower extremities may be even higher in women with coexisting risk factors (e.g. obesity, thrombophilia or acquired APS)[22;23]. Women with APS are at high risk of recurrent thrombosis[24], and this risk may even be higher in pregnant women[21]. A retrospective comparison of the overall risk of recurrence of VTE revealed risk of 11% per 100 patient-years during pregnancy and 3.7% in the non-pregnant state (the risk ratio for VTE during pregnancy was 3.5 with 95% confidence interval (CI) 1.6-7.8)[25]. Although a clear association between APAs and vascular events has been described, the data from a cohort study did not support that aCL antibodies affect vascular mortality[26].

5. Catastrophic APS

Catastrophic APS (CAPS), also known as "Asherson's syndrome") is an unusual (<1%) variant of APS, which is characterised by rapid appearance of multiple thromboses (mainly small-vessel thrombosis) that lead to multiorgan failure[27]. It is an acute, life-threatening, complication which may occur both in non-pregnant and pregnant women[28].

Diagnostic algorithms which have been proposed include the occurence of new thromboses in at least three different organs in less than a week[29]. In patients with a history of APS or persistent APA-positivity as described in the guidelines, a diagnosis of definite CAPS is made if the patient has new thrombosis in at least three organs, with micro-thrombosis confirmed by biopsy[29]. If only two organs are affected, or if confirmation with biopsy is not available, a diagnosis of probable CAPS is made. If the patient does not have a history of APS or persistent APA-positivity, APA-positivity must be confirmed twice with at least 12 weeks apart[29].

Disseminated intravascular coagulation occurs in approximately 25% of patiens with CAPS[30]. In more than 50% of the cases, catastrophic events are triggered by infections, trauma or surgery, anticoagulation withdrawal, malignancies, lupus "flares" or obstetric complications[28].

CAPS may infrequently appear during pregnancy after a Caesarean section or fetal loss[28]. The HELLP syndrome (hemolysis, elevated liver enzymes, low platelets) may be part of the catastrophic syndrome[31]. Bone marrow necrosis and a refractory HELLP syndrome have been reported in a woman with catastrophic APS. The fetus died in spite of termination of pregnancy[32]. A retrospective study comprised 15 cases of catastrophic APS in pregnancy or puerperium. APS was primary in 7 while 8 had SLE or lupus-like disease. In 8 of 15 cases (53%) the catastrophic syndrome were associated with HELLP syndrome. Six cases (43%) occurred in the puerperium and 1 after fetal death[28].

Laboratory testing

Transient occurrence of APA may not be associated with increased risk for clinical events. Therefore, it is essential that a positive test for APA is repeated after at least 12 weeks to confirm diagnostic citeria[7].

LA assays are functional assays based on one of several phospholipid-dependent clotting tests[10]. LA seems to be the most specific test for APS[33]. LA is strongly associated with fetal loss at more than 10 weeks' gestation. In a metaanalysis on women without autoimmune disease, LA was associated with late recurrent fetal loss (at least 2 fetal losses) with odds ratio 7.8 (95% CI 2.3-26.5)[34]. Positive tests for APAs are found in 2% of the general population and in 30-40% of patients with SLE[12;35]. In general obstetric clinics the prevalence of APAs has been reported to be between 2.7% and 7%[36].

aCL antibodies are detected by enzyme linked immunoabsorbent assays (ELISAs) that measure anti-β2GP1 antibody dependent IgG and IgM aCL antibodies[2;7;37]. The aCL ELISA test has high sensitivity, but low specificity[8] and skill and experience are necessary in interpreting the results[4]. Despite international efforts to standardize laboratory testing significant variation in the performance of APS antibody assays in laboratories remains a critical problem[2].

In 1990 three independent groups reported that aCL antibodies were directed against the plasma protein β2GP1(38-40). Several commercial ELISA assays for the detection of anti-β2GP1 antibodies of IgG and IgM type have later been developed. However, the laboratory detection of APAs by ELISA tests has been flawed by lack of standardisation and disconcordant results between manufacturers and laboratories[41]. The European Forum on Antiphospholipid Antibodies have published methodological analyses and proposals for the performance of these assays[42;43].

To exclude the presence of APAs, both clotting-based assays for LA and ELISA tests for anti-β2GP1/aCL should be performed[7]. LA-testing should be performed according to guidelines published as an official communication of the Scientific Standardization Committee of the International Society on Thrombosis and Haemostasis[44]. The latest consensus on classification criteria for APS states that cut-off for positive aCL and/or anti-β2GP1 tests should be >99th percentile of the titres in a reference group or, for aCL antibodies, should be present in medium or high titre (>40 IgG or IgM phospholipid units)[7].

6. Thrombocytopenia in patients with APS

APS related thrombocytopenia is defined by a platelet count less than $100 \cdot 10^9/L$, confirmed twice 12 weeks apart, and is found in approximately 20% of patients with APS and in more than 40% of patients who have APS associated with underlying SLE(45). A minority of patients have thrombocytopenia with platelets less than $50 \cdot 10^9/L$(45). APS-associated thrombocytopenia is an autoimmune phenomenon and its relation to thrombotic risk is poorly characterized. However, thrombocytopenia does not appear to reduce thrombotic risks in patients with APS(45).

7. Distinguishing APS from other prothrombotic and thrombocytopenic conditions

The differential diagnosis in patients presenting with thrombocytopenia includes thrombotic thrombocytopenic purpura (TTP), heparin-induced thrombocytopenia (HIT) and DIC(45). Distinguishing these conditions can be challenging. Diagnosing APS requires documentation of persistent APA antibodies in combination with compatible clinical features of thrombosis or pregnancy morbidity. However, APA antibodies have been documented in TTP and other thrombotic microangiopathies including haemolytic uremic syndrome and HELLP syndrome(16), as well as in cases of HIT. Patients with TTP present with microangiopathic hemolytic anaemia, typically manifesting with schistocytes on the blood smear and evidence of hemolysis, which is not a typical feature in APS. Measurement of the ADAMTS-13 metalloprotease, if available, may be helpful in these situations given that TTP is associated with ultra-large von Willebrand factor multimers that result from a deficiency in ADAMTS-13. If the patient is under medication with heparin, HIT must be considered. Notably, false-positive HIT antigen tests can be distinguished from true HIT antibodies by using enzyme immunoassays for PF4/heparin complexes tested with heparin excess or with use of functional assays(46). Patients with DIC typically have negative tests for APAs, frequently with evidence of thrombocytopenia, coagulopathy and thrombotic or hemorrhagic complications(45). Patients with severe DIC have low platelet count, fibrinogen and antithrombin (consumption coagulopathy).

8. Thrombotic microangiopathic hemolytic anaemia (TMHA) and APS

The term thrombotic microangiopathic hemolytic anaemia (TMHA) was introduced by Symmers in 1952 to describe clinical disorders related to the presence of localised or diffuse microvascular thrombosis(47). TMHA is characterised by thrombocytopenia, microangiopathic hemolytic anaemia (as indicated by erythrocyte fragmentation on peripheral blood smears) accompanied by a negative Coombs' test, fever, neurological symptoms, and kidney involvement(48). Several reports have pointed out the relationship of TMHA with the presence of APAs(48). SLE was the first autoimmune disease in which the association of TMHA with APA was recognised(48). There is evidence to support the hypothesis that TMHA might be a manifestation of APS(48).

9. APS, preeclampsia and the HELLP syndrome

A systematic literature search for the association of aCL antibodies with preeclampsia generated 68528 abstracts and 64 full-text articles (7). Inclusion criteria were cohort-, case-control or controlled cross-sectional-studies comprising women with no autoimmune diseases but with IgG or IgM aCL antibody of at least 20 units, or both, with preeclampsia as endpoint. Twelve studies were included in a meta-analysis. The study comprised publications from before 2006 (when new criteria were established) and thus did not consider the latest antiphospholipid criteria when addressing aCL cut-off levels in the final analysis[7]. Different methods of diagnosing preeclampsia were used in these 12 publications. The severity of preeclampsia was not stated in 7 of the publications. Pooled OR for association of aCL antibodies with preeclampsia was 2.9 (95% CI 1.4-5.9)[5]. Pooled OR for aCL antibodies and severe preeclampsia was 11.2 (95 % CI 2.7-46.8). It was concluded that moderate-to-high levels of aCL antibodies were associated with preeclampsia. There was, however, insufficient evidence to advocate use of aCL antibodies as predictors of preeclampsia[5].

Branch and Khamashta reported in 2003 that in women with SLE and prior thrombosis the median rate of preeclampsia was 32% ranging up to 50%; that of preterm births ranged from 32% to 65%[2]. One study suggested that the second trimester Doppler ultrasound examination may be the best predictor of late pregnancy outcome in SLE and/or the APS[49].

Women with APAs seem to have increased risk of developing a HELLP syndrome[31;50-52]. One series, that comprised 75 pregnancies with primary or secondary APS, included 7 women who had 8 episodes of HELLP[53]. A retrospective analysis of 16 episodes of HELLP complicating APS comprised 15 women. APS was primary in 9 women and secondary in 6 cases[31]. The HELLP syndrome was complete in 10 episodes and partial in 6, occurring in the second trimester (44%) in 7 cases (the earliest at 18 weeks' gestation), and 12.5% at 18-20 weeks[31]. The outcome was 8 live births, 2 stillbirths and 6 fetal deaths[31]. Backos *et al.* reported two cases of a HELLP syndrome in a series of 150 pregnancies in women with recurrent miscarriages and APAs[54]. In a placebo controlled study of intravenous immunoglobulin treatment for APS, Branch *et al.* observed that 6 out of 16 women with APA developed severe preeclampsia and/or HELLP[55]. In a literature review of well described cases of HELLP complicating APS, HELLP occurred before 27 weeks' gestation in most cases. The HELLP syndrome occurred as early as the 8th week of gestation[56]. Thus, HELLP appears to develop earlier in women with APS than in women in the general population. The condition also tends to be more severe[31].

In the cases of HELLP syndrome associated with APS published by Le Thi Thoung *et al.* no case of liver infarction was observed[31]. Pauzner *et al.*, on the other hand, found liver infarcts to be almost always associated with APS in women with a HELLP syndrome[56]. Pauzner *et al.* also reviewed 30 pregnancies in 28 women with pregnancy-associated hepatic infarcts. APA were present in 15 of 16 patients with available data, 16 had typical HELLP syndrome. Almost all patients with hepatic infarcts were APA positive in addition to suffering from complete or atypical HELLP syndrome. Hepatic infarcts occurred at all stages of pregnancy(57). In APA positive women the HELLP syndrome usually occurs during the second trimester of pregnancy; one-third of these develop hepatic infarcts[58].

10. Pathogenesis of APS

Habitual abortions (defined as ≥3 spontaneous consecutive pregnancy losses) affect 1-2% of women in reproductive age. Up to 5% of women in reproductive age have ≥2 recurrent abortions[59]. APA antibodies have also been implicated in first trimester miscarriage[60]. Deleterious effects of APA antibodies in women with recurrent abortions is extended to pre-embryonic and embryonic losses[30]. APA may impair both trophoblast invasion in the decidua and the spiral arteries and the placental hormone production and cause utero-placental insufficiency and fetal loss[30].

Serbie *et al.* examined the products of consumption from early pregnancy failures in women with recurrent fetal loss to investigate the mechanism of pregnancy loss[61]. There were 31 primary APS-positive, 50 APA-negative, 34 aneuploid and 20 control cases with termination of pregnancy for social reasons at 6-14 weeks gestation. Chorionic villous morphology and frequency of intervillous thrombosis were not different among groups. Normal decidual and endovascular trophoblast invasion in the spiral ateries was identified significantly less frequent in primary APA-positive cases (24%), compared with controls (75%), aneuploid (53%), or APA-negative cases (61%; Z=-3.0, P <0.01)(61). Chorionic villous morphology and intervillous thrombosis were not different among the groups. Normal decidual and endovascular trophoblast invasion in spiral ateries was identified significantly less frequent in primary APA-positive cases (24%), than in controls (75%), aneuploid (53%), or APA-negative cases (61 %). It was concluded that defective decidual and spiral atery endovascular trophoblast invasion, rather than excessive intervillous thrombosis, is the most frequent histological abnormality in primary APA-positive women with early pregnancy loss[61]. In recurrent miscarriage with APAs, 20-60% of the aborted foetuses are chromosomally abnormal, and chromosomal anomalies as cause of fetal loss must be considered also in APA positive patients[4;62;63].

There is a variety of mechanisms by which APA antibodies may cause pregnancy loss. APA antibodies may interfere with the normal *in vivo* function of phospholipids or phospholipid-binding proteins that are crucial to regulation of coagulation[2]. Tissue factor (TF), the major cellular initiator of the coagulation protease cascade, plays important roles in both thrombosis and inflammation[64]. *In-vitro* studies have shown that certain APAs, specifically those directed against β2GP1, induce expression of TF[37;65]. APAs also dysregulate the fibrinolytic system by cross-linking with annexin II (profibrinolytic endothelial cell surface receptor) on the endothelial cell surface inducing increased expression of TF[64]. Autoantibodies have a causative role in monocyte TF expression. Growing evidence suggests that APA-dependent induction of TF activity on circulating blood monocytes is an important mechanism of hypercoagulability in APS[64]. TF acting as an pro-inflammatory molecule enhances neutrophil activity which may cause trophoblast injury, placental dysfunction and damage to the embryo[64]. Activated neutrophiles release reactive oxygen species and proteolytic enzymes leading to decidual damage[64]. Complement C3 and C5 play a role in APA-induced thrombosis[64]. *In vitro* and animal studies have shown that APAs can bind directly to trophoblasts cells and cause cellular injury, defective extravillous cytotrophoblast (EVT) invasion (in the decidua and spiral arteries), and induce a local inflammatory response as a result of activation of complement[8]. Activation of complement and recruitment of inflammatory cells within the decidual tissues are necessary steps in APA-induced pregnancy loss[66].

The negative effect of APS on pregnancy is most likely tied to abnormal placental function[2]. Adverse pregnancy outcomes in women with APS may result from poor placental perfusion due to localised thrombosis, perhaps through interference by APA antibodies with trophoblastic annexin V[30].

Some investigators have found narrowing of spiral arteries, intimal thickening, acute atherosis and fibrinoid necrosis in the placenta of women with fetal loss associated with APS. Others have found extensive placental necrosis, infarctions and thrombosis[2]. APAs may activate endothelial cells as indicated by increased expression of adhesion molecules, secretion of cytokines, and production of arachidonic acid metabolites[2].

The pathogenesis of APA-mediated thrombosis probably involves several pathogenic mechanisms including thrombogenic microparticles derived from maternal endothelial cells, platelets and trophoblasts[67]. Other mechanisms are inhibition of the natural antithrombotic proteins, such as protein C, TF pathway inhibitor, annexin V, activation of the complement system and impairment of fibrinolysis which regulate thrombus remodelling and dissolution[68].

Vitamin D is essential for calcium and bone mineralism, but is also a mediator of many other effects such as modulation of the immune response, being able to combat certain microorganisms[69]. Vitamin D deficiency has been reported to be common among patients with APS and is associated with clinically defined thrombotic events. Vitamin D deficiency (serum level ≤ 15 ng/ml) occured in 50% of cases with APS compared to 30% of control subjects significantly correlating with thrombosis, neurological and ophthalmic manifestations, pulmonary hypertension, *livedo reticularis* (a vascular condition characterized by purplish mottling of the skin) and skin ulcers[69]. An inverse correlation between vitamin D levels and thrombosis was found in this cohort[69]. Vitamin D is a potent inhibitor of the anti-β2GPI antibody-mediated expression of TF induced by endothelial cells[69]. Thus, vitamin D deficiency might be associated with decreased inhibition of TF expression and increased coagulation in APS.

Studies have also shown that inflammatory mechanisms in the placental bed may contribute to APS[64]. Some studies suggest that APA induce a pro-coagulant response in endothelial cells and monocytes through interaction with toll-like receptor- 4 (TLR-4)[64].

11. Therapeutic options

Over a long period treatment of APS included low-dose aspirin either alone or combined with prednisone, unfractioned heparin or low molecular weight heparin (LMWH), intravenous immunoglobulin infusion or plasma exchange[36]. Warfarin crosses the placenta and is teratogenic in the first trimester[8]. Women, who are on long- term warfarin treatment because of previous thrombosis, should switch to heparin when trying to conceive or when pregnancy is confirmed[8]. In high risk groups, such as women with mechanical heart valves, warfarin may be used in pregnancy, but only after organogenesis (6th-12th week) because of high risk of fetal malformations[3]. Warfarin treatment is however, also associated with spontaneous abortions, prematurity and CNS abnormalities[70]. As warfarin cross the placenta and subsequently affect fetal coagulation, there is a risk for bleeding complications in the fetus and during birth[71].In the Cochrane review by Empson *et al.* it was concluded that a combination therapy with heparin and aspirin may reduce pregnancy loss in women with APA by 54%[36]. Heparin combined with aspirin reduced the pregnancy loss more than aspirin alone (relative risk (RR) 0.46; 95% CI 0.29-0.71)[36]. In the trials of prednisone and aspirin, no benefit was shown, rather a significant increase in prematurity (RR 4.83; 95% CI 2.85-8.21)[36]. In addition, prednisone was also associated with a 3.5-fold (95% CI 1.5-8.2) greater risk of gestational diabetes than aspirin alone, heparin and aspirin, or placebo[72-74]. Prednisone appears to have no role in the treatment of recurrent pregnancy loss associated with APA antibodies[36].

Current management of APS in pregnancy generally includes heparin combined with aspirin. LMWHs are at least as effective as unfractioned heparin and are safer[21;71]. The rationale of this combination is that aspirin may inhibit APA mediated hypercoagulopathy in the intervillous space of the placenta while heparin may prevent APA from interfering with cytotrophoblast migration and promote blastocyst implantation in addition to prevention of venous thrombosis[75].

Prolonged heparin treatment may induce osteoporosis. Recently, there has been a move towards low molecular weight heparin because of the advantages of daily dosing and a perception that it may have less effect on bone mineral density than heparin[36].

The pregnancy- associated prothrombotic changes in the coagulation system are maximal immediately after delivery[21]. Despite lack of controlled studies regarding duration of anticoagulation, it is well accepted that persistent APA-positive women require post-partum anticoagulation. Therefore, it is desirable to continue LMWH during labor or delivery in women receiving antenatal thromboprophylaxis[21]. The duration of recommendations range from 3-5 days[21], to 6-8 weeks[76] and up to 12 weeks[77].

12. Use of anticoagulants in lactating women

Heparin and LMVHs are not secreted into breast milk and can be safely given to nursing mothers. Warfarin is safe after delivery and for breast feeding, althogh it requires close monitoring, frequent visits to an anticoagulant clinic and carries an increased risk of postpartum hemorrhage and perineal hematoma compared with LMWH [21]. Warfarin does not induce an anticoagulant effect in the breast-fed infant. Therefore, the use of warfarin in women who require postpartum anticoagulation therapy is safe and these women should be encoraged to breast feed[78].

No randomised controlled trials have investigated prevention in women with a history of late miscarriage, fetal death and IUGR. Most obstetricians would consider treatment with low-dose aspirin and prophylactic dose of (low molecular weight) heparin in such cases. In women with APA antibodies, and a history of severe preeclampsia, at least low dose aspirin (75-80 mg once a day) is recommended[79]. Glucorticoids, cytotoxic agents, and intravenous immunoglobulin have no confirmed benefit and should not be used to treat pregnant women with APS[79].

13. Contraception after birth

Oral estrogen coating contraceptives increase the maternal thrombotic risk of women with APAs and SLE[80]. Therefore, intrauterine devices are probably more appropriate. However, progesterone-only contraceptives do not increase the risk of thrombosis[81]. If a woman with

APS wants to be pregnant again, pre-conceptional treatment deserves consideration[42]. Some women with APS may need life-long warfarin treatment.

14. References

[1] de LB, Mertens K, de Groot PG. Mechanisms of disease: antiphospholipid antibodies-from clinical association to pathologic mechanism. Nat Clin Pract Rheumatol 2008 Apr;4(4):192-9.

[2] Branch DW, Khamashta MA. Antiphospholipid syndrome: obstetric diagnosis, management, and controversies. Obstet Gynecol 2003 Jun;101(6):1333-44.

[3] Ahmed K, Darakhshan A, Au E, Khamashta MA, Katsoulis IE. Postpartum spontaneous colonic perforation due to antiphospholipid syndrome. World J Gastroenterol 2009 Jan 28;15(4):502-5.

[4] Carp HJ. Antiphospholipid syndrome in pregnancy. Curr Opin Obstet Gynecol 2004 Apr;16(2):129-35.

[5] do Prado AD, Piovesan DM, Staub HL, Horta BL. Association of anticardiolipin antibodies with preeclampsia: a systematic review and meta-analysis. Obstet Gynecol 2010 Dec;116(6):1433-43.

[6] Tincani A, Andreoli L, Chighizola C, Meroni PL. The interplay between the antiphospholipid syndrome and systemic lupus erythematosus. Autoimmunity 2009 May;42(4):257-9.

[7] Miyakis S, Lockshin MD, Atsumi T, Branch DW, Brey RL, Cervera R, et al. International consensus statement on an update of the classification criteria for definite antiphospholipid syndrome (APS). J Thromb Haemost 2006 Feb;4(2):295-306.

[8] Cohen D, Berger SP, Steup-Beekman GM, Bloemenkamp KW, Bajema IM. Diagnosis and management of the antiphospholipid syndrome. BMJ 2010;340:c2541.

[9] Serrano F, Nogueira I, Borges A, Branco J. Primary antiphospholipid syndrome: pregnancy outcome in a portuguese population. Acta Reumatol Port 2009 Jul;34(3):492-7.

[10] Cervera R, Piette JC, Font J, Khamashta MA, Shoenfeld Y, Camps MT, et al. Antiphospholipid syndrome: clinical and immunologic manifestations and patterns of disease expression in a cohort of 1,000 patients. Arthritis Rheum 2002 Apr;46(4):1019-27.

[11] Hamilton ME. Superior mesenteric artery thrombosis associated with antiphospholipid syndrome. West J Med 1991 Aug;155(2):174-6.

[12] Harris EN, Gharavi AE, Hughes GR. Anti-phospholipid antibodies. Clin Rheum Dis 1985 Dec;11(3):591-609.

[13] Brey RL. Antiphospholipid antibodies in young adults with stroke. J Thromb Thrombolysis 2005 Oct;20(2):105-12.

[14] Coull BM, Levine SR, Brey RL. The role of antiphospholipid antibodies in stroke. Neurol Clin 1992 Feb;10(1):125-43.

[15] Clinical and laboratory findings in patients with antiphospholipid antibodies and cerebral ischemia. The Antiphospholipid Antibodies in Stroke Study Group. Stroke 1990 Sep;21(9):1268-73.

[16] Uthman I, Khamashta M. The abdominal manifestations of the antiphospholipid syndrome. Rheumatology (Oxford) 2007 Nov;46(11):1641-7.

[17] Si-Hoe CK, Thng CH, Chee SG, Teo EK, Chng HH. Abdominal computed tomography in systemic lupus erythematosus. Clin Radiol 1997 Apr;52(4):284-9.
[18] Raval M, Paul A. Cerebral Venous Thrombosis and Venous Infarction: Case Report of a Rare Initial Presentation of Smoker's Polycythemia. Case Rep Neurol 2010;2(3):150-6.
[19] Csepany T, Bereczki D, Kollar J, Sikula J, Kiss E, Csiba L. MRI findings in central nervous system systemic lupus erythematosus are associated with immunoserological parameters and hypertension. J Neurol 2003 Nov;250(11):1348-54.
[20] Lindqvist P, Dahlback B, Marsal K. Thrombotic risk during pregnancy: a population study. Obstet Gynecol 1999 Oct;94(4):595-9.
[21] Royal College of Obstetricians and Gynaecologists. Thromboprophylaxis during pregnancy, labour and after vaginal delivery. Guideline 2004; http://www.blackwellpublishing.com/medicine/bmj/nnf5/pdfs/uk guidelines/ENOXAPARIN.
[22] McColl MD, Ramsay JE, Tait RC, Walker ID, McCall F, Conkie JA, et al. Risk factors for pregnancy associated venous thromboembolism. Thromb Haemost 1997 Oct;78(4):1183-8.
[23] Simpson EL, Lawrenson RA, Nightingale AL, Farmer RD. Venous thromboembolism in pregnancy and the puerperium: incidence and additional risk factors from a London perinatal database. BJOG 2001 Jan;108(1):56-60.
[24] Khamashta MA, Cuadrado MJ, Mujic F, Taub NA, Hunt BJ, Hughes GR. The management of thrombosis in the antiphospholipid-antibody syndrome. N Engl J Med 1995 Apr 13;332(15):993-7.
[25] Pabinger I, Grafenhofer H, Kyrle PA, Quehenberger P, Mannhalter C, Lechner K, et al. Temporary increase in the risk for recurrence during pregnancy in women with a history of venous thromboembolism. Blood 2002 Aug 1;100(3):1060-2.
[26] Endler G, Marsik C, Jilma B, Schickbauer T, Vormittag R, Wagner O, et al. Anti-cardiolipin antibodies and overall survival in a large cohort: preliminary report. Clin Chem 2006 Jun;52(6):1040-4.
[27] Asherson RA. The catastrophic antiphospholipid syndrome. J Rheumatol 1992 Apr;19(4):508-12.
[28] Gomez-Puerta JA, Cervera R, Espinosa G, Asherson RA, Garcia-Carrasco M, da Costa IP, et al. Catastrophic antiphospholipid syndrome during pregnancy and puerperium: maternal and fetal characteristics of 15 cases. Ann Rheum Dis 2007 Jun;66(6):740-6.
[29] Erkan D, Espinosa G, Cervera R. Catastrophic antiphospholipid syndrome: updated diagnostic algorithms. Autoimmun Rev 2010 Dec;10(2):74-9.
[30] Levine JS, Branch DW, Rauch J. The antiphospholipid syndrome. N Engl J Med 2002 Mar 7;346(10):752-63.
[31] Le Thi TD, Tieulie N, Costedoat N, Andreu MR, Wechsler B, Vauthier-Brouzes D, et al. The HELLP syndrome in the antiphospholipid syndrome: retrospective study of 16 cases in 15 women. Ann Rheum Dis 2005 Feb;64(2):273-8.
[32] Sinha J, Chowdhry I, Sedan S, Barland P. Bone marrow necrosis and refractory HELLP syndrome in a patient with catastrophic antiphospholipid antibody syndrome. J Rheumatol 2002 Jan;29(1):195-7.

[33] Carreras LO, Forastiero RR, Martinuzzo ME. Which are the best biological markers of the antiphospholipid syndrome? J Autoimmun 2000 Sep;15(2):163-72.
[34] Opatrny L, David M, Kahn SR, Shrier I, Rey E. Association between antiphospholipid antibodies and recurrent fetal loss in women without autoimmune disease: a metaanalysis. J Rheumatol 2006 Nov;33(11):2214-21.
[35] Love PE, Santoro SA. Antiphospholipid antibodies: anticardiolipin and the lupus anticoagulant in systemic lupus erythematosus (SLE) and in non-SLE disorders. Prevalence and clinical significance. Ann Intern Med 1990 May 1;112(9):682-98.
[36] Empson M, Lassere M, Craig JC, Scott JR. Recurrent pregnancy loss with antiphospholipid antibody: a systematic review of therapeutic trials. Obstet Gynecol 2002 Jan;99(1):135-44.
[37] Amengual O, Atsumi T, Khamashta MA, Hughes GR. The role of the tissue factor pathway in the hypercoagulable state in patients with the antiphospholipid syndrome. Thromb Haemost 1998 Feb;79(2):276-81.
[38] Galli M, Comfurius P, Maassen C, Hemker HC, de Baets MH, van Breda-Vriesman PJ, et al. Anticardiolipin antibodies (ACA) directed not to cardiolipin but to a plasma protein cofactor. Lancet 1990 Jun 30;335(8705):1544-7.
[39] Matsuura E, Igarashi Y, Fujimoto M, Ichikawa K, Koike T. Anticardiolipin cofactor(s) and differential diagnosis of autoimmune disease. Lancet 1990 Jul 21;336(8708):177-8.
[40] McNeil HP, Simpson RJ, Chesterman CN, Krilis SA. Anti-phospholipid antibodies are directed against a complex antigen that includes a lipid-binding inhibitor of coagulation: beta 2-glycoprotein I (apolipoprotein H). Proc Natl Acad Sci U S A 1990 Jun;87(11):4120-4.
[41] Urbanus RT, de Groot PG. Antiphospholipid antibodies--we are not quite there yet. Blood Rev 2011 Mar;25(2):97-106.
[42] Reber G, Tincani A, Sanmarco M, de MP, Boffa MC. Proposals for the measurement of anti-beta2-glycoprotein I antibodies. Standardization group of the European Forum on Antiphospholipid Antibodies. J Thromb Haemost 2004 Oct;2(10):1860-2.
[43] Tincani A, Allegri F, Sanmarco M, Cinquini M, Taglietti M, Balestrieri G, et al. Anticardiolipin antibody assay: a methodological analysis for a better consensus in routine determinations--a cooperative project of the European Antiphospholipid Forum. Thromb Haemost 2001 Aug;86(2):575-83.
[44] Pengo V, Tripodi A, Reber G, Rand JH, Ortel TL, Galli M, et al. Update of the guidelines for lupus anticoagulant detection. Subcommittee on Lupus Anticoagulant/Antiphospholipid Antibody of the Scientific and Standardisation Committee of the International Society on Thrombosis and Haemostasis. J Thromb Haemost 2009 Oct;7(10):1737-40.
[45] Lim W. Antiphospholipid antibody syndrome. Hematology Am Soc Hematol Educ Program 2009;233-9.
[46] Pauzner R, Greinacher A, Selleng K, Althaus K, Shenkman B, Seligsohn U. False-positive tests for heparin-induced thrombocytopenia in patients with antiphospholipid syndrome and systemic lupus erythematosus. J Thromb Haemost 2009 Jul;7(7):1070-4.
[47] Symmers WS. Thrombotic microangiopathic haemolytic anaemia (thrombotic microangiopathy). Br Med J 1952 Oct 25;2(4790):897-903.

[48] Espinosa G, Bucciarelli S, Cervera R, Lozano M, Reverter JC, De La Red G, et al. Thrombotic microangiopathic haemolytic anaemia and antiphospholipid antibodies. Ann Rheum Dis 2004 Jun;63(6):730-6.
[49] Le Thi HD, Wechsler B, Vauthier-Brouzes D, Duhaut P, Costedoat N, Andreu MR, et al. The second trimester Doppler ultrasound examination is the best predictor of late pregnancy outcome in systemic lupus erythematosus and/or the antiphospholipid syndrome. Rheumatology (Oxford) 2006 Mar;45(3):332-8.
[50] Wada Y, Sakamaki Y, Kobayashi D, Ajiro J, Moro H, Murakami S, et al. HELLP syndrome, multiple liver infarctions, and intrauterine fetal death in a patient with systemic lupus erythematosus and antiphospholipid syndrome. Intern Med 2009;48(17):1555-8.
[51] Haram K, Trovik J, Sandset PM, Hordnes K. Severe syndrome of hemolysis, elevated liver enzymes and low platelets (HELLP) in the 18th week of pregnancy associated with the antiphospholipid-antibody syndrome. Acta Obstet Gynecol Scand 2003 Jul;82(7):679-80.
[52] Haram K, Bjorge L, Sandset PM. Successful preconceptional prophylactic treatment with combined acetyl salicylic acid and low-molecular heparin (Fragmin) in a case of antiphospholipid-antibody syndrome with prior life-threatening hemolysis, elevated liver enzymes and low-platelet syndrome: a case report. Acta Obstet Gynecol Scand 2005 Dec;84(12):1213-4.
[53] Huong DL, Wechsler B, Bletry O, Vauthier-Brouzes D, Lefebvre G, Piette JC. A study of 75 pregnancies in patients with antiphospholipid syndrome. J Rheumatol 2001 Sep;28(9):2025-30.
[54] Backos M, Rai R, Baxter N, Chilcott IT, Cohen H, Regan L. Pregnancy complications in women with recurrent miscarriage associated with antiphospholipid antibodies treated with low dose aspirin and heparin. Br J Obstet Gynaecol 1999 Feb;106(2):102-7.
[55] Branch DW, Peaceman AM, Druzin M, Silver RK, El-Sayed Y, Silver RM, et al. A multicenter, placebo-controlled pilot study of intravenous immune globulin treatment of antiphospholipid syndrome during pregnancy. The Pregnancy Loss Study Group. Am J Obstet Gynecol 2000 Jan;182(1 Pt 1):122-7.
[56] Pauzner R, Dulitzky M, Carp H, Mayan H, Kenett R, Farfel Z, et al. Hepatic infarctions during pregnancy are associated with the antiphospholipid syndrome and in addition with complete or incomplete HELLP syndrome. J Thromb Haemost 2003 Aug;1(8):1758-63.
[57] Asherson RA, Galarza-Maldonado C, Sanin-Blair J. The HELLP syndrome, antiphospholipid antibodies, and syndromes. Clin Rheumatol 2008 Jan;27(1):1-4.
[58] Tsirigotis P, Mantzios G, Pappa V, Girkas K, Salamalekis G, Koutras A, et al. Antiphospholipid syndrome: a predisposing factor for early onset HELLP syndrome. Rheumatol Int 2007 Dec;28(2):171-4.
[59] Blumenfeld Z, Brenner B. Thrombophilia-associated pregnancy wastage. Fertil Steril 1999 Nov;72(5):765-74.
[60] Stone S, Khamashta MA, Poston L. Placentation, antiphospholipid syndrome and pregnancy outcome. Lupus 2001;10(2):67-74.

[61] Sebire NJ, Fox H, Backos M, Rai R, Paterson C, Regan L. Defective endovascular trophoblast invasion in primary antiphospholipid antibody syndrome-associated early pregnancy failure. Hum Reprod 2002 Apr;17(4):1067-71.
[62] Ogasawara M, Aoki K, Okada S, Suzumori K. Embryonic karyotype of abortuses in relation to the number of previous miscarriages. Fertil Steril 2000 Feb;73(2):300-4.
[63] Takakuwa K, Asano K, Arakawa M, Yasuda M, Hasegawa I, Tanaka K. Chromosome analysis of aborted conceptuses of recurrent aborters positive for anticardiolipin antibody. Fertil Steril 1997 Jul;68(1):54-8.
[64] Girardi G, Mackman N. Tissue factor in antiphospholipid antibody-induced pregnancy loss: a pro-inflammatory molecule. Lupus 2008 Oct;17(10):931-6.
[65] Zhou H, Wolberg AS, Roubey RA. Characterization of monocyte tissue factor activity induced by IgG antiphospholipid antibodies and inhibition by dilazep. Blood 2004 Oct 15;104(8):2353-8.
[66] Girardi G, Berman J, Redecha P, Spruce L, Thurman JM, Kraus D, et al. Complement C5a receptors and neutrophils mediate fetal injury in the antiphospholipid syndrome. J Clin Invest 2003 Dec;112(11):1644-54.
[67] Pierangeli SS, Chen PP, Raschi E, Scurati S, Grossi C, Borghi MO, et al. Antiphospholipid antibodies and the antiphospholipid syndrome: pathogenic mechanisms. Semin Thromb Hemost 2008 Apr;34(3):236-50.
[68] Krone KA, Allen KL, McCrae KR. Impaired fibrinolysis in the antiphospholipid syndrome. Curr Rheumatol Rep 2010 Feb;12(1):53-7.
[69] Agmon-Levin N, Blank M, Zandman-Goddard G, Orbach H, Meroni PL, Tincani A, et al. Vitamin D: an instrumental factor in the anti-phospholipid syndrome by inhibition of tissue factor expression. Ann Rheum Dis 2011 Jan;70(1):145-50.
[70] van Driel D., Wesseling J, Sauer PJ, Touwen BC, van d, V, Heymans HS. Teratogen update: fetal effects after in utero exposure to coumarins overview of cases, follow-up findings, and pathogenesis. Teratology 2002 Sep;66(3):127-40.
[71] Bates SM, Greer IA, Pabinger I, Sofaer S, Hirsh J. Venous thromboembolism, thrombophilia, antithrombotic therapy, and pregnancy: American College of Chest Physicians Evidence-Based Clinical Practice Guidelines (8th Edition). Chest 2008 Jun;133(6 Suppl):844S-86S.
[72] Cowchock FS, Reece EA, Balaban D, Branch DW, Plouffe L. Repeated fetal losses associated with antiphospholipid antibodies: a collaborative randomized trial comparing prednisone with low-dose heparin treatment. Am J Obstet Gynecol 1992 May;166(5):1318-23.
[73] Laskin CA, Bombardier C, Hannah ME, Mandel FP, Ritchie JW, Farewell V, et al. Prednisone and aspirin in women with autoantibodies and unexplained recurrent fetal loss. N Engl J Med 1997 Jul 17;337(3):148-53.
[74] Silver RK, MacGregor SN, Sholl JS, Hobart JM, Neerhof MG, Ragin A. Comparative trial of prednisone plus aspirin versus aspirin alone in the treatment of anticardiolipin antibody-positive obstetric patients. Am J Obstet Gynecol 1993 Dec;169(6):1411-7.
[75] Allahbadia GN, Allahadia SG. Low molecular weight heparin in immunological recurrent abortion- the incredible cure. J Assist Reprod Genet 2005;20:82-90.
[76] Derksen RH, Khamashta MA, Branch DW. Management of the obstetric antiphospholipid syndrome. Arthritis Rheum 2004 Apr;50(4):1028-39.

[77] Erkan D. The relation between antiphospholipid syndrome-related pregnancy morbidity and non-gravid vascular thrombosis: a review of the literature and management strategies. Curr Rheumatol Rep 2002 Oct;4(5):379-86.
[78] Ginsberg JS, Greer I, Hirsh J. Use of antithrombotic agents during pregnancy. Chest 2001 Jan;119(1 Suppl):122S-31S.
[79] Giannakopoulos B, Krilis SA. How I treat the antiphospholipid syndrome. Blood 2009 Sep 3;114(10):2020-30.
[80] Duarte C, Ines L. Oral contraceptives and systemic lupus erythematosus: what should we advise to our patients? Acta Reumatol Port 2010 Apr;35(2):133-40.
[81] Erkan D, Patel S, Nuzzo M, Gerosa M, Meroni PL, Tincani A, et al. Management of the controversial aspects of the antiphospholipid syndrome pregnancies: a guide for clinicians and researchers. Rheumatology (Oxford) 2008 Jun;47 Suppl 3:iii23-iii27.

11

Update on Antiphospholipid Antibody Syndrome Management

Rocco Manganelli, Salvatore Iannaccone,
Serena Manganelli and Mario Iannaccone
AORN 'S.G. Moscati', Avellino
Italy

1. Introduction

The anthiphospholipid syndrome (APS) is characterized by a high risk of venous and arterial thrombosis and by complications during pregnancy, especially recurrent miscarriages. The thrombotic event is caused by a complex interaction between antiphospholipid antibodies (aPLs) and endothelium and platelets. Inflammation may play a role in the pathology of APS even though the consensus of Sydney (Miyakis et al., 2006) requires the absence of vascular inflammation signs for the diagnosis of APS. However, the complement system has recently been involved in the pathogenesis of fetal losses in animal models and, interestingly, the protective role of heparin in such cases could be due to the complement inhibition rather than to anticoagulation. The treatment of APS is based on antiplatelet drugs (aspirin) and anticoagulants (both heparins and vitamin K antagonists). In the acute phase the treatment is in general very similar to that of non-APS thrombosis, that is with unfractionated heparin (UFH) therapy followed by oral anticoagulation. However, APS treatment remains problematic due to lack of standardized laboratory tests and of randomized controlled trials (RCTs).

2. Prophilaxis of thromboembolism

2.1 Secondary prophylaxis of vascular thrombosis

The risk of thrombotic recurrences is lower if the venous district, rather than the arterial one, is involved. The key issue in the antithrombotic management of APS patients concerns whether arterial and venous events should receive the same intensity of therapy. According to Ruiz-Irastorza review we can treat lower-risk patients with conventional anticoagulation in order to reach Target International Ratio (INR) values between 2.0 and 3.0, reserving high-intensity anticoagulation (INR > 3.0) to patients with arterial thrombosis or venous thrombotic recurrences (Ruiz-Irastorza et al., 2007). On the contrary Lim argues in his systematic review that high-intensity anticoagulation (INR: 3.0-4.0) is not better than conventional anticoagulation in protecting patients with first thrombotic venous event and non-cerebral arterial thrombosis (Lim et al., 2006). The conclusions are based on two RCTs (Crowther et al.,2003; Finazzi et al.,2005) that are susceptible to criticism as: 1. recruitment mainly concerns venous thromboses, with the exception of strokes and recurrent thrombosis, the sample is not representative of the APS population. 2. In the high-intensity anticoagulation arms, the warfarin dose is often subtherapeutic with frequent thrombotic recurrences with INR < 3.0. Cerebral thromboses are the most frequent arterial events of APS. The risk of new cerebral thromboses is addressed by the prospective Antiphospholipid Antibodies and Stroke Study (APASS) (Levine et al., 2006), that showed no difference in the comparison between a single antiplatelet (aspirin 325 mg/day) and a single anticoagulant (warfarin: INR 1.4 - 2.8). In this study the extension of the results to the APS population is questionable, as the analysis of aPLs is made on a single sample at the time of enrolment, while for the diagnosis of APS it is essential to have at least two measurements taken at a distance of some time. A recent small Japanese RCT (Okuma et al., 2009), that instead only enrolled patients with definite diagnosis of APS according to the consensus of Sydney, shows that the combination of conventional anticoagulation plus low-dose aspirin (LDA) (100 mg/day) is more effective than aspirin used on its own. In conclusion, we believe that the prevention of arterial thromboses requires either anticoagulation at INR 3.0-4.0 or a combined treatment. Apart from the debate regarding the intensity of anticoagulation, there is a general agreement upon it being maintained indefinitely, even if some authors argue that a finite treatment can be performed if the first episode of venous thromboembolism occurs in the context of a transient and reversible risk factor (surgery, prolonged immobilization, pregnancy, estrogen therapy) (Giannakopoulos & Krillis, 2009).

2.1.1 Prophylaxis of APS obstetric complications

The pregnancy morbidity of APS includes maternal thromboses, spontaneous abortions before the 10th week and late obstetric complications (fetal deaths, premature births caused by preeclampsia or placental insufficiency). Pregnant women with aPLs positivity should be stratified in order to perform the optimal treatment: A. Women with ascertained APS and previous thrombosis, B. Pregnant women with a history of recurrent miscarriages, C. Pregnant women with a history of fetal deaths > 10 weeks and premature births <34 weeks. A. Women with ascertained APS and previous thrombotic event, possibly already on warfarin therapy, should undergo combination therapy with LDA (75-100mg/day) plus therapeutic doses of unfractionated heparin (UFH) (subcutaneously every 8-12 h) or low molecular weight heparin (LMWH) (e.g. enoxaparin 1 mg/kg subcutaneously every 12 h). During pregnancy, warfarin must be stopped between the 6th and the 12th week due to its teratogenicity, and also afterwards it can cause fetal hemorrhage. B. Women with a history of recurrent miscarriages should be treated with a combination therapy of LDA plus prophylactic doses of UFH (5000-7500 IU subcutaneously every 12 h) or LMWH in prophylactic doses (e.g., enoxaparin 1 mg/kg/day). C. Women with a history of fetal deaths >10 weeks and premature births <34 weeks should be treated with a combination therapy of LDA plus prophylactic/intermediate doses of UFH (e.g., 7500-10000 IU subcutaneously every 12 h) or LDA plus LMWH usually in prophylactic doses (e.g., enoxaparin 1 mg/kg every 24 hours). These treatment patterns derive from meta-analysis and expert guidelines (Empson et al., 2005; Bates et al.,2008) . There is not indisputable evidence that anticoagulation with heparins works better than aspirin alone and it has not even been established which is more effective between UFH or LMWH. In fact, if on the one hand RCTs have shown a reduction in the number of pregnancy losses with a combination of UFH-LDA, on the other hand other RCTs, that used LMWH-LDA, do not show a clear superiority. There are many observational studies in favor of the effectiveness of LDA alone.

Moreover, the PARIS Collaborative Group meta-analysis (Askie et al.,2007) shows that the pregnancy outcome in women at high risk of preeclampsia treated with LDA, is similar to that of the general population, after 20 weeks of gestation. Two pilot studies show no differences when comparing the LDA-UFH to the LDA-LMWH combination therapy (Noble et al., 2005; Stephenson et al., 2004). In order to clarify controversies, a trial with three arms is strongly needed: 1. UFH versus LDA, 2. LMWH versus LDA, 3. LDA alone (Mehdi et al.,2010)

2.1.2 Primary prophylaxis of vascular thrombosis

The group of subjects with aPLs positivity in absence of clinical APS manifestations (aPLs carriers), includes asymptomatic carriers, patients with SLE, and pregnant women aPL-positive without a history of obstetric complications and/or thrombosis. Only some of the aPLs carriers will progress towards overt APS and we still do not know why some will develop the thrombotic event and others will not. The role played by additional risk factors, both congenital and acquired, is also under investigation. It is clear, however, that the elimination of reversible risk factors and the prophylaxis during high risk periods, such as prolonged immobilization and surgery, are paramount in the primary prophylaxis of thrombosis. In asymptomatic carriers, for whom the risk of thrombosis is very low (<1%), a prophylactic use of aspirin is not justified. In the APLASA RCT (Erkan et al., 2007), aspirin at 81 mg/day did not prove superior to placebo in preventing the first thrombotic event in asymptomatic individuals persistently aPL-positive. Thus, the approach based on thrombotic risk stratification is reasonable in healthy carriers, reserving the LDA prophylaxis to individuals with additional risk factors (hypertension, diabetes, hypercholesterolemia, smoking, estrogen therapy) and/or immunological high risk profile (high aPLs titre, especially lupus anticoagulant (LA) and 'multiple' positivity: aCL, LA, β2GPI). The risk of thrombosis in both SLE patients and pregnant women carriers, is on the other hand higher (3-4% and 3-7% respectively). These categories will benefit from LDA prophylaxis as demonstrated by several observational studies (Hereng et al., 2008 ; Erkan et al.,2001) . No randomized studies show that hydroxychloroquine, a drug that reduces platelet activation aPL-induced, has also an added prophylactic value in SLE patients (Kaiser et al., 2009).

3. Management of cardiac diseases in APS

3.1 Introduction

APL antibodies are associated with a wide spectrum of cardiac manifestations that include accelerated atherosclerosis, ischemic coronary artery disease (CAD), valve abnormalities, intracardiac thrombosis, pulmonary hypertension (PH).

3.1.1 Atherosclerosis and APS

Ischemic coronary artery disease in APS is largely due to atherosclerosis. The fact that the population of APS patients does not show an increased prevalence of Framingham 'traditional' risk factors when compared to the general population suggests that other 'non-traditional' risk factors, such as aPLs, might facilitate the development of atherosclerosis. Carotid intimal-medial thickness (IMT) detected by B-mode ultrasounds, is a known predictor of coronary artery disease and stroke in adults. An increased frequency of higher IMT in patients with APS indicates that they are more likely to incur in atherosclerotic events. Ames (Ames et al., 2002) found that anticardiolipin antibodies (aCLs) independently predict the extension of IMT in the carotid arteries, while other authors (Vlachoyiannopoulos et al., 2003) failed to demonstrate such predictive role of aCLs. Ankle-brachial pressure index (ABPI), another marker of atherosclerotic risk, is abnormally high in APS, but no correlation with aPLs has been found (Baron et al., 2005). In conclusion, it is commonly acknowledged that a correlation between aPLs and atherosclerosis exists. APLs may play a role in atherogenesis due to procoagulant and proinflammatory effects on endothelial cells and/or their interference on LDL and HDL metabolism.

3.2 Management of coronary artery disease

The correlation between APS and coronary artery disease (CAD) is not well established. Vaarala's prospective study on a cohort of 4081 healthy middle-aged men found that a high level of aCLs constituted an independent risk factor with relation to myocardial infarction (MI) or cardiac death, with high prevalence in patients younger than 45 (22%) (Vaarala et al., 1995). It is therefore useful to recommend aPLs screening to infarcted patients under 45 in the absence of obvious risk factors. In previous studies the association between aPLs and MI has not been demonstrated. Anticoagulation with warfarin is usually prescribed to patients who have experienced coronary thrombotic occlusion. Petri in the Hopkins Lupus cohort highlighted the protective role of hydroxychloroquine due to the reduction of the lupus disease activity, the antiplatelet effect, the reduction of aPLs, and the lipid-lowering effect (Petri, 2000). Moreover, high homocysteine levels may be involved in APS-related thrombosis, suggesting a potential role of folic acid. Obviously, we need to identify and treat traditional cardiovascular risk factors in APS patients, including hypercholesterolemia with use of HMG-CoA inhibitors, cholesterol-lowering agents with anti-inflammatory properties. In conclusion, the Consensus Committee for treatment of cardiac diseases in APS (Lockshin et al., 2003), recommends an extensive use of statins, folic acid, B vitamins and hydroxychloroquine.

3.3 Management of valve abnormalities

Valve abnormalities in the form of vegetation and/or thickening similar to Libman-Sacks endocarditis, are the most common cardiac manifestation in APS (~ 35%). They are defined by the "coexistence of aPLs along with echocardiografic detection of lesions and/or regurgitation and/or stenosis of mitral and/or aortic valve or any combination of the above" (Miyakis et al., 2006). Although anticoagulation do not cure valve vegetations, treatment is recommended in order to prevent valve thrombosis and arterial thromboembolism. Valve vegetations are in fact associated with cerebral involvement, especially stroke but also epilepsy, migraine and cognitive dysfunction. Use of aspirin is appropriate in asymptomatic patients. Administration of corticosteroids is controversial, and some authors advise against their use, considering them ineffective or even capable of further compromising valve functionality. It has been suggested that aPLs cross-react with antigens on the surface of valves, roughly as in the case of rheumatic fever, leading to inflammation and thrombosis of valve leaflets. On the hypothesis that inflammation is the initial event of valve damage, Petri recommends a short course of corticosteroids with follow-up 2D cardiac echocardiograms to determine the rate of corticosteroid taper (Petri, 2004). A small minority of APS patients (~ 5%) develop a valve disease that is severe enough to require surgical therapy including commisurotomy, annuloplasty and biological or mechanical valve replacement. Mechanical valve replacement may be a better option compared to bioprothesis due to the fact that patients are already anticoagulated and that mechanical valves last longer.

3.4 Management of intracardiac thrombosis

Intracardiac thrombi are a rare complication of APS. They may occur in all cardiac chambers but mainly in the right heart and are a dangerous source of systemic embolization. Erdogan's series showed mural thrombi in 13% of cases in the absence of local conditions favoring blood stasis, and thrombi were treated with aggressive anticoagulation and surgical excision (Erdogan et al., 2005). There are no studies comparing medical, surgical or mixed treatments. The Committee Consensus recommends to start warfarin therapy as soon as a thrombus is detected, and to consult the cardiac surgeon when appropriate (Miyakis et al., 2006).

3.5 Management of anticoagulation in cardiopulmonary bypass surgery

APS patients undergoing cardiac surgery show very high perioperative morbility and mortality rates due to thromboembolic events, especially cerebrovascular ones, to bleeding, acute biventricular failure and multiple organ failure caused by catastrophic APS triggered by surgery. Colli showed a 50% morbility rate and a 22% mortality rate in nine patients who underwent heart valve surgery (Colli et al., 2010). Safe and effective anticoagulation during cardiopulmonary bypass (CPB) surgery depends largely on adequate monitoring of coagulation parameters, but that is a challenging task because of the aPLs interference with in vitro hemostasis tests. Furthermore, the contact of blood with extracorporeal surfaces during CPB stimulates the coagulation cascade. APLs prevent the binding of coagulation proteins to the phospholipid surfaces, resulting in prolonged activated partial thromboplastin time (aPTT) and/or activated clotting time (ACT). In these circumstances anti-Xa factor monitoring is the gold standard laboratory test to be used. When treating venous thromboembolism, the target range of anti-Xa activity is 0.6 ± 1.0 u/ml ± 1. Anti- Xa levels of 1.5 ± 2.0 u/ml ± 1 are considered therapeutic for CPB. However, it is difficult to tune the implementation of anti- Xa assays to CPB, due to the time constraints of the latter (Koniari et al., 2010). Some authors have therefore suggested to double the ACT baseline value, on an empirical basis, to more than 999 seconds, while others (East et al., 2000) proposed a preoperative set-up of heparin-celite/ACT titration curves in order to assess the effect of aPL antibodies on ACT monitoring. There is no consensus in literature on the best way to ensure adequate intraoperative anticoagulation but heparin is routinely administered for its safety profile and the broader clinical experience. In the six case report Weiss refers to, unfractionated heparin was administered at doses ranging from 357U/Kg to 775U/Kg, without any intraoperative complications due to ineffective anticoagulation (Weiss et al., 2008). One patient suffered from postoperative bleeding, and in all cases target ACT was higher than 550 seconds. Other therapeutic strategies, such as the one based on the use of bivalirudin, have been performed on APS patients with heparin-induced thrombocytopenia.

Bivalirudin is a direct thrombin inhibitor that produces an effective attenuation of thrombus formation due to its particular action. In fact bivaluridin not only inhibits the active site of the thrombin, but it also recognizes its fibrinogen-binding site, preventing the activation of both the fluid-phase thrombin and the fibrin-bound thrombin. In the case of bleeding due to excessive anticoagulation, protamine sulfate should be continuously administered in small intravenous doses, e.g. 50 mg/h (Gorki et al., 2008), until the bleeding is reduced. Antifibrinolytic drugs, aprotinin or plasmin inhibitors, which are commonly used to stop the bleeding, are not usually given because of the potential risk of postoperative thrombosis. In two cases, however, epsilon-aminocaproic acid was administered without incurring in any subsequent complication. In conclusion, antithrombotic perioperative strategies, which must be agreed upon with the hematologist, should be identified in all APS patients undergoing cardiac surgery.

3.6 Management of myocardial dysfunctions

It is debated whether APS patients may experience a systolic or diastolic dysfunction unrelated to hypertension, valve heart disease or CAD. Isolated autoptic studies in subjects who died of heart failure, showed diffuse cardiomiopathy with microthrombosis of small intramyocardial arterioles with surrounding microinfarctions without vasculitis, suggesting a direct thrombotic effect of aPLs. Myocardial thrombothic microangiopathy has been found in catastrophic APS patients who suffered from MI with a normal angiographic profile of coronary arteries. Echocardiographic studies have shown the presence of primitive diastolic dysfunction despite the absence of systolic dysfunction or other cardiac disease. In a cross-sectional study (Tektonidou et al., 2001) the echocardiographic parameters reflecting right ventricular dysfunction (prolonged deceleration time, isovolumetric relaxation time, E/A ratio-parameters) were associated with high titers of aCLs. As in other cardiac diseases, the diastolic dysfunction may in some cases anticipate overt left ventricular failure. We do not know what treatment is effective in preventing myocardial dysfunctions and therefore the treatment administered should be the one recommended by the systolic and diastolic heart failure guidelines.

3.7 Management of Pulmonary Hypertension

See 4.3 Pulmonary Hypertension

4. Management of lung diseases

4.1 Introduction

A wide variety of pulmonary manifestations are found in APS patients. The most frequent ones are Pulmonary embolism (PE) and Pulmonary hypertension (PH), while the less common ones include Acute respiratory distress syndrome (ARDS) and Diffuse alveolar hemorrhage (DAH).

4.2 Acute pulmonary embolism. Treatment

Acute pulmonary embolism is the most frequent pulmonary complication (40%) and in about half the cases is preceded by deep venous thrombosis (DVT). Its treatment does not differ from the one adopted on non-APS patients: acute anticoagulation with unfractionated or low molecular weight heparins, followed by long-term oral warfarin. In the event of adverse reactions or other contraindications to heparin, the use of direct thrombin inhibitors in the acute phase (e.g. intravenous hirudin and its derivative bivaluridin) or Xa factor inhibitors (fondaparinux) is recommended (Tapson & Humbert, 2007). In patients with recurrent PE due to persistent DVT of the legs, the placement of inferior vena cava filters may be performed. Thrombolytic therapy, as in all patients with acute PE, is indicated in the case of hemodynamic instability associated with acute right ventricular failure. As previously discussed when debating the intensity of anticoagulation, it seems reasonable to recommend an international normalized ratio (INR) between 2.5 and 3.5.

4.3 Pulmonary Hypertension

4.3.1 Preliminary remarks

Pulmonary Hypertension (PH) is a serious condition with significant morbidity and mortality rates, which has a frequency of 3.5% in primary APS and of 1.8% in APS with SLE. PH in APS develops as a result of: A - acute pulmonary embolism, B - mitral/aortic valvulopathy in Libman-Sacks endocarditis, and C - in the absence of identifiable lung or cardiac disease (Idiophatic pulmonary hypertension). A - Chronic thromboembolic pulmonary hypertension (CTEPH) develops in about 3% of subjects who experienced an episode of acute PE with relation to incomplete resolution of acute clotting, leading to an endothelial damage triggering a series of remodeling events with in situ development of microthrombi (Hoeper et al., 2006). B - In the Libman-Sacks endocarditis, non-bacterial vegetations cause valvular regurgitation, high left heart filling pressures that lead over time to passive pulmonary venous hypertension. C - The association of aPLs with Idiophatic pulmonary hypertension (IPAH) is mentioned in studies regarding small series of patients: in 24 patients, mainly SLE ones, aPLs were found in 68% of cases (Asherson et al., 1990). The role of aPLs in the IPAH pathogenesis is unknown but they may induce the production of endothelin-1 (ET-1), a powerful vasoconstrictor, in some patients.

4.3.2 Pulmonary Hypertension. Treatment

Chronic anticoagulation, necessary to prevent the formation of new thromboemboli, is paramount in PH, but the treatment of choice remains the pulmonary thromboendoarterioctomy (PTE) introduced by Jamieson (Jamieson et al., 2003). The surgical procedure requires a very complex technique performed in cardiopulmonary bypass with intermittent circulatory arrest that allows the surgeon the full view of the thromboembolic material and its dissection. PTE should be performed early in the course of the illness when pulmonary vascular resistance, measured via right heart catheterization, is still not irreversibly high, as mortality is related to the degree of preoperative vascular resistance. If a high resistance persists after surgery, that is a sign of strongly negative outcome. For this reason some authors suggest to perform PTE only if a significant improvement in pulmonary vascular resistance (> 50%) is expected after surgery (Dartevelle et al., 2004). In patients who are ineligible for surgery, the literature produced between 1990 and 2000 reported variable success rates with relation to vasodilator therapy with calcium channel blockers or with long-term infusion of epoprostenol (prostacyclin). From a general point of view, we have drugs for the treatment of pulmonary arterial hypertension (PAH), approved by the United States Food and Drug Administration (FDA), that antagonize the three pathogenic mechanisms of PAH: 1. endothelin receptor antagonists (relative excess of ET-1), 2. phosphodiesterase-5 inhibitors and 3. prostacyclin analogues (relative deficit of nitric oxide and prostaglandins). Bosentan, a non selective oral endothelin receptor antagonist, is used to improve exercising capacity in IPAP and in PH depending on either scleroderma or congenital systemic-to-pulmonary shunts of the Eisenmenger's syndrome, but its application in other forms of secondary pulmonary hypertension is uncertain. Pulmonary venous hypertension caused by valve abnormalities in Libman-Sacks endocarditis, requires the implementation of the usual measures aimed at reducing pulmonary congestion, first of all the administration of diuretics.Valve replacement may be necessary if left ventricular dysfunction becomes severe. Anticoagulation is recommended to prevent valve thrombosis and subsequent systemic embolic phenomena, but the treatment does not fix valvular lesions (See 3.3 - Management of valve abnormalities).

4.4 Acute respiratory distress syndrome (ARDS). Treatment

ARDS is a form of non-cardiogenic pulmonary edema that occurs in the setting of normal atrial and ventricular filling pressures. It is defined by the presence of bilateral pulmonary infiltrates with a partial pressure arterial oxygen (PaO2) to fraction of inspired oxygen (FiO2) ratio below 200 , and it is most frequently reported in catastrophic APS. In the early stages of ARDS, the alveolar capillary membrane permeability is increased, causing the passage of red cells and neutrophils into the alveoli. The migration of immunoglobulins and aPLs into the alveoli has also been demonstrated, suggesting the key role of aPLs in driving the ARDS process. On the other hand, it is possible to assume that the 'cytokine storm' found in CAPS is the main event increasing capillary permeability with neutrophils migration. The management of ARDS patients consists, apart from anticoagulation, of high doses of steroids and, occasionally, of pulses of cyclophosphamide and plasmapheresis (Stojanovic, 2006).

4.5 Diffuse alveolar hemorrhage. Treatment

Diffuse alveolar hemorrhage (DAH) shows widespread alveolar infiltrates determining dyspnea, cough, fever, hypoxemic respiratory failure with hemoptysis found in 70 % of cases. The histological lesion at the basis of DAH is pulmonary capillaritis, in which the migration of neutrophils into the interstitium causes necrosis and damage to capillary integrity, with intra-alveolar red cell extravasation. Such migration may be caused either by aPLs, through the up-regulation of endothelial cell adhesion molecules, or by the C5a complement fraction that activates neutrophils. Treatment is the same as in ARDS,with corticosteroid and cyclophosphamide immunosuppression representing an important therapeutic tool. It starts with the administration of high doses of corticosteroids (IV methylprednisolon 1g/d for 3-5 days) and cyclophosphamide pulse therapy is used if recurrence occurs after the cessation of steroids. Almost all DAH patients already treated with corticosteroids improve after the addition of cyclophosphamide (Deane & West, 2005). In refractory cases, IV immunoglobulins and plasma exchange may be used. In the case of hemoptysis, it may be necessary to suspend anticoagulation and resume treatment as soon as lung conditions improve.

5. Management of kidney diseases in APS

5.1 Introduction

Renal manifestations in APS depend on the involvement of intrarenal small vessels, causing APS nephropathy (APSN), and of large extrarenal vessels.

5.1.1 APS nephropathy

APS nephropathy is a well defined clinicopathological entity characterized by a vasoocclusive disorder of the kidney microcirculation. It includes acute lesions in form of Thrombotic Microangiopathy (TMA) with mesangiolysis and/or double contours of the glomerular wall, variously associated with chronic lesions (fibrous intimal hyperplasia, focal cortical atrophy, arteriolosclerosis, tubular thyroidization) (Nochy et al.,1999). The prevalence of microangiopathic thrombotic lesions causes acute kidney failure often associated with malignant hypertension and nephrotic or sub-nephrotic proteinuria. Chronic lesions are associated with moderate hypertension, chronic kidney failure and mild proteinuria. Fibrous Intimal Hyperplasia (FIH) shows intimal thickening by myofibroblastic cells leading over time to arteriolar occlusion due to fibrous projections and organized thrombi. Focal Cortical Atrophy (FCA) is characterized by focal areas of fibrosis and retraction of the subcapsular cortex on ischemic basis. The described lesions are found in primary APS, in secondary APS with SLE nephritis, with TMA being especially observed in catastrophic APS. In SLE patients with aPLs, APSN occurs in a very high percentage (39.5%) (Tektonidou et al., 2004) while it is present in just 4.3% of SLE patients without aPLs. APSN in addition to SLE represents an additional risk factor for renal morbidity, hypertension and interstitial fibrosis, the last two being well known prognostic indicators of kidney function. During catastrophic APS, kidneys are the organs most frequently involved (71%) (Cervera et al., 2009), resulting in acute renal failure, severe hypertension, proteinuria and hematuria.

5.1.2 Involvement of extrarenal vessels

Hypertension is commonly observed in both primary and secondary APS, and is frequently associated with livedo reticularis. Uncontrolled hypertension can be caused by renal artery stenosis (RAS) or, less commonly, by renal infarctions (Alchi et al., 2010). RAS shows two angiographic patterns: generally smooth, non-critical stenosis in the mid-portion of the renal artery and, rarely, more proximal atherosclerotic-like lesions. The nature of RAS in APS remains unclear, but the good response to anticoagulation with recovery of renal function and normalization of blood pressure, suggests the existence of a thrombotic basis (Godfrey et al., 2000). Finally, both primary APS and aPL-positive patients with SLE nephritis, especially those who are LA positive, are prone to develop thrombosis of the renal veins and inferior vena cava, associated with nephrotic range proteinuria.

5.2 Treatment

The management of renal manifestations of APS depends mainly on the identification of specific complications, either intra- or extrarenal, and it is similar to the general treatment of APS. The basic principles of the treatment are as follows: A - general measures to reduce renal damage progression, B - treatment of APS nephropaty, C - treatment of extrarenal vascular occlusions/stenosis, D - treatment of kidney failure in CAPS. A - In an attempt to slow down the decrease of the glomerular filtration rate, we should identify and address the factors that contribute to kidney damage, with particular relation to hypertension. Symptomatic treatment is based on the inhibition of the renin-angiotensin system, whose role in the genesis of renal injury is largely acknowledged. ACE inhibitors and AT1 receptor antagonists are the elective therapeutic remedies. The blocking effect of the renin-angiotensin system results in a specific renoprotective action (Fogo, 2001), in a containment of proteinuria and in a better control of hypertension. The mean arterial pressure should be kept within the 90 mm/Hg value. Other forms of renal protection include general measures of containment of the vascular risk and,where indicated, a low dietary protein intake, usually with serum creatinine > 2- 2,5 mg/dl. B - Treatment of APS nephropathy is based on anticoagulation with heparins and warfarin. Although there are no evaluation studies on anticoagulant therapy in aPL-associated nephropathy, anticoagulation with warfarin should be lifelong, because the risk of recurrent thrombotic events exceeds the risk of bleeding. Immunosuppressive agents are not used in primary APSN because they do not prevent thrombosis, even though a few reports showed beneficial effects, perhaps on the basis of a decrease in the aPL-induced inflammatory response. For instance, cyclophosphamide (500 mg/m^2 IV monthly for twelve months) or azathioprine (2.0 mg/kg/day) and steroids were administered by Korkmaz with some effectiveness in patients with moderate renal insufficiency (creatinine: 1.0-2.7 mg/dl) and variable proteinuria (0.6-10.1 g/24 h), in combination with warfarin (to ensure an INR > 2.5) (Korkmaz et al., 2003). The immunosuppressive treatment is mandatory in patients with APS nephropaty associated with SLE nephritis, where warfarin is administered with corticosteroids and cytotoxics, usually cyclophosphamide and azathioprine. Mycophenolate mofetil has recently proved more effective than cyclophosphamide in inducing remission of severe lupus nephritis with fewer side effects, and it might represent a viable alternative to azathioprine in maintenance therapy (Zhu et al., 2007). C – Occlusive and/or stenotic complications regarding extrarenal vessels are treated with unfractionated or low molecular weight heparins followed by oral anticoagulation with warfarin. With relation to RAS, anticoagulant therapy may play a role in stabilizing or improving stenosis and in preventing restenosis after angioplasty. Some reports showed that anticoagulation with INR >3 may reverse arterial stenosis and achieve subsequent clinical improvement (Sangle et al., 2005; Ben-Ami et al., 2006). D - First-line APSN therapy associated with catastrophic APS is based on a combination of corticosteroids plus IV immunoglobulins and/or plasma exchange (see 8.- Management of Catastrophic APS). We think that IV immunoglobulin or plasma exchange may also play a role in acute forms of APSN supported by TMA unresponsive to anticoagulation, and that extracorporeal immune-absorption procedures, that selectively remove IgG molecules, may represent a viable alternative to traditional apheretic techniques.

6. Management of thrombocytopenia in APS

6.1 Introduction

Thrombocytopenia, defined by a platelet (PLT) count of less than 100-150 x $10^9/L$, is one of the main features of APS, found in ~ 25% of PAPS patients and in ~ 40% of cases of APS with SLE. Furthermore, primary immune thrombocytopenia (PIT) and APS have in common aPL autoantibodies, suggesting a similar pathophisiology. Liebman's review reported six studies - published between 1994 and 2006 – that showed a very frequent (~ 50%) detection of aPLs in PIT (Liebman, 2007). Those papers showed no correlation between aPLs titre and severity of thrombocytopenia (PLT count <50 $x10^9/L$). Two of them established a relation between aPLs and rates of thrombotic events, albeit with discordant results. In Stasi's study no thrombotic event was revealed at median follow-up of 31 months (Stasi et al.,1994), while Diz-Kucukkaya found that aPLs positivity, specifically LA positivity, is an important thrombotic risk factor (Diz-Kucukkaya et al., 2001). In fact 60% of aPL-positive patients, but none of the aPL-negative, developed thrombotic events at the five-year follow-up. The mechanism of thrombocytopenia in APS is unknown and most authors state it is immune-mediated and not due to a consumptive process.

6.2 Treatment

Thrombocytopenia associated with APS is usually moderate (> 50 $x10^9/L$), it shows no clinical manifestations and rarely requires interventions. Treatment is indicated when thrombocytopenia is marked (<30 $x10^9/L$) and symptomatic with bleeding. Therapeutic options include steroids, intravenous immunoglobulins (IVIG), immunosuppressive agents (azathioprine, cyclophosphamide) (Lim, 2009). The employment of newer agents such as rituximab, and exceptionally the practice of splenectomy, should be considered in case of failure of conventional therapies. In the absence of clinical trials or guidelines, Galli suggested that treatment regimes of APS thrombocytopenia should be similar to those of PIT, due to their shared features and pathophisiology (Galli et al., 1996) . We extrapolated the following therapeutic patterns, with the relevant drug dosages, from the recent International Consensus Report on the Investigation and Management of Primary Immune Thrombocytopenia (Provan et al., 2010). *First-line therapy*: 1 - Glucorticoids are the standard initial treatment. Prednisone is usually administered in doses of 0.5-2mg/kg/d. Administration of dexamethasone 40 mg/day (equivalent to 400 mg of prednisone a day) for 4 days every 2-4 wk for 1-4 cycles, produces sustained response on the PLT count. Parenteral administration of high-dose methylprednisolon (30 mg /kg/d for 7 d) followed by oral steroids, is also effective . 2 - IV immunoglobulins: IVIG treatment shows a quicker response in PIT compared to corticosteroids. The standard regimen includes the infusion of 0.4 g/kg/d for 4-5 days, but we are more likely to obtain a PLT increase using high doses of 1g/Kg/d for 1 or 2 days. Rare but dangerous toxicities include kidney failure and thrombosis. *Second-line treatment options:* 1 - immunosuppressive agents are used in order to achieve an increase of the PLT count considered hemostatic for the individual patient. Azathioprine is administered at doses of 1-2 mg/kg/d (maximum 150 mg/d), and it shows fewer side effects compared to other immunosuppressants: weakness, sweating, increased transaminases, neutropenia with infection, pancreatitis. Cyclophosphamide may be administered either orally (1-2 mg/kg/d) or IV (0.3-1g/Kg for 1-3 doses every 2-4 weeks). Toxicity is mild to moderate and it includes neutropenia, nausea and vomiting, deep leg venous thrombosis. 2 – Rituximab is usually given at doses of 375 mg/m^2 every week for 4 weeks. In PIT, Rituximab causes a PLT count response in approximately 64% of patients, with a response duration ranging from five to 48 months. The efficacy of rituximab in the treatment of APS patients with thrombocytopenia is still to be determined and only a few studies can be found in literature (Ames et al., 2007; Trappe et al., 2006; Ahn et al., 2005). The most common side effects are infusion-related, such as fever, chills, headache, rash, bronchospasm and hypotension, mostly occurring during the first infusion. After the administration of rituximab, peripheral B cell levels show a dramatic decrease, returning to near baseline from 6 to 12 months after completion of therapy. Despite such B-cell depletion, a decrease in serum immunoglobulin levels is only found in a minority of patients. Rituximab should not be used in patients with active B hepatitis, because of the risk of hepatitis activation. 3 - Splenectomy is a viable treatment option in thrombocytopenic patients, as approximately 20% of them show a very low PLT count, despite medical treatment and pheresis. Eleven out of fifty-five APS patients with thrombocytopenia required a splenectomy in a retrospective study (Galindo et al., 1999), that reported a high rate of successful long term response. In view of the potential risk of post-splenectomy arterial thrombosis, intervention should be reserved to severe and symptomatic forms of thrombocytopenia, unresponsive to more conventional treatment. Finally, literature cites isolated cases of thrombocytopenia in APS with good therapeutic response to danazol, aspirin, dapsone, chloroquine.

6.3 Treatment of bleeding complications

Bleeding is considerably less frequent than thrombosis, as shown by the Italian Registry of Antiphospholipid Antibodies, which takes into account 319 patients: only 4 out of 80 of thrombocytopenic subjects suffered major bleeding events. Finazzi, revising the same Registry, found 32% of thrombotic events, but no bleeding, in 44 patients with a PLT count between 100-150 $x10^9/L$. (Finazzi, 1997). In the 32 patients with a PLT count $< 50 \times 10^9/L$, bleeding was observed in 6%, and thrombosis in 9% of cases, indicating the possibility of thrombosis in spite of severe thrombocytopenia. In accordance with Lim's review, we report the following practical recommendations regarding the treatment of active hemorrhages (Lim, 2009). Bleeding occurring in the central nervous, gastrointestinal or genitourinary system often requires a rapid increase of the PLT count. In some cases, it is sufficient to switch from the steroid to the immunoglobulin therapy, but it seems more appropriate to adopt a combination treatment with corticosteroids and IVIG. Platelet transfusions, leading to a post-transfusional PLT increase of about 20 $x10^9/L$, may be associated. Antifibrinolytic agents, such as oral or IV tranexamic acid (1 g, three times a day) and episilon-aminocaproic acid (1-4 g every 4-6 hours) may be useful in preventing recurrent bleeding. On the other hand, if bleeding is due to the anticoagulant treatment, therapy should be temporarily discontinued administering the relevant antidotes (protamine sulfate for heparin, vitamin K for warfarin), and practising the transfusional support (fresh plasma for heparin and warfarin, prothrombin concentrated complexes for warfarin). In patients with severe thrombocytopenia and high thrombotic risk, the PLT count should be brought to at least 30-50 $x10^9/L$, for anticoagulation to be adequately performed. It does not seem useful to reduce the intensity of anticoagulation in those cases, as we infer from data regarding secondary prevention of deep vein thrombosis that low doses of warfarin are not protective.

7. Management of dermatological diseases in APS

7.1 Introduction

The skin appears to be an important target organ for aPLs and 40% of the patients may present cutaneous features as a major complaint. Skin lesions may be sorted according to their seriousness in 'major' (widespread cutaneous necrosis and/or digital gangrene) and 'minor' (e.g. livedo reticularis, superficial thrombophlebitis, pseudo-vasculitis lesions, circumscribed ulcerations, subungual splinter hemorrhages). Major ones are caused by non inflammatory thrombosis of small arteries of the dermis and subcutaneous fat. The most frequent (17.5% to 40%) and typical skin manifestation is livedo in both its reticularis and racemosa versions, characterized by a purplish reticular or mottled skin pattern consisting of regular unbroken circles (livedo reticularis) or irregular circles (livedo racemosa), that is irreversible even after rewarming. Livedo racemosa has a more generalized location, being widespread all over the trunk, limbs and buttocks. The distinctive skin color of livedo is related to the reduced blood flow and the oxygen tension caused by vasoconstriction. Some authors state that livedo racemosa is a predictor of systemic thrombotic events, as there is evidence of a strong association between the former and cerebrovascular/ocular ischemic events, arterial thrombosis, migraine, epilepsy and renal artery stenosis (Toubi et al., 2005). The association of livedo with Sneddon's syndrome, typically affecting women before or during their middle age, is debated.This syndrome shows widespread livedo that precedes the onset of stroke by several years, and many authors found that 40%-50% of the patients affected are aPL-positive (Frances et al., 1999). The relationship between livedo and arterial thrombosis suggests a possible common role played by endothelial cells. In fact, many aPLs interact with the phospholipid-protein complexes on the surface of endothelial cells, therefore leading to the production of procoagulant substances such as tissue factor (TF), plasminogen activator inhibitor-1 and endothelin-1. This interaction between aPLs and endothelial cells may cause the vasoconstriction typical of livedo racemosa (Amengual et al., 1999).

7.2 Treatment

The treatment of patients with cutaneous manifestations should take into account the kind of skin lesion and the overall clinical situation. In the absence of RCTs regarding prophylaxis and therapy of dermatological lesions, treatment remains empirical. Digital gangrene and skin necrosis are the major thrombotic events requiring full anticoagulation with heparin (Rossini et al., 2002). Should lesions persist despite anticoagulation, some reports suggest alternative treatments (iloprost, tissue plasminogen activator, gammaglobulins, corticosteroids, plasma exchange and immunosuppressive therapy) (Frances et al., 1989; Srinivasan et al., 2001; Zahavi et al., 1993). Major cutaneous lesions may appear particularly serious in the context of multiorgan thrombotic occlusion during catastrophic APS in which combined treatments are required (see 8.- Management of Catastrophic APS). Frances recommends long-term anticoagulation with INR targeted to 2.5 for the prophylaxis of severe skin lesions (Frances, 2010). In patients who have 'minor' cutaneous manifestations with no other systemic features, e.g. circumscribed ulcers or pseudovasculitis lesions, the administration of low doses (75 mg/d) of aspirin may be useful, although anticoagulant therapy must be adopted if lesions persist or worsen (Asherson et al., 2006). In any case, removal of the necrotic tissue and local antiseptic therapy are paramount for the reduction of the infective risk. Livedo racemosa resists to anticoagulant or antiplatelet therapies, as it appears and extends in spite of them. In the European APS cohort (Cervera et al., 2002), where most patients were anticoagulated, livedo appeared in 26 cases during the five-year follow-up. Livedo is less evident in tanned areas, but it is known that exposure to sunlight is not recommended for SLE patients with APS. In view of the thrombotic risk in aPL-positive patients with livedo, it is important to reduce or remove other provoking factors, therefore men are advised to stop smoking and women not to use contraceptive pills containing estrogens. For the same reason, those patients should be properly screened in order to detect silent cerebral ischemia and/or kidney illnesses, and warfarin therapy should be adopted if needed. Even though low doses of aspirin are commonly prescribed to patients with livedo and no systemic features, its effectiveness in the prevention of strokes remains doubtful.

8. Management of catastrophic APS

8.1 Introduction

In 1992 Asherson described a potentially life-threatening variant of APS called catastrophic APS (CAPS), and subsequently named Asherson's syndrome (Asherson, 1992). It is characterized by multiple organ failure due to thrombothic microangiopathy (TMA) involving several organs, either simultaneously or in rapid sequence: brain, heart, kidneys, lungs, gastrointestinal tract. In 35% of cases it is possible to identify a triggering factor, which is mainly an infection or sepsis originating from the respiratory, urinary, gastrointestinal tracts.A pathogenic link between infections and CAPS has been acknowledged and its rationale is based on the theory of molecular mimicry, according to which β2GPI peptides share the aminoacid sequence and conformational structure with common bacteria and viruses. As common microbial structures represent the natural ligand for toll-like receptors (TLRs), it has been argued that ß2GPI might interact with TLRs and that anti-ß2GPI antibodies recognizing the molecule might cross-link it together with TLRs (Espinosa et al., 2007). Ultimately, TLRs intracellular signaling pathway leads to a proinflammatory and prothrombotic phenotype of endothelial cells, respectively through the production of proinflammatory cytokines and adhesions molecules, and the up regulation of the tissue factor. Other triggering factors of CAPS are the withdrawal or the administration of low doses of anticoagulants, invasive or surgical procedures, cancer, lupus flares, obstetric complications.

8.2 Treatment

CAPS appears in less than 1% of APS patients and carries a high mortality rate. Although there are no RCTs for this rare syndrome, the CAPS International Registry, accessible via the Web, provides us with important clinical, prognostic and therapeutic data. We can see that the CAPS mortality rate went to 33% between 2001 and 2005, down from 50% in the years before 2000 (Bucciarelli et al., 2006), and that may be due to the early treatment of triggering factors and even more to the improvement of first-line therapy, which should always include anticoagulation, corticosteroids and plasma exchange. This is in accordance with the International Consensus on CAPS management guidelines (Asherson et al., 2003) that recommends: effective anticoagulation with IV heparin, plus high doses of steroids, plus IV Immunoglobulins (IVIG) and/or plasma exchange (PE). The following are some considerations on the use of A. corticosteroids, B. immunoglobulins and C. plasma exchange with relation to this syndrome: A. Corticosteroids interact with the cytoplasmic receptor, and the resulting steroid receptor complex neutralizes Nuclear Factor-kB (NF-kB), which in turn activates transcription genes for the synthesis of pro-inflammatory molecules (TNF-α, interleukins-1 and 2, cyclooxygenase-2 and intercellular adhesion molecules (ICAM). Moreover, corticosteroids partly neutralize activator protein-1, triggering the transcription of several genes involved in the synthesis of pro-inflammatory proteins. There is evidence of NF-kB playing an important role in states, such as sepsis and ARDS, frequently associated with

CAPS. Consequently, the inhibition of NF-kB and the down regulation of the cytokines, both corticosteroid-induced, are beneficial in reducing host-derived tissue injury and organ dysfunctions when treating CAPS. B. IV immunoglobulins, that are immunomodulating agents, perform several activities. These include block of pathological autoantibodies, modulation of complement activation, clearance of pathological IgG and suppression of pathogenic cytokines. IVIG contain anti-idiotypic antibodies capable of recognizing and specifically suppressing different autoantibodies. That might explain both the short term neutralization of the aPLs pathogenic role and the long term decrease in the aPLs titre. (Vora and al., 2006). C. The effectiveness of plasma exchange therapy is widely acknowledged, although both the replacement fluid to be used (whether albumin solutions or fresh frozen plasma) and the timing and frequency of treatments, are still debated (Uthman et al., 2005). The guidelines recommend the use of fresh frozen plasma (FFP), especially in the presence of thrombotic microangiopathic hemolitic anemia (e.g. schistocytes). In fact thrombotic microangiopathies (TTP, HUS, HELLP syndrome) have in common with CAPS similar hematological manifestations (aPL positivity, thrombocytopenia, microangiopathic hemolitic anemia) and triggering factors (e.g. infections, drugs) (Asherson, 2007). Moreover such conditions, including HELLP syndrome at post-partum period, may require similar treatment with plasma exchange, using fresh frozen plasma instead of albumin reinfusion. (Szczepiorkowski et al., 2007). Although the exact mechanism of plasma exchange is still unknown, it has been demonstrated that PE is effective in removing IgG-CL, anti-β2GPI, cytokins, complement and TNF-α. We propose the use of IV methylprednisolon at doses of 1g/d for 3-5 consecutive days, followed by oral steroid at a dose equivalent to 1mg/Kg/d of prednisone; IV Immunoglobulins at 1g/Kg/d for two days ; plasma exchange with reinfusion of FFP not inferior to the volume of plasma, for at least 3-5 days. In the absence of clinical improvement, other therapies should be provided: cyclophosphamide in SLE flares, prostacyclin or fibrinolytics or defibrotide. In CAPS patients with severe thrombocytopenia resistant to other forms of treatment, the administration of rituximab may be useful, as the direct inhibition of B-lymphocytes contributes to the decrease of the aPLs titre and the subsequent platelet activation (Erre et al., 2008). Finally, the objectives to be aggressively pursued in the management of CAPS are essentially four: 1 - addressing the triggering factors (adoption of antibiotic therapy in the event of infection and surgical toilet of the infection sources), 2 - maintenance of effective anticoagulation, also when CAPS is associated with thrombocytopenia, 3 - suppression and/or removal of cytokine excess, 4 - adoption of intensive care measures when necessary. Such strategy plays an essential role in the survival of CAPS patients whose mortality, as shown by the CAPS registry data analysis regarding 112 patients, is due to: neurologic involvement (mainly stroke) (27.2%); cardiac involvement (mainly cardiac failure) (19.8%); infections (mainly bacterial sepsis) (19.8%); multi organ failure (17.3%); pulmonary involvement (mainly ARDS) (9.8%); abdominal involvement, including liver failure and acute abdomen, in four patients (Espinosa et al., 2008). The presence of SLE is the only prognostic factor predicting a higher mortality (59% vs 37.9%) regardless of clinical manifestations, number of organs involved, laboratory parameters and treatment adopted (Bayraktar et al., 2007).

9. Conclusions

In APS patients, the current therapeutic standard is oral anticoagulation aimed at preventing thrombotic events. Warfarin or coumarin inhibit the synthesis of vitamin K-dependent clotting factors (FII, FVII, FIX, FX) and of anticoagulant plasma proteins C and S. The INR target should be kept between 2 and 3 in case of first venous thrombotic event, while it should be higher than 3 in case of arterial thrombosis and/or recurrent venous thrombosis. In women with obstetric complications treatment is based on the use of aspirin and heparin. The treatment of choice for patients suffering from acute thromboembolic event is the administration of unfractionated heparin which, through the activation of ATIII, indirectly inhibits thrombin formation and inactivates Xa factor. Alternatively, we can use LMWH, whose binding to ATIII causes above all of all the inactivation of Xa factor, and then of thrombin to a lesser extent. LMWHs have a more predictable pharmacological effect and they induce thrombocytopenia less frequently, due respectively to their weaker binding with plasma proteins and with platelets. Anticoagulation may be ineffective or even contraindicated under certain clinical circumstances. In fact, some manifestations of APS, such as cardiac valvular disease, livedo reticularis and thrombocytopenia, are unresponsive to anticoagulation. Moreover, some patients experience thromboembolic events despite anticoagulation, while others do not tolerate full doses of warfarin because of its hemorrhagic side effects. Additional drugs have been introduced over the years in order to overcome such problems. Their therapeutic use has been found following experimental evidence, tested in vitro and/or on animal models, that revealed the pathogenic effects of aPL/β2GPI complexes both on hemostatic reactions and on the activation of cellular elements (endothelials cells, monocytes , platelets), also clarifying the role of B cells in the aPLs synthesis. We think that clinical experiences based on thrombin-inhibitors, on hydrossycloroquine, statins and B-cell depletion therapy (e.g. rituximab) have been so far the most interesting ones and we can assume they will be consistently adopted in the management of APS. In particular dabigatran, a new direct thrombin-inhibitor, usually prescribed at a dose of 150 mg twice a day for the prophylaxis of post-operative venous thromboembolism, could represent a viable alternative to warfarin. Dabigatran is administered orally and does not require anticoagulation monitoring, although we need clinical studies validating its use in APS patients. Hydroxyicloroquine, which directly inhibits the binding of aPL/β2GPI complexes to phospholipid surfaces, has the advantage of not causing bleeding, and therefore it is useful in patients showing hemorrhagic side effects caused by warfarin. Hydroxyicloroquine can also be used, in view of its antiplatelet effect, in those patients who have experienced thrombotic recurrences despite anticoagulation. It is usually administered at doses of 400-800 mg/d and, because of its potential retinal toxicity , ophtalmic examination is essential prior to therapy. Controlled studies regarding the effectiveness and safety of its use have not been produced yet. Statins are an additional tool in the APS treatment due to their anti-atherosclerotic and anti-inflammatory effect, only partially depending on the relevant cholesterol decrease. Experimental studies indicate that they may act by reducing the aPL-induced endothelial activation, by blocking NF-kB pathway and the subsequent synthesis of adhesion molecules and IL-6, and by reversing the up-regulation of the tissue factor (Espinosa & Cervera; 2010). In addition, it has been shown that rosuvastatin is effective in reducing venous thromboembolic events in non-APS patients but also in this case we do not have clinical data indicating that statins prevent the formation of thrombi in APS patients. The experience with rituximab is still limited although encouraging reports, mainly dealing with the recovery of thrombocytopenia, have recently been published. We are currently waiting for the results of the ongoing Pilot Study of Rituximab for the anticoagulation-resistant manifestations of APS (RITAPS). This open-label trial will assess safety and efficacy of rituximab in those manifestations of APS which prove unresponsive to anticoagulation. In conclusion, despite promising results provided by the aforementioned treatments, we feel that well-designed randomized trials are still needed.

10. References

Ahn ER, Lander G, Bidot CJ, Jy W, Ahn YS. Long-term remission from life-threatening hypercoagulable state associated with lupus anticoagulant (LA) following rituximab therapy.Am J Hematol. 2005 Feb;78(2):127-9.

Alchi B, Griffiths M, Jayne D.What nephrologists need to know about antiphospholipid syndrome. Nephrol Dial Transplant. 2010 Oct;25(10):3147-54.

Amengual O, Atsumi T, Khamashta MA. Tissue factor in antiphospholipid syndrome: shifting the focus from coagulation to endothelium. Rheumatology Oxford 2003;42:1029-31.

Ames PR, Margarita A, Delgado Alves J, et al. Anticardiolipin antibody titre and plasma homocysteine level independently predict intima media thickness of carotid arteries in subjects with idiopathic antiphospholipid antibodies. Lupus 2002;11(4):208–14.

Ames PR, Tommasino C, Fossati G, Scenna G, Brancaccio V, Ferrara F.Limited effect of rituximab on thrombocytopaenia and anticardiolipin antibodies in a patient with primary antiphospholipid syndrome.Ann Hematol. 2007 Mar;86(3):227-8.

Asherson RA, Higenbottam TW, Dinh Xuan AT, Khamashta MA, Hughes GR. Pulmonary hypertension in a lupus clinic: experience with twenty-four patients. J Rheumatol. 1990;17:1292-1298.

Asherson RA, Cervera R, de Groot PG, Erkan D, Boffa MC, Piette JC, Khamashta MA, Shoenfeld Y; Catastrophic Antiphospholipid Syndrome Registry Project Group Catastrophic antiphospholipid syndrome: international consensus statement on classification criteria and treatment guidelines. Lupus. 2003;12(7):530-4.

Asherson RA, Frances C, Iaccarino L, et al. The antiphospholipid antibody syndrome: diagnosis, skin manifestation and current therapy. Clin Exp Rheumatol 2006;24:S46-51.

Asherson RA. New subset of the antiphospholipid syndrome in 2006: ''PRE-APS'' (probable APS) and microangiopathic antiphospholipid syndromes (''MAPS''). Autoimmun Rev 2006; 6:76–80. Society for Apheresis. J Clin Apher 2007;22:106-75.

Asherson RA. The catastrophic antiphospholipid syndrome. J Rheumatol 1992;19:508–12.

Askie LM, Duley L, Henderson-Smart DJ, Stewart LA, on behalf of the PARIS Collaborative Group. Antiplatelet agents for prevention of pre-eclampsia: a meta-analysis of individual patient data. Lancet 2007; 369: 1791–98.

Baron MA, Khamashta MA, Hughes GR, et al. Prevalence of an abnormal ankle–brachial index in patients with primary antiphospholipid syndrome: preliminary data. Ann Rheum Dis 2005;64(1):144–6.

Bates SM, Greer IA, Pabinger I, Sofaer S, Hirsh J. Venous thromboembolism, thrombophilia, antithrombotic therapy, and pregnancy: American College of Chest Physicians Evidence-Based Clinical Practice Guidelines (8th edn). Chest 2008; 133: 844S–86S.

Bayraktar UD, Erkan D, Bucciarelli S, Espinosa G, Asherson R; Catastrophic Antiphospholipid Syndrome Project Group. The clinical spectrum of catastrophic antiphospholipid syndrome in the absence and presence of lupus.J Rheumatol. 2007 Feb;34(2):346-52.

Ben-Ami D, Bar-Meir E, Shoenfeld Y. Stenosis in antiphospholipid syndrome: a new finding with clinical implications. Lupus 2006: 466–472

Bucciarelli S, Espinosa G, Cervera R, Erkan D, Gómez-Puerta JA, Ramos-Casals M, Font J, Asherson RA; European Forum on Antiphospholipid Antibodies. Mortality in the catastrophic antiphospholipid syndrome: causes of death and prognostic factors in a series of 250 patients. Arthritis Rheum. 2006 Aug;54(8):2568-76.

Cervera R, Piette JC, Font J, et al. Antiphospholipid syndrome: clinical and immunologic manifestations and patterns of disease expression in a cohort of 1,000 patients. Arthritis Rheum 2002; 46: 1019–1027

Cervera R, Bucciarelli S, Plasín MA et al. Catastrophic Antiphospholipid Syndrome (CAPS) Registry Project Group (European forum on antiphospholipid antibodies). Catastrophic antiphospholipid syndrome(CAPS): descriptive analysis of a series of 280 patients from the "CAPS Registry." J Autoimmun 2009; 32: 240–245

Colli A, Mestres CA, Espinosa G, Plasín MA, Pomar JL, Font J, Cervera R: Heart valve surgery in patients with the antiphospholipid syndrome: analysis of a series of nine cases. Eur J Cardiothorac Surg 2010, 37(1):154-8.

Crowther MA, Ginsberg JS, Julian J et al. A comparison of two intensities of warfarin for the prevention of recurrent thrombosis in patients with the antiphospholipid antibody syndrome. N. Engl. J. Med. 349(12),1133-1138 (2003).

Dartevelle P, Fadel E, Mussot S, et al. Chronic thromboembolic pulmonary hypertension. Eur Respir J. 2004;23:637-648.

Deane KD, West SG.Antiphospholipid antibodies as a cause of pulmonary capillaritis and diffuse alveolar hemorrhage: a case series and literature review. Semin Arthritis Rheum. 2005 Dec;35(3):154-65.

Diz-Küçükkaya R, Hacihanefioğlu A, Yenerel M, Turgut M, Keskin H, Nalçaci M, Inanç M.Antiphospholipid antibodies and antiphospholipid syndrome in patients presenting with immune thrombocytopenic purpura: a prospective cohort study. Blood. 2001 Sep 15;98(6):1760-4.

East Chr, Clements F, Mathew J, et al. Antiphospholipid Syndrome and Cardiac Surgery: Management of anticoagulation in two Patients. Anesth Analg 2000, 90:1098-101.

Empson M, Lassere M, Craig J, Scott J. Prevention of recurrent miscarriage for women with antiphospholipid antibody or lupus anticoagulant. Cochrane Database Syst Rev 2005; 18: CD002859.

Erdogan D, Goren MT, Diz-Kucukkaya R, Inanc M.Assessment of cardiac structure and left atrial appendage functions in primary antiphospholipid syndrome: a transesophageal echocardiographic study. Stroke. 2005 Mar;36(3):592-6.

Erkan D, Merrill JT, Yazici Y, Sammaritano L, Buyon JP, Lockshin MD. High thrombosis rate after fetal loss in antiphospholipid syndrome: effective prophylaxis with aspirin. Arthritis Rheum 2001; 44: 1466–67.

Erkan D, Harrison MJ, Levy R, et al. Aspirin for primary thrombosis prevention in the antiphospholipid syndrome: a randomized, double-blind, placebo-controlled trial in asymptomatic antiphospholipid antibody-positive individuals. Arthritis Rheum 2007;56:2382–2391

Erre GL, Pardini S, F aedda R, Passiu G. Effect of rituximab on clinical and laboratory features of antiphospholipid syndrome: a case report and a review of literature. Lupus. 2008;17:50-5.

Espinosa G, Cervera R, Asherson RA. Catastrophic antiphospholipid syndrome and sepsis. A common link?J Rheumatol. 2007 May;34(5):923-6.

Espinosa G, Bucciarelli S, Asherson RA, Cervera R. Morbidity and mortality in the catastrophic antiphospholipid syndrome: pathophysiology, causes of death, and prognostic factors. Semin Thromb Hemost. 2008 Apr;34(3):290-4.

Espinosa G, Cervera R. Recent trends in the management of antiphospholipid syndrome (Hughes syndrome).Drugs Today (Barc). 2010 Jan;46(1):39-47.

Finazzi G. The Italian Registry of Antiphospholipid Antibodies. Haematologica. 1997;82:101-105.

Fogo AB. Fibrose rénale et système rénine-angiotensine. Actualites Nephrologiques Jean Hamburger 2001; 31: 73-88.

Finazzi G, Marchioli R, Brancaccio V et al.: A randomized clinical trial of high-intensity warfarin vs. conventional antithrombotic therapy for the prevention of recurrent thrombosis in patients with the antiphospholipid syndrome (WAPS). J. Thromb. Haemost. 3(5),848-853 (2005).

Frances C, Tribout B, Boisnic S, et al. Cutaneous necrosis associated with the lupus anticoagulant. Dermatologica 1989; 178: 194–2011

Frances C, Papo T, Wechsler B, Laporte JL, Biousse V, Piette JC. Sneddon syndrome with or without antiphospholipid antibodies: a comparative study in 46 patients. Medicine 1999; 78: 209–219.

Frances C.Dermatological manifestations of Hughes' antiphospholipid antibody syndrome.Lupus. 2010 Aug;19(9):1071-7.

Galindo M, Khamashta MA, Hughes GR.Splenectomy for refractory thrombocytopenia in the antiphospholipid syndrome.Rheumatology (Oxford). 1999 Sep;38(9):848-53.

Galli M, Finazzi G, Barbui T. Thrombocytopenia in the antiphospholipid syndrome. Br J Haematol. 1996 Apr;93(1):1-5.

Giannakopoulos B, Krilis SA: How I treat the antiphospholipid syndrome. Blood 114(10),2020-2030 (2009).

Godfrey T, Khamashta MA, Hughes GR. Antiphospholipid syndrome and renal artery stenosis. QJM 2000; 93: 127–129

Gorki H, Malinovski V, Stanbridge RDL: The antiphospholipid syndrome and heart valve surgery. Eur J CardioThorac Surg 2008, 33:168-18.

Hereng T, Lambert M, Hachulla E, et al. Influence of aspirin on the clinical outcomes of 103 anti-phospholipid antibodies-positive patients. Lupus 2008; 17: 11–15.

Hoeper MM, Mayer E, Simonneau G, Rubin LJ. Chronic thromboembolic pulmonary hypertension. Circulation. 2006 Apr 25;113(16):2011-20.

Jamieson SW, Kapelanski DP, Sakakibara N, Manecke GR, Thistlethwaite PA, Kerr KM,et al. Pulmonary endarterectomy: experience and lessons learned in 1,500 cases.Ann Thorac Surg. 2003 Nov;76(5):1457-62; discussion 1462-4.

Kaiser R, Cleveland C, Criswell L. Risk and protective factors for thrombosis in systemic lupus erythematosus: results from a large, multi-ethnic cohort. Ann Rheum Dis 2009; 68: 238–41.

Koniari I, Siminelakis SN, Baikoussis NG, Papadopoulos G, Goudevenos J, Apostolakis E.Antiphospholipid syndrome; its implication in cardiovascular diseases: a review. J Cardiothorac Surg. 2010 Nov 3;5:101.

Korkmaz C, Kabukcuoglu S, Isiksoy S et al. Renal involvement in primary antiphospholipid syndrome and its response to immunosuppressive therapy. Lupus 2003; 12: 760–765

Levine SR, Brey RL, Tilley BC, et al, APASS Investigators. Antiphospholipid antibodies and subsequent thrombo-occlusive events in patients with ischemic stroke. JAMA 2004; 291: 576–84.

Liebman H.Other immune thrombocytopenias. Semin Hematol. 2007 Oct;44(4 Suppl 5):S24-34.

Lim W, Crowther MA, Eikelboom JW. Management of antiphospholipid antibody syndrome: a systematic review. JAMA 2006; 295: 1050–57.

Lim W. Antiphospholipid antibody syndrome.Hematology Am Soc Hematol Educ Program.2009:233-9

Lockshin M, Tenedios F, Petri M, et al. Cardiac disease in the antiphospholipid syndrome: recommendations for treatment. Committee consensus report. Lupus 2003;12(7):518–23.

Mehdi AA, Uthman I, Khamashta M. Treatment of antiphospholipid antibody syndrome Int J Clin Rheumatol 2010 5(2): 241-54

Miyakis S, Lockshin MD, Atsumi T, Branch DW, Brey RL, Cervera R, et al. International consensus statement on an update of the classification criteria for definite antiphospholipid syndrome (APS). J Thromb Haemost. 2006 Feb;4(2):295-306.

Noble LS, Kutteh WH, Lashey N, et al. Antiphospholipid antibodies associated with recurrent pregnancy loss: prospective, multicenter, controlled pilot study comparing treatment with low-molecularweight heparin versus unfractionated heparin. Fertil Steril 2005; 83: 684–90

Nochy D, Daugas E, Droz D, Beaufils H, Grunfeld JP, Piette JC, et al. The intrarenal vascular lesions associated with primary antiphospholipid syndrome. J Am Soc Nephrol1999; 10: 507–518

Okuma H, Kitagawa Y, Yasuda T, Tokuoka K, Takagi S. Comparison between single antiplatelet therapy and combination of antiplatelet and anticoagulation therapy for secondary prevention in ischemic stroke patients with antiphospholipid syndrome Int J Med Sci. 2009 Dec 5;7(1):15-8.

Petri M. Hopkins lupus cohort. 1999 update. Rheum Dis Clin North Am 2000;26(2): 199–213

Petri MA. Classification criteria for antiphospholipid syndrome: the case for cardiac valvular disease. J Rheumatol. 2004 Dec;31(12):2329-30.

Provan D, Stasi R, Newland AC, Blanchette VS, Bolton-Maggs P, Bussel JB et al: International consensus report on the investigation and management of primary immune thrombocytopenia. Blood. 2010 Jan 14;115(2):168-86.

Rossini J, Roverano S, Graf C, Paira S. Widespread cutaneous necrosis associated with antiphospholipid antibodies: report of four cases. J Clin Rheumatol 2002; 8: 326–331.

Ruiz-Irastorza G, Hunt BJ, Khamashta MA. A systematic review of secondary thromboprophylaxis in patients with antiphospholipid antibodies. Arthritis Rheum 2007; 57: 1487–95.

Sangle SR, D'Cruz DP, Abbs IC et al. Renal artery stenosis in hypertensive patients with antiphospholipid (Hughes) syndrome: outcome following anticoagulation. Rheumatology (Oxford) 2005; 44: 372–377

Srinivasan SK, Pittelkow MR, Cooper Jr LT. Recombinant tissue plasminogen activator for the treatment of cutaneous infarctions in antiphospholipid antibody syndrome: a case report. Angiology 2001; 52: 635–639.

Stasi R, Stipa E, Masi M, Oliva F, Sciarra A, Perrotti A, Olivieri M, Zaccari G, Gandolfo GM, Galli M, et al.Prevalence and clinical significance of elevated antiphospholipid antibodies in patients with idiopathic thrombocytopenic purpura.Blood. 1994 Dec 15;84(12):4203-8.

Stephenson MD, Ballem PJ, Tsang P, et al. Treatment of antiphospholipid antibody syndrome (APS) in pregnancy: a randomized pilot trial comparing low molecular weight heparin to unfractionated heparin. J Obstet Gynaecol Can 2004; 26: 729–34.

Stojanovich L.Pulmonary manifestations in antiphospholipid syndrome.Autoimmun Rev. 2006 May;5(5):344-8

Szczepiorkowski ZM, Bandarenko N, Kim HC, et al. Guidelines on the use of therapeutic apheresis in clinical practice: evidence-based approach from the Apheresis Applications Committee of the American Society for Apheresis. J Clin Apher 2007;22:106-75.

Tapson VF, Humbert M.Incidence and prevalence of chronic thromboembolic pulmonary hypertension: from acute to chronic pulmonary embolism.Proc Am Thorac Soc. 2006 Sep;3(7):564-7.

Tektonidou MG, Ioannidis JP, Moyssakis I, et al. Right ventricular diastolic dysfunction in patients with anticardiolipin antibodies and antiphospholipid syndrome. Ann Rheum Dis 2001;60(1):43–8.

Tektonidou MG, Sotsiou F, Nakopoulou L et al. Antiphospholipid syndrome nephropathy in patients with systemic lupus erythematosus and antiphospholipid antibodies: prevalence, clinical associations, and long-term outcome. Arthritis Rheum 2004; 50: 2569–2579

Toubi E, Krause I, Fraser A, et al. Livedo reticularis is a marker for predicting multi-system thrombosis in antiphospholipid syndrome. Clin Exp Rheumatol 2005;23:499-504.

Trappe R, Loew A, Thuss-Patience P, Dörken B, Riess HSuccessful treatment of thrombocytopenia in primary antiphospholipid antibody syndrome with the anti-CD20 antibody rituximab--monitoring of antiphospholipid and anti-GP antibodies: a case report.Ann Hematol. 2006 Feb;85(2):134-5.

Uthman I, Shamseddine A, Taher A.The role of therapeutic plasma exchange in the catastrophic antiphospholipid syndrome. Transfus Apher Sci 2005;33:11-7.

Vaarala O, Manttari M, Manninen V, et al. Anti-cardiolipin antibodies and risk of myocardial infarction in a prospective cohort of middle-aged men. Circulation 1995;91:23–7.

Vlachoyiannopoulos PG, Kanellopoulos PG, Ioannidis JP, et al. Atherosclerosis in premenopausal women with antiphospholipid syndrome and systemic lupus erythematosus: a controlled study. Rheumatology (Oxford) 2003;42(5):645–51.

Vora SK, Asherson RA, Erkan D. Catastrophic antiphospholipid syndrome. J Intensive Care Med. 2006 May-Jun;21(3):144-59.

Weiss S, Nyzio JB, Cines D, Detre J, Milas BL, Narula N, Floyd TF.Antiphospholipid syndrome: intraoperative and postoperative anticoagulation in cardiac surgery.J Cardiothorac Vasc Anesth. 2008 Oct;22(5):735-9.

Zahavi J, Charach G, Schafer R, Toeg A, Zahavi M. Ischemic necrotic toes associated with antiphospholipid syndrome and treated with iloprost. Lancet 1993; 342: 862.

Zhu B, Chen N, Lin Y, Ren H, Zhang W, Wang W, Pan X, Yu H. Mycophenolate mofetil in induction and maintenance therapy of severe lupus nephritis: a meta-analysis of randomized controlled trials. Nephrol Dial Transplant. 2007 Jul;22(7):1933-42.

Section 4

Conclusion

12

Antiphospholipid Syndrome – An Evolving Story of a Multisystemic Disease

Silvia S. Pierangeli[1,*], Rohan Willis[1], Brock Harper[2] and E. Nigel Harris[3]
[1]*Antiphospholipid Standardization Laboratory, Division of Rheumatology, Department of Internal Medicine, University of Texas Medical Branch, Galveston, TX*
[2]*Division of Rheumatology. Department of Internal Medicine, University of Texas Medical Branch, Galveston, TX*
[3]*University of the West Indies, Kingston*
[1,2,3]*USA*
[4]*Jamaica*

1. Introduction

Antiphospholipid syndrome (APS) is an autoimmune multisystemic disorder characterized clinically by recurrent thrombosis and pregnancy morbidity and serologically by the presence of antiphospholipid antibodies (aPL) including anticardiolipin (aCL) and anti-β2 glycoprotein I (anti-β2GPI) antibodies and lupus anticoagulant (LA) [1].

Historically, aPL antibodies were classified based on the clinical laboratory test in which they were detected, i.e. LA and aCL antibodies. It is now widely accepted that aPL antibodies are a heterogenous group of antibodies that react with a myriad of phospholipids (PLs), PL-protein complexes and PL binding proteins. The main antigenic target of these antibodies is recognized to be $\beta_2$glycoprotein I (β_2GPI), which along with prothrombin accounts for more than 90% of the antibody binding activity in APS patients. Other potentially significant antigenic targets include tissue plasminogen activator (tPA), phosphatidylserine (PS), plasmin, annexin 2, activated protein C (APC), thrombin, antithrombin (AT) and annexin A5 [2,3].

In the general population, APS is the most common cause of acquired thrombophilia and is a recognized risk factor for the development of deep vein thrombosis (DVT) with or without pulmonary embolism, new strokes in individuals below the age of 50 and recurrent fetal loss [4]. The prevalence of DVT occurrence in the general population is estimated at 2-5%, 15 - 20% associated with APS, suggesting that the prevalence of venous thrombosis associated with APS may be as high as 0.3-1% of the general population [4]. APL antibodies are present in 30-40% of systemic lupus erythematosus (SLE) patients and up to a third of these patients (10-15% of SLE patients) have clinical manifestations of APS, especially venous or arterial thromboses [5,6].

* Corresponding Author

The APS related thrombotic events range in severity from the relatively benign superficial thromophlebitis to myocardial infarction, stroke and catastrophic APS (CAPS) [7]. APS also accounts for a significant proportion of recurrent pregnancy loss in SLE patients, indeed, aPL are now regarded as the most frequent acquired risk for a treatable cause of recurrent pregnancy loss and for pregnancy complications (early and severe pre-eclampsia) [5,8].

The first description of aPL antibodies dates back to 1952, when Moore *et al* described patients suffering from SLE with a persistently false positive VDRL flocculation test for syphilis, a test based on the detection of antibodies against cardiolipin (CL) extracted from beef heart [7]. In the same year, Conley et al [8,9] described two SLE patients with a peculiar circulating inhibitor of coagulation [10]. These "anticoagulants" could inhibit *in vitro* coagulation assays, but did not influence the activity of coagulation factors and were not associated with a bleeding diathesis. Feinstein and Rapaport introduced the term LA to describe this phenomenon in 1972 [10]. Although the relation between thrombosis and the presence of these anticoagulants in SLE patients was already noticed in 1963 [11], it took until 1980 before the association between LA and thrombosis was widely recognized [12]. As LA was found to be associated with a persistently false positive syphilis test, this led to the development of an aCL immunoassay and the establishment of the association between thrombosis and aCL anticardiolipin [13]. From this time on, patients presenting with thrombosis and/or pregnancy loss in combination with persistently positive aCL antibodies and/or circulating LA were considered to have the APS [14,15]. Subsequently, patients with systemic lupus erythematosus (SLE) and related connective tissue diseases (CTD) that had abnormal LA tests, were labeled as 'secondary' APS (SAPS) in the presence of these conditions and 'primary' (PAPS) in their absence [16]. A study of patients with SLE showed that aCL positivity preceded the onset of a more severe form of SLE, as well as SLE complicated with thrombosis, pregnancy loss and thrombocytopenia [5]. However, studies have found no difference between PAPS and SAPS with respect to the clinical complications, the timing of those complications, the prognosis or frequency of positive aCL, LA or other autoantibody tests. In addition, management of PAPS and SAPS is the same and prognosis does not appear to differ [17].

2. Traditional and non-traditional manifestations of APS

APS is classically characterized by vascular thromboses or obstetric morbidity in association with the presence of aPL antibodies [1]. Vascular thromboses include venous thromboses resulting clinically in deep venous thrombosis and/or pulmonary emboli while arterial thromboses may present with ischemia affecting limbs, cerebral vascular accidents or transient ischemic attacks and small-vessel thrombosis may result in cutaneous ulceration [1,18]. Presence of thrombosis should be confirmed with a diagnostic angiogram, Doppler ultrasound, pulmonary scintigraphy, histopathology or computed tomography (CT) or magnetic resonance imaging (MRI) of the brain depending on the clinical context [1].

In a longitudinal cohort of patients with APS, transient ischemic attacks (TIA)s and cerebrovascular accidents (CVA)s were the most common thrombotic events occurring in 2.4% and 2.3% respectively of patients with established APS followed by pulmonary embolism and deep venous thrombosis over a period of 5 years [18].

Obstetric manifestations of APS include fetal loss with loss after 10 weeks of gestation being more strongly associated with APS, placental insufficiency potentially resulting in decreased gestational weight or fetal distress and preterm delivery and development of pre-eclampsia and frank eclampsia [1]. Early pregnancy loss occurs in 17.1% and late pregnancy loss occurs in 6.7% of pregnancies in women with established APS while 35% of successful pregnancies were premature and 13.7% had intrauterine growth restriction [18].

Catastrophic APS (CAPS) is the rare but life-threatening development of wide-spread intravascular thrombosis seen in less than 1% of patients with APS [18-20]. Patients present acutely with multi-organ system failure, evidence of small vessel thrombosis and presence of positive aPL antibodies [19,20]. Death occurs in approximately 45% of patients during the acute event with primary causes being cerebral involvement, cardiac involvement, infections, multiorgan failure, pulmonary involvement and abdominal involvement [20]. Infection is the most common trigger identified in CAPS being present in approximately 20% of patients [20].

Patients with APS may also develop manifestations not included in the classification criteria. Neurologic symptoms other than strokes or TIAs including chorea, dementia, transverse myelitis, multiple sclerosis and epilepsy have been attributed to APS although studies are contradictory [1,18,21]. Livedo reticularis occurs more commonly in APS and may progress to livedo vasculitis with purpuric lesions, nodules and painful ulcerations [1,18,22]. Presence of livedo reticularis appears to carry an increased risk of arterial thrombosis, CVA and pregnancy loss [22].

Thrombocytopenia is the most common hematologic manifestation, occurring in over 30% of patients with APS [22]. Cardiac involvement frequently manifests as valvular disease with presence of mitral or tricuspid valve thickening or regurgitation and presence of valvular vegetations [19]. APS is also associated with a thrombotic microangiopathy of the renal arterioles and glomeruli known as APS nephropathy, which leads to hypertension, nephrotic range proteinuria, hematuria and progressive renal insufficiency [1].

3. Current diagnostic algorithms

a. "Criteria" aPL tests.

Current classification criteria for definite APS require the use of three "standardized" laboratory assays to detect aPL antibodies. These assays include aCL, both IgG and/or IgM by enzyme-linked immunosorbent assay (ELISA), the anti-β_2GPI IgG and/or IgM by ELISA and the LA [1]. These tests, when positive, represent criteria for diagnosis when at least one of the two major clinical manifestations (thrombosis or pregnancy losses) is present according to the revised Sapporo criteria (Table 1).

Laboratory testing for aPL antibodies is one of the most problematic areas in the field of APS. The confirmation of diagnosis of the APS relies on laboratory tests, since clinical manifestations such as thrombosis and pregnancy losses may occur for many reasons not related to the presence of aPL antibodies. Most importantly, patients with APS who have experienced thrombosis and/or pregnancy losses need a specific therapy that is often life-long and must be personalized, requiring careful monitoring of additional risk factors to prevent recurrences of APS manifestations. Given the potential serious side effects of anticoagulant therapy, a solid diagnosis is essential in planning management.

a)Lupus anticoagulant (LAC)	Positive on two or more occasion at least 12 weeks apart, detected according to the guidelines of ISTH
b)Anticardiolipin (aCL) antibody	Positive for IgG or IgM isotype in serum or plasma, present in medium and high titer on two or more occasions, at least 12 weeks apart, measured by standardized ELISA.
c)Anti-β_2GPI antibody	Positive for IgG or IgM isotype (in titer > the 99th percentile) on two or more occasions, at least 12 weeks apart measured by standardized ELISA

Miyakis et al J Thromb Haemost 2006; 4; 295-306.

Table 1. Laboratory Criteria for APS (Revised Sapporo Criteria).

Although international consensus guidelines for the determination of LA have been published and revised, the existence of "standardized" tests for detection of aCL and anti-β_2GPI has remained elusive. Furthermore, despite over 7000 publications related to the clinical use of aPL antibody tests, a consensus on clinical recommendations has been difficult to achieve. This difficulty appears related to sub-optimal design in clinical studies and a lack of laboratory standardization in areas such as the following: 1) units of measurement, 2) calibration curves, 3) determination of cut-off values, and 4) laboratories not performing the tests according to established guidelines. Significant inter-assay and inter-laboratory variation in the results of both aCL and anti-β_2GPI testing still exists, affecting the consistency of the diagnosis of APS [23].

Over the years, international workshops have worked hard to standardize the laboratory test in this area. These workshops include the APL European forum, the Australasian Anticardiolipin Working Party (AAWP), the College of American Pathologists (CAP), the National External Quality Assessment Scheme (NEQAS), and the Standardization Subcommittee (SSC) on lupus anticoagulant and phospholipid-dependent antibodies of the International Society of Thrombosis and Hemostasis (ISTH). While some laboratories can obtain reliable testing results, there is still wide inter-laboratory variation despite all the efforts at standardization. This situation may result from laboratories performing aPL assays with their own protocols or using commercial kits that do not conform to the proposed guidelines for these tests. Furthermore, standardization of tests or re-evaluation of standardization is important since APS is related to serious complications like thrombosis and pregnancy loss; missing a diagnosis because of laboratory variability could have serious medical consequences. The use of semi- or fully-automated analyzers and commercial kits instead of in-house assays poses additional challenges to the process of standardization [23].

To address the challenges on aPL testing described above, an international *"Criteria aPL Task Force"* (Task Force) of researchers and scientific leaders in the field was formed prior to the 13th International Congress on Antiphospholipid Antibodies in Galveston, TX, April 2010 (APLA 2010). The "Criteria" aPL Task Force was further divided into three subgroups, which were charged by the APLA 2010 Congress Chair to address, in an evidence-based manner, various topics related to the testing of aCL, anti-β_2GPI and LA. To accomplish its mission, the Criteria aPL Task Force considered published information, the results of a survey distributed among APLA 2010 congress attendees and the discussions that occurred during a special preconference workshop at APLA 2010. On the basis of this approach, the

Task Force reached several conclusions and proposed recommendations discussed below and summarized in Table 2; this information has recently been published [24-26].

Subgroup1 International Consensus Guidelines on assay performance of aCL and anti-β_2GPI assay.	**Conclusions** Development of International Consensus Guidelines for aCL and anti-β_2GPI assays including pre-analytical, analytical and post-analytical considerations. *(Lakos G et al. Arthritis Rheum 2011 Sep 27. doi: 10.1002/art.33349)*
Subgroup 1 Guidelines on use of calibrator for aCL/ anti-β_2GPI assays and selection and preparation of reference material	**Conclusions:** a) Tests to be reported in GPL/MPL units if monoclonal antibodies are used as a calibrator. b) Levels of secondary calibrators should be meticulously defined prior to use. c) Evaluation of the performance of various monoclonal and polyclonal antibodies in order to identify optimal material for standardization. d) Establishment of international units for measurement for anti-β_2GPI antibodies (work in progress) *(Pierangeli S et al. Clin Chim Acta. 2011 Oct 15. [Epub ahead of print])*
Subgroup 2 Review of the Updated ISTH SCC guidelines on the use of Lupus anti-coagulant (LAC) for diagnosis.	**Conclusions:** a) Weak LAC does not predict behavior in vivo. b) Consideration of false-positive results with the use of phospholipid -diluting agent. c) Additional lab testing to differentiate LAC from factor inhibitors, if clinically indicated. d) An inter-laboratory study to validate the statement about integrated test and not requiring performance of "mixing" tests e) LAC to be tested 2-3 weeks after warfarin discontinuation f) Clinicians to contact reference laboratories to discuss specific issues related to LAC and results interpretation.
Subgroup 3 Role of aPL as "risk factors".	**Conclusions:** a) Develop collaborations with existing large, population-based, prospective cohorts with available data on thrombosis and/or pregnancy outcomes to examine the value of aPL-SCORE. b) Full panel of currently available aPL test should be performed and if possible new tests like anti- PS/PT, anti-β_2GPI domain I, annexin A5 should also be evaluated

Table 2. "CRITERIA" aPL Task Force Recommendations.

b. "Non-Criteria" aPL Tests.

As indicated above, the revised classification criteria for the diagnosis of APS include the positivity of at least one of the three 'Criteria' aPL tests [1]. However, the use of these tests may not guarantee full sensitivity and specificity to confirm a diagnosis of APS. In clinical practice, there are indeed many 'false positives' with aPL tests, especially the aCL ELISA, which can give positive results in clinical conditions besides APS; these conditions include infectious disease (i.e., syphilis), malignancy and other autoimmune diseases. On the other hand, there are patients with a clinical pattern strongly suggestive of APS, but persistently negative for 'Criteria' tests. In addition the "criteria" aPL tests may not identify the "pathogenic" subpopulations of aPL.

Several autoantibodies have been demonstrated to bind directly to negatively charged phospholipids other than CL (individually or as a phospholipid mixture) or to other proteins in the coagulation cascade (i.e., prothrombin and/or phosphatidylserine-prothrombin complexes); antibodies can also interfere with anticoagulant activity of the annexin A5. However, the clinical and diagnostic utility of these newly developed assays as well as their standardization requires much further study. In some cases, these new assays lack standardization and there are not international units of measurements.

A "Non-Criteria" aPL Task Force assembled prior to APLA 2010 was charged by the Congress Chair to address, in an evidence-based manner, the status of various new tests being developed for confirmation of diagnosis of APS. The results and recommendations of that task force have been recently published elsewhere [27].

4. Antigenic targets of antiphospholipid antibodies: Phospholipids and phospholipid binding proteins

As stated previously, aPL represent a heterogenous group of antibodies with reactivity to not only PLs but also proteins, in particular those able to bind and form complexes with PLs [2]. Historically, serological activity against cardiolipin (CL) (Figure 1a), an anionic PL found in mitochondrial membranes, was one of the earliest key descriptive features of APS and although still important is overshadowed by β_2GPI, which is now recognized as the main antigenic target of pathogenic aPL [2]. Indeed, β_2GPI along with prothrombin (PT) account for more than 90% of the antibody binding activity in APS patients and it is unsurprising that antibodies against these 2 abundant proteins involved in hemostasis are most consistently associated with LA activity [28]. β_2GPI consists of five contiguous domains (Figure 1b), the first proposed to be the binding site for pathogenic anti-β_2GPI antibodies and the fifth the binding site for anionic and hydrophobic phospholipids such as phosphatidylserine (PS), lyso (bis) phosphatidic acid (LBPA), and CL exposed on cell surfaces and protein receptors [2,29]. The role that apoptosis plays in the exposure of these phospholipids on the cell surface and the subsequent interaction with β_2GPI has been proposed as a possible mechanism for the production of pathogenic aPL in APS patients [30]. An interesting pathogenic role for oxidized low-density lipoprotein (ox-LDL)/β_2GPI complexes bound by aPL in the initiation and progression of atherogenesis has been described [31,32].

Several models have been put forward for pathogenic anti-β_2GPI Abs complexed with β_2GPI activating monocytes, ECs, trophoblasts and platelets via simultaneous binding to PLs and candidate protein receptors to induce production of tissue factor and proinflammatory cytokines [33-36]. *In vivo* and in *in vitro* studies have demonstrated the role of annexin A2 (AnnA2), in association with Toll-like receptor 4 (TLR4) and/or apolipoprotein ER2'

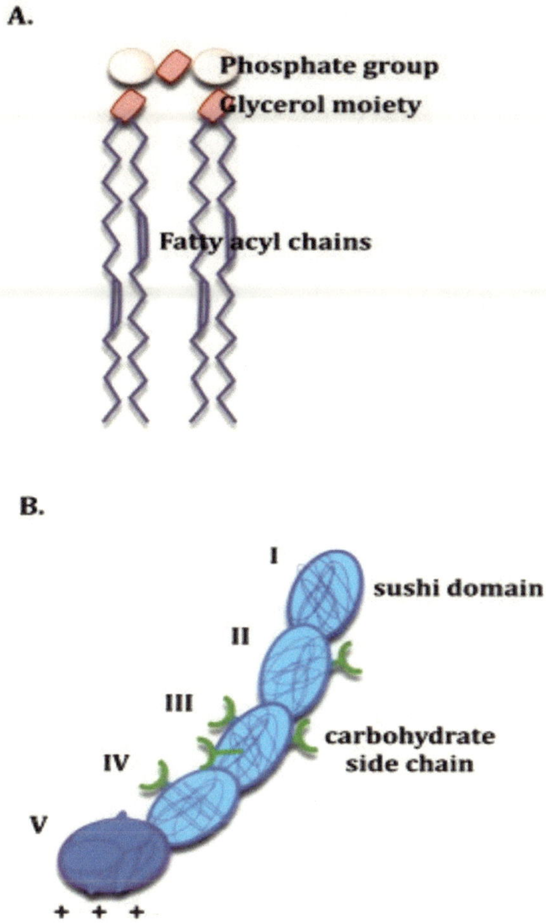

Pierangeli et al.

Fig. 1. Schematic representation of Cardiolipin and of β_2Glycoprotein I.
A. Cardiolipin structure contains 2 negatively charged phosphate head groups, 3 glycerol moieties and 4 fatty acyl chains
B. β2-glycoprotein I structure consists of 5 contiguous sushi domains. The first 4 consisting of 60 amino acids and the fifth consisting of 80 amino acids and more positive charged amino acids

(ApoER2′) that act as co-receptors containing intracellular signaling domains, in the activation of ECs, monocytes and cells of the decidua and trophoblast [37-39]. Candidate receptors on platelets include ApoER2′ and the glycoprotein Ibα (GPIbα) subunit of the GPIb-V-IX receptor and Sikara et al have demonstrated a putative role for platelet factor 4 (PF4) in the stabilization and binding of dimeric β_2GPI /anti-β_2GPI complexes to platelet membranes [40,41].

Many serine proteases that function in maintaining hemostasis are targets of autoantigens in APS patients. These include activated protein C (APC), prothrombin, antithrombin (AT) and many coagulation factors including factors IXa, IIa and II [42]. There is evidence to suggest that antibodies directed against AnnA5, an abundant cationic protein that functions as a natural anticoagulant especially in placental tissue, can cause placental thrombosis and fetal resorption in mice, although there is conflicting evidence of the significance of these antibodies in APS patients [43,44]. A recently described protein antigenic target, vimentin, has been suggested to play a putative role in platelet and leukocyte activation in APS patients but further characterization of the role of this cytoskeletal protein is necessary [45].

5. Origins of APS: Infection-associated APS and molecular mimicry

The failure of normal T cell tolerance mechanisms seems to be an important component for the development of autoimmunity in several diseases. In APS, there is evidence to suggest that *molecular mimicry* can induce production of pathogenic APL antibodies, presumably because of a breakdown in normal peripheral tolerance mechanisms [46]. Although aPL were first characterized by their ability to bind CL, it is now well accepted that these antibodies recognize various PL and protein antigenic complexes [1,2].

Indeed, efforts to induce high titer production of pathogenic aPL in animal models succeeded only after immunization with heterologous β_2GPI rather than pure phospholipids [47]. This led researchers to believe that perhaps *in vivo* binding of foreign PL-binding proteins resembling β_2GPI to self phospholipids in APS patients may lead to the formation of immunogenic complexes, against which aPL antibodies are produced. Gharavi *et al* in 1999 synthesized a 15 amino acid peptide, GDKV, which spanned an area of the fifth domain of β_2GPI known to be a major PL-binding site of the molecule, and demonstrated the peptide's ability to induce pathogenic aPL and anti-β_2GPI antibody production in mice [48]. A monoclonal antibody with aPL and anti-β_2GPI activity generated from these GDKV-immunized mice was shown to be pathogenic using *in vivo* models for thrombus enhancement and microcirculation [49]. The resulting search for candidate peptides in microorganisms that exhibited functional and sequence similarity to the PL-binding domain of β_2GPI produced the peptides TIFI and VITT from cytomegalovirus (CMV), TADL from adenovirus (AdV) and SGDF from *Bacillus subtilis*. All these peptides had strong similarities with GDKV and induced high titers aPL and anti-β_2GPI production in mice. Subsequent *in vivo* and *in vitro* experiments confirmed the pathogenicity of antibodies induced in TIFI-immunized mice [50-52].

Further supporting evidence for molecular mimicry as a possible mechanism for APS development was provided by a study evaluating the APS-related pathogenic potential of microorganisms carrying sequences related to a hexapeptide, TLRVYK, known to be specifically recognized by a pathogenic monoclonal anti-β_2GPI Ab [53]. Following immunization with *Haemophilus influenzae, Neisseria gonorrhoeae* or tetanus toxoid; high titers of antibodies of anti-peptide (TLRVYK) and anti-β_2GPI activity were observed in BALB/c mice. These affinity-purified antibodies were then infused into naive mice at day 0 of pregnancy. At day 15, these mice had significant thrombocytopenia, prolonged activated partial thromboplastin times (aPTT) and increased frequency of fetal loss compared to controls [53].

Infections are thought perhaps to be the most prominent environmental trigger for aPL production and APS development. Syphilis was the first infectious disease recognized to be linked to aPL production and this infectious type aPL is for the most part non-pathogenic

[54]. However, several subsequent reports have shown that many other infections not only trigger aPL production but are associated with the development of APS manifestations as well [55,56]. CMV, parvovirus B19, Human immunodeficiency virus (HIV), Hepatitis B and C viruses, Human T-cell lymphoma/leukemia virus (HTLV) and Varicella Zoster Virus (VZV) are just a few of the infectious agents that have reported associations with aPL production and APS manifestations [56]. A recent study has demonstrated that protein H of *Streptococcus pyogenes* can bind β_2GPI, inducing conformational changes, exposing hidden epitopes and in so doing then enable production of anti-β_2GPI antibodies [57].

Rauch *et al* have recently put forward a hypothesis regarding the dual role of the innate immune system in the initiation and progression of APS based on their work. This hypothesis highlights the central part played by toll-like receptors (TLRs), especially TLR4, in inducing a break in tolerance, aPL production and epitope spread to several autoantigens [58]. Utilizing lupus prone mice treated with CMV derived peptides in the presence of TLR7 or TLR9 agonists and other lupus prone mice deficient in TLR7 or both TLR7 and TLR9, our group has demonstrated for the first time that both these TLRs are involved in aPL production in β_2GPI immunized mice [59].

6. Genetics of APS

Animal models and family and population studies have been used to highlight genetic associations with APS disease characteristics and the occurrence of aPL antibodies in patients. In 1992 Hashimoto *et al* described an animal model of lupus associated APS in NZW x BXSB F1 (W/B F1) male mice that displayed spontaneous production of IgG aCL antibodies which exhibit co-factor (β_2GPI) dependent binding to cardiolipin [60]. Interestingly, analysis of the genes utilized in the production of pathogenic aCL in these mice showed preferential usage of certain V_H (variable region of heavy immunoglobulin chain) and V_K (variable region of kappa light immunoglobulin chain) genes, whereas other non-pathogenic aCL utilize random V gene combinations possibly indicating that pathogenic aCL production in these mice is antigen driven rather than germiline encoded [61]. Genome-wide analysis using microsatellite markers in these mice and their progeny revealed that the generation of each disease character was controlled by two independently segregating major dominant alleles producing full expression as a complementary gene action. Although there was complete genetic concordance between the occurrence of antiplatelet Abs and thrombocytopenia, other disease characteristics were independently controlled by different combinations of two dominant alleles suggesting that no single genetic factor can explain the pathogenesis of APS [62]. Papalardo et al have recently shown, using MHCII deficient mice and MHCII deficient mice transgenic for human MHCII haplotypes, that MHCII is necessary for producing aPL after immunization with β_2GPI and certain haplotypes are more effective than others [63].

Since 1980, several studies have described families with high incidences of primary APS associated with LA, aCL and other autoantibodies [64-66]. The most consistent HLA associations in families with APS are HLA-DR4 and DRw53; other less consistent associations include DR7, DQw3, DQw7, A30, Cw3 and B60 [67-70]. In non-familial population studies HLA-DR4 and DRw53 were also consistently associated with APS disease characteristics in addition to DR7 and DQB1*0302 [71-73].

The occurence of aCL antibodies has been reported in association with DRB1*09 in Japanese patients with APS secondary to SLE and with C4A or C4B null alleles in black American populations. However, patients in the Hopkins Lupus Cohort who were homozygous for C4A deficiency had a lower frequency of aCL and LA than patients without this deficiency [74-76]. Other less consistent non-familial HLA associations with APS include DRB1*04, DQB1*0301/4, DQB1*0604/5/6/7/8/9, DQA1*0102 and DQA1*0301/2 [73,77-79]. Several non-HLA genes associations with increased autoantibody production and risk of thrombosis have been described in APS patients. Perhaps the most profound is a polymorphism in domain 5 of β_2GPI, valine instead of leucine at position 247, which is found more frequently in patients with APS than matched controls and is associated with anti-β_2GPI production and increased risk for arterial thrombosis in these patients [80]. Other less established genetic associations with increased thrombosis in APS include the factor V Leiden mutation, the G20210A prothrombin mutation (F2 G20210A) and protein C and S deficiencies [81].

7. Pathogenic effects of antiphospholipid antibodies: What we have learned from *In Vivo* animal models?

a. Animal Models of Thrombosis and Endothelial Cell Activation

Based on the observation that patients with aCL antibodies appear to get thrombi at intermittent intervals, our group hypothesized that these antibodies might only enhance the thrombotic process after another inciting agent initiated it. With this in mind, Pierangeli *et al* [82] turned to a mouse model of thrombosis devised by Stockmans *et al* [83] and modified by Barker *et al* [84] that enables measurement of the dynamics of thrombus formation after this is induced by a standardized injury. In a series of experiments, this group of investigators found that CD1 male mice, injected with purified immunoglobulins (4 IgG, 3 IgM, 2 IgA preparations) or with affinity purified aCL antibodies (2 IgG and 2 IgM) had significantly larger and more persistent thrombi compared to mice immunized with immunoglobulins from healthy humans. The effect of these Ig preparations was also dose-dependent [85]. In collaboration with Dr Pojen Chen (UCLA, Los Angeles, Ca), the group showed also that human monoclonal aCL antibodies derived from a patient with the APS had thrombogenic properties *in vivo* [86]. Similarly, mice producing aCL antibodies after immunization with β_2GPI or human aPL antibodies also had thrombogenic properties *in vivo* [87]. Furthermore, murine monoclonal aPL and a monoclonal antibody obtained by immmunization with the phospholipid-binding domain of β_2GPI, also showed thrombogenic properties in their model [48]. The results of studies utilizing this model showed for the first time that aPL antibodies significantly enhance thrombus formation in mice.

Subsequently, Jankowski *et al* and Fischetti *et al* demonstrated the thrombogenic effects of monoclonal and polyclonal anti-β_2GPI in hamsters and rats respectively [88,89]. More recently, Arad and colleagues showed in an animal model that affinity purified anti-β_2GPI antibodies induce thrombosis in mice in a dose-dependent manner [90]. Hence, several investigators have underscored and confirmed the causal relationship between the presence of these autoantibodies and thrombo-embolic complications. In all these models, a priming effect (injury, endotoxin, etc.) was needed to induce thrombus formation in addition to aPL antibodies injected passively into the animals or induced by active immunization. Not only did these models demonstrate "enhanced" thrombus formation compared to controls but also they mimicked what happens in actual APS patients, in whom thrombus formation follows a triggering event (trauma, immobilization, infection, etc).

Antibody mediated endothelial cell activation and injury have been identified as potential factors that may be involved in the pathogenesis of thrombosis by aPL. The relationship between endothelial cell activation and the thrombotic diathesis in APS could be explained by a procoagulant state of the activated endothelium or by the adherence of mononuclear cells accompanied by the increased expression of adhesion molecules, such as intercellular adhesion molecule-1 (ICAM-1), vascular cell adhesion molecule-1 (VCAM-1) and E-selectin (E-sel). Pierangeli *et al* have utilized a unique animal model of microcirculation that allows one to examine and measure changes in adhesiveness of leukocytes in the microcirculation of an isolated cremaster muscle in mice [34], as an indication of EC activation *in vivo* (Figure 2). These parameters include rolling and sticking of leukocytes and diapedesis of white blood cells into the tissue from the blood vessel, etc. Utilizing this model, those investigators first showed that polyclonal aPL antibodies significantly enhance adhesion of leukocytes to endothelium *in vivo* and that this correlated with enhanced thrombosis [34,91]. These effects were observed utilizing some human and some murine monoclonal aPL antibodies [92].

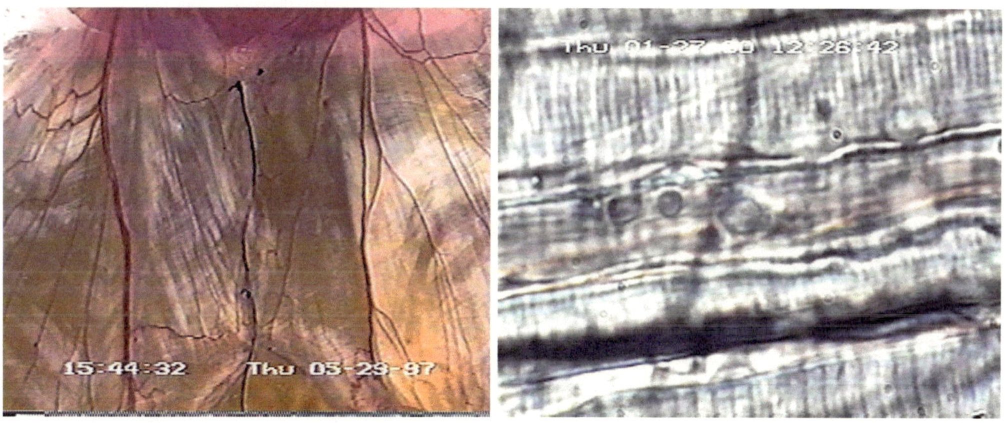

A. B.

Pierangeli et al.

Fig. 2. In Vivo Model of Endothelium Activation. Mice are injected with aPL antibodies or control immunoglobulin twice at 0 and 48 hours. At 72 hours the cremaster muscle of anesthetized mice (A) is isolated and the adhesion of leukocytes in 5 postcapillary venules is assessed (B). Adhesion is defined as leukocytes that remained stationary for at least 30 seconds.

In summary, these animal models of thrombosis and endothelial cell activation have not only been useful in demonstrating the pathogenic effects of aPL antibodies and their causative role in inducing APS morbidity, but have also been instrumental in dissecting the intracellular mechanisms involved, in identifying cellular receptors activated by aPL antibodies *in vivo* and in testing potential new treatments for APS (discussed in detail in other sections of this chapter) [37,39,51,93-105].

b. Animal Models of Pregnancy Loss in APS.

Considerable progress has also been made in developing an *in vivo* model of pregnancy loss related to aPL antibodies in the last 20 years. Gharavi *et al* first reported that MRL/lpr mice with IgG aCL antibodies had smaller litter sizes than controls [106]. However, these lupus prone mice produce autoantibodies with multiple specificities and have other clinical abnormalities (such as kidney disease), which may account for pregnancy loss.

In 1990, Branch *et al* reported that Balb/c mice passively immunized with immunoglobulins from patients with the APS had nearly 100% fetal wastage compared to mice passively immunized with immunoglobulins from patients with normal human immunoglobulins [107]. Subsequently, experiments demonstrated that passive immunization of mice with polyclonal or monoclonal IgG aCL antibodies resulted in significant fetal resorption [108]. Furthermore, Gharavi and colleagues showed that if aCL antibodies are induced in PL/J mice (autoimmune prone mice) the animals showed an increase rate of fetal resorption [109].

Fishman and colleagues reported that production of IL-3 and GM-CSF is decreased in splenocytes derived from their mouse models [110] and that intra-peritoneal administration of recombinant IL-3 to pregnant mice resulted in abrogation of fetal loss and thrombocytopenia.

More recently Girardi *et al* utilized that mouse model to demonstrate the involvement of complement activation in aPL-mediated pregnancy morbidity utilizing various mice deficient in complement components [96,111]. Furthermore, that group of investigators showed that heparin prevents pregnancy loss in mice injected with aPL due to the complement inhibitory properties of the drug and not to its anticoagulant effects [112].

8. Direct proinflammatory and prothrombotic effects of antiphospholipid antibodies on platelets, monocytes and endothelial cells

The activation of platelets, endothelial cells and monocytes via direct binding of aPL antibodies plays an important role in the creation of a proinflammatory and prothrombotic phenotype in APS patients. Binding of dimeric β_2GPI/anti-β_2GPI complexes to platelets is dependent on exposure of anionic phospholipids, especially phosphatidylserine (PS), on platelets, which occurs after stimulation by agonists such as thrombin, collagen, and adenosine diphosphate (ADP) [113,114]. Pathogenic aPL enhance the expression of GPIIb/IIIa, a major fibrinogen receptor, on platelets and our group has shown that in GPIIb/IIIa deficient (β_3-null) mice and mice treated with a monoclonal anti-GPIIb/IIIa antibody there is reduced aPL-mediated thrombus formation [115,116]. Our group has also demonstrated that the major intracellular signaling pathway activated by aPL binding to platelets is the p38 mitogen activated protein kinase (MAPK) pathway and that subsequent phosphorylation of cytosolic phospholipase A2 (cPLA2) results in thromboxane B2 (TXB2) production. After initial activation through the p38 MAPK pathway, other MAPK pathways in platelets, such as ERK-1 (p44 MAPK) and ERK-2 (p42 MAPK), have a potential secondary role in signaling [116].

The adhesion molecules VCAM-1, ICAM-1 and E-sel have been shown to be upregulated in ECs activated by aPL [34,117,118]. Utilizing ICAM-1, VCAM-1, E-sel and P-selectin (P-sel) knockout mice, our group demonstrated the importance of ICAM-1, E-sel, P-sel and VCAM-

1 in promoting leukocyte adhesion and thrombus formation mediated by human polyclonal and monoclonal aPL antibodies [91]. Many groups have also demonstrated the upregulation of tissue factor (TF) expression and micro-particle formation with associated increases in interleukin-6 (IL-6) and IL-8 secretion in ECs and monocytes treated with aPL [119-122]. López-Pedrera *et al.* showed that aPL could induce TF in monocytes by activating the phosphorylation of mitogen-activated protein kinase/extracellular regulated kinase (MEK-1/ERK) protein, and the p38 mitogen-activated protein kinase (MAPK)-dependent nuclear translocation and activation of nuclear factor kB (NFkB)/Rel proteins [123]. Increased surface expression of both vascular endothelial growth factor (VEGF) and Flt-1 on monocytes and elevated plasma levels of VEGF in APS patients suggests that TF upregulation in monocytes may occur as a result of stimulation of the Flt-1 tyrosine kinase receptor by VEGF [33]. Many researchers have provided evidence that upregulated TF mRNA and antigen expression and TF pathway activation plays a key role in APS thrombotic manifestations. Indeed, our group found in an ongoing clinical trial, that mean serum levels of soluble TF, tumor necrosis factor-α (TNFα) and VEGF were significantly elevated in APS patients compared to controls and treatment with fluvastatin, a statin with efficacy in treating APS, resulted in significant decreases of these pro-inflammatory markers in most APS patients [124].

Role of complement in aPL-mediated thrombosis.

Complement inhibitors are now being tested in patients with inflammatory, ischemic and autoimmune diseases [125-127]. The C5 component of complement is cleaved to form products with multiple proinflammatory effects and thus represents an attractive target for complement inhibition in immune-mediated inflammatory diseases. Furthermore, C5a is the most potent anaphylotoxin and a powerful chemotaxin for neutrophils and monocytes, with the ability to promote margination, extravasation and activation of these cells. In addition, C5b-9 can also stimulate the release of multiple proinflammatory molecules and may well play an important role in inflammation apart form its lytic function. Thus, blocking C5b-9 as well as C5a generation may be required for optimal inhibition of the inflammatory response.

At the same time, inhibition of the complement cascade at the level of C5 does not impair the generation of C3b through the classical and alternative pathways, preserving C3b-mediated opsonization of pathogenic microorganisms as well as solubilization of immune complexes, needed in a normal immune response. For this reason, therapeutic strategies that include C5a and its receptor are considered an especially promising approach to complement inhibition. For example, therapy with anti-C5 monoclonal antibody (MoAb) has proven effective in preventing collagen-induced arthritis in mice and in ameliorating established disease. In other studies anti-C5a MoAb improved endothelial dysfunction in cardiopulmonary bypass [125,126,128]. Furthermore, an anti-human-C5 MoAb is in phase II studies in patients with rheumatoid arthritis and in phase I studies in patients with active lupus nephritis [125].

In our own studies anti-C5 MoAb reversed aPL-induced thrombophilia and endothelial cell activation in mice [129]. A complement C5a receptor antagonist peptide: AcPhe [Ornithine-Pro-D-cyclohexylananine-Trp-Arg] (C5aR-AP) has specific anti-C5a effects in rats and has been shown to have potent *in vivo* anti-inflammatory activities in murine models of endotoxic shock, renal ischemia-reperfusion injury and the Arthus reaction [130-133]. C5aR-

AP has also been demonstrated to inhibit effects of C5a on human polymorphonuclear cells and human vascular ECs [132]. Coversin (rEV576), a C5 inhibitor isolated from the saliva of the tick *Ornithodoros moubata,* was recently shown by our group to significantly inhibit venous thrombosis in the presence of aPL in a mouse model [134]. Coversin has proven to be an effective therapeutic agent in preclinical models of myasthenia gravis, Guillain Barré syndrome, sepsis and asthma and our results indicate a potential therapeutic role for coversin in primary thromboprophylaxis and in preventing the extension of acute venous thrombosis in APS patients [134-136].

9. Thrombotic and non-thrombotic effects of aPL antibodies associated with pregnancy morbidity

Given the prothrombotic nature of the disease, impairment of maternal-fetal blood exchange as a result of thrombus formation in the uteroplacental vasculature was thought to be the main pathogenic mechanism underlying pregnancy morbidity in APS [137]. However, there is evidence to suggest that placental thrombosis is only partially responsible for APS pregnancy morbidity. Despite placental thrombosis and infarction being demonstrated in some APS patients with first and second trimester abortions, histological evidence of thrombosis in the uteroplacental circulation cannot be demonstrated in the majority of placentas from APS patients [138-140]. IgG fractions from LA positive APS patients can however induce a procoagulant phenotype with significant increases in thromboxane synthesis in placental explants from normal human pregnancies [141]. Interestingly, Rand *et al* have reported significantly lower levels of annexin A5, an important anticoagulant during pregnancy, covering the intervillous surfaces of placentas in women with aPL when compared to controls [142]. *In vitro* studies have also demonstrated displacement of annexin A5 from trophoblast and endothelial cell monolayers by aPL antibodies while murine studies have demonstrated the necessity of this protein in maintaining placental integrity [43,143]. Anti-annexin A5 antibodies have been reported in APS patients at frequencies up to 30% and several studies have demonstrated the association of these Abs with recurrent fetal loss in APS patients [44,144].

There is growing evidence for a direct effect of aPL antibodies on trophoblasts supported by the fact that β_2GPI and anionic PLs are normally expressed on the outer leaflet of trophoblast membranes under physiological conditions due to high levels of tissue remodeling, also explaining the placental tropism of aPL antibodies[145]. *In vitro* studies utilizing murine and human monoclonal aPL antibodies and polyclonal IgG antibodies from APS patients have demonstrated β_2GPI dependent binding of these antibodies to trophoblast monolayers [146,147]. These aPL antibodies have been shown to react with syncytiotrophoblast and to prevent intertrophoblast fusion, trophoblast invasiveness and hCG secretion [146,148,149]. Finely tuned regulation of cell surface adhesion and signaling molecule expression, activation of matrix metalloproteinases (MMPs), angiogenesis and spiral artery transformation characterizes the complex and dynamic process that is placentation [150]. Induction by aPL antibodies of abnormal trophoblast expression of particular integrins and cadherins potentially affecting decidual invasion has been demonstrated *in vitro* [151]. Anti-β_2GPI monoclonal antibodies can inhibit the proliferation of a human choriocarcinoma cell line and extravillous trophoblast differentiation *in vitro* and endometrial biopsy samples from APS patients with recurrent abortions have shown impaired endometrial differentiation [148,152]. Inhibition of endometrial angiogenesis by aPL antibodies has been demonstrated in a recent study assessing *in vitro* human endometrial endothelial cell (HEEC) angiogenesis and *in vivo* angiogenesis in a murine model. Human polyclonal IgG aPL antibodies were shown to significantly decrease the number and total length of tubule formation, VEGF and MMP production and NF-κB DNA binding activity in HEEC and to reduce new vessel formation in inoculated mice [153].

There is extensive evidence for an inflammatory component to the pathology associated with pregnancy morbidity in APS patients. Polyclonal and monoclonal β_2GPI dependent aPL antibodies can bind stromal decidua cell monolayers and induce a pro-inflammatory phenotype characterized by increased ICAM-1 expression and TNFα secretion [154]. Diminished expression of the complement regulatory protein DAF (decay accelerating factor) has been demonstrated in endometrial biopsy samples from APS patients with recurrent pregnancy loss underscoring the importance of complement activation [152]. Pregnant mice inoculated with human IgG aPL antibodies from APS patients with obstetric APS manifestations had increased rates of fetal resorption, fetal growth retardation and extensive placental damage characterized by recruitment of neutrophils, upregulated TF and TNF-α secretion, decidual focal necrosis and apoptosis, loss of fetal membrane elements and complement deposition [96]. These effects were abrogated in mice given inhibitors of classical and alternative complement pathways and in mice that were C3, C4 or factor B deficient pointing to the involvement of all complement pathways in aPL mediated pregnancy morbidity [155,111]. Additional murine studies have demonstrated the importance of C5a-C5a receptor interactions, especially on neutrophils and monocytes, in inducing TF production, oxidative damage, diminished VEGF levels and subsequent placental hypoperfusion and injury, fetal growth restriction and resorption [111,156,157].

10. Current and potential new treatments for APS-associated clinical manifestations

The cornerstone of treatment for APS remains conventional anticoagulation. Patients who have experienced a venous thromboembolic event (VTE) and are positive for an aPL antibody should be treated with an initial course of unfractionated heparin (UFH), low molecular weight heparin (LMWH) or pentasaccharide followed by warfarin [158]. The initial target intensity of oral anticoagulation is a goal international normalized ratio (INR) of 2.0-3.0 [158]. Patients that suffer an arterial thrombotic event on this regimen should be treated with higher intensity anticoagulation with a goal INR of >3.0 or standard intensity oral anticoagulation (INR 2.0-3.0) in combination with low dose aspirin (LDA). Patients who are intolerant of oral anticoagulation (e.g. inability to achieve and maintain target INR, excessive anticoagulation or adverse effect of warfarin) may be treated with long-term LMWH [159]. Patients who are pregnant should not be treated with warfarin therapy due to potential teratogenicity; rather use of LDA in combination with heparin (Rai, 1998) or LMWH [160,161].

The therapeutic management as well as the prevention of recurrent thrombosis in APS has been focused on utilizing anti-thrombotic medications. Recurrences, despite seemingly adequate treatment, have been reported and the use of oral anticoagulation at a relatively high INR for a long period of time has been associated with a high risk of bleeding, with the need for frequent monitoring and patient compliance with diet and lifestyle to optimize the therapy. Moreover, still debated is the approach to patients with aPL antibodies without a previous thrombotic event. Some physicians would recommend prophylaxis with low dose aspirin although there are no evidence-based data supporting that low dose aspirin alone is sufficient for primary thrombosis prophylaxis [162]. It is well known that aPL antibodies might be persistently present in the serum of APS patients for long periods of time, but thrombotic events do occur only occasionally. It has been suggested that aPL antibodies (*first hit*) increase the thrombophilic threshold (i.e. induce a prothrombotic/ proinflammmatory phenotype in endothelial cells), but that clotting takes place only in the presence of a *second hit* or triggering event (i.e.: an infection, a surgical procedure, use of estrogens, prolonged immobilization, etc) [89]. Current treatments of thrombosis in APS are directed towards modulating the final event or "second hit". Treatments that modulate early effects of aPL antibodies on target cells – i.e. monocytes or endothelial cells - (*first hit*) would be more beneficial and potentially less harmful than current treatments.

Barriers to the development of new drugs for APS include the multifactorial nature of thrombosis, controversies about the strength of association between aPL antibodies and thrombotic events, and the fact that the mechanisms of aPL-induced thrombosis are not well understood. In the long-term management of APS patients, controlled studies with warfarin alternatives and the new anticoagulant agents (such as oral direct and indirect thrombin inhibitors) as well as newer therapeutic agents are vital. However, it is possible that the current "antithrombotic" approach to aPL-positive patients will be replaced by an "immunomodulatory" approach in the future as our understanding of the mechanisms of aPL-mediated thrombosis grows. Understanding the molecular mechanisms triggered by aPL antibodies and identifying biomarkers released as a consequence of cellular activation may help to design new ways to treat clinical manifestations in APS. Based on data from mechanistic *in vitro* and *in vivo* studies, new targeted treatments may be proposed including: specific inhibition of tissue factor, blocking binding of the aPL antibodies to target cells (i.e.: platelets, endothelial cells, monocytes, trophoblasts, etc), using p38 MAPK inhibitors, NF-κB inhibitors or GPIIb/IIIa inhibitors, abrogating the activation of complement, or targeting cytokines such as IL-6 and TNF-α. Most of these have been discussed in other sections of this chapter (Table 3). Clinical trials are needed to demonstrate whether any of those new therapies are safe and efficacious in APS patients [98,100-103,163-167].

Statins, hydroxychloroquine and rituximab in APS.

Three FDA approved drugs – statins, hydroxychloroquine (HCQ) and rituximab – are also being considered as possible new treatments for APS-associated clinical manifestations based on the effects of these drugs on *in vitro* and *in vivo* animal studies.

a. Statins in APS.

Statins are potent inhibitors of cholesterol synthesis in the mevalonate pathway. In the general population, clinical trials of statin therapy have demonstrated beneficial effects in primary and secondary prevention of coronary heart disease as well as ischemic stroke [168]. However, their beneficial effects are only partially explained by their ability to lower cholesterol levels. Pleiotropic effects of statins have been reported, which include decreasing the expression of CAMs in monocytes and affecting leukocyte /endothelial interactions, down-regulating inflammatory cytokines in endothelial cells or increasing fibrinolytic activity 169-171].

Target or Medication	Supportive Evidence Based on In Vitro and/or Animal Studies	Supportive Evidence Based on aPL(+) Human Studies
Tissue Factor (TF)	Dilazep inhibitis aPL-induced TF upregulation in monocytes and endothelial cells (EC)	No
Nuclear Factor (NF)-κB	NF-κB inhibition decreases aPL-induced upregulation of TF in EC and aPL-enhanced thrombosis in mice	No
P38 Mitogen Activated Protein Kinase (MAPK)	P38MAPK inhibition decreases aPL-induced upregulation of TF in EC, platelet activation, and aPL-enhanced thrombosis in mice	No
Platelet Glycoprotein (GP) Receptors	GP receptor antagonists decrease the aPL-mediated enhancement of platelet activation and abrogate aPL-induced thrombus formation in mice	No
Hydroxychlor-oquine (HCQ)	HCQ decreases aPL-induced platelet activation, inhibits aPL-mediated thrombosis in mice, and protects aPL-induced displacement of Annexin A5 from phospholipids bilayers	Possibly protective against thrombosis in lupus patients A trial will be started Spring 2012
Statins	Statins reverse aPL-induced endothelial cell activation and TF upregulation, and abrogates enhanced thrombus formation in mice	Statins decrease pro-inflammatory and pro-thrombotic markers (pilot data, small number of patients)
β_2GPI and/or anti-β_2GPI binding to Target Cells	Peptides that mimic domains of β_2GPI or β_2GPI receptor blockers (e.g., anti-annexin A2, anti-TLR4, aPOER2 antagonists) inhibit aPL-induced EC activation and/or aPL-mediated thrombosis in mice.	No
Complement	Anti-C5 monoclonal antibody decreases aPL-mediated thrombus formation in mice; anti- C5aRA peptide inhibits aPL-mediated thrombosis and TF expression in mice	No
B Cells	B-cell activating factor (BAFF) blockage can prevent the disease onset in antiphospholipid syndrome mouse model	Rituximab is effective for non-criteria aPL manifestations based on the anecdotal reports

Table 3. Potential Immunomodulatory Approaches in Antiphospholipid-Antibody (aPL) Positive Patients.

There have been numerous publications recently on the benefit of statins in the medical community following the recent results from the JUPITER study, in which patients with normal LDL levels of less than 130 mg/dL and elevated C-reactive protein (CRP), levels greater than 2.0 mg/dL, receiving rosuvastatin 20 mg daily experienced significant reduction in cardiovascular events, non-fatal myocardial infarction, and non-fatal stroke [172].

Studies have suggested that fluvastatin has beneficial effects on aPL-mediated pathogenic effects. First, one study showed that fluvastatin prevented the expression of CAMs and IL-6 in EC treated with aPL antibodies [173]. Subsequently, Ferrara *et al* showed that the thrombogenic and pro-inflammatory effects of aPL antibodies *in vivo* could be abrogated in mice fed with fluvastatin for 15 days [97] and this effect was independent of the cholesterol lowering effects of the drug. The same group of investigators then showed that fluvastatin inhibited the effects of aPL antibodies on tissue factor expression on endothelial cells *in vitro* at doses utilized to reduce cholesterol levels in patients [174]. Furthermore, Martinez *et al.* demonstrated that rosuvastatin decreases VCAM-1 expression by human umbilical vein endothelial cells (HUVEC) exposed to APS serum in an *in vitro* model [175].

Subsequently, Murthy *et al* examined whether proinflammatory/prothrombotic markers are elevated in patients with aPL antibodies and whether treatment with fluvastatin has an effect on those. (Clinical Trials.gov Identifier: NCT00674297). The preliminary analysis of this ongoing pilot study showed that fluvastatin 40 mg daily for 3 months significantly reduced the pro-inflammatory and prothrombotic biomarkers IL-6, IL-1β, sTF, sICAM-1, sVCAM-1 and E-selectin in persistently aPL-positive patients with or without SLE [176]. Furthemore, utilizing proteomic analysis, Cuadrado *et al* have shown that inflammatory proteins can be reversed following one month of treatment with fluvastatin [177].

In summary, although statins have been used in primary and secondary cardiovascular disease prevention, no conclusive data exist for thrombosis prevention in aPL-positive patients. Based on data available, it is conceivable that statins may be beneficial in reversing upregulation of TF, CAMs and inflammatory cytokines in EC and monocytes. Upon successful completion of clinical trials, in theory, statins might even replace warfarin and antiplatelet agents in prevention of recurrent arterial and venous thrombosis, thus eliminating the risk of hemorrhagic complications associated with warfarin and enabling better life style in these patients. Statins may also serve as an alternative treatment in APS patients who experience thrombosis despite adequate anticoagulation with warfarin or with antiplatelet agents, or in those with thrombocytopenia in whom warfarin is contraindicated. Finally, statins would be an appealing prophylactic therapy in patients with high levels of aPL antibodies and without a history of thrombosis. Statins are teratogenic and therefore their use in pregnancy is contraindicated. Side effects must be closely monitored, including elevated liver function tests and potential hyperglycemia and diabetes mellitus. The use of statins in the management of patient with APS needs to be further delineated in well-designed mechanistic and clinical studies.

b. Hydroxychloroquine

Hydroxychloroquine (HCQ) is an antimalarial drug, although the precise mechanism of its anti-inflammatory action is not known. In addition to its anti-inflammatory effects, there are immunomodulatory effects of HCQ that include increasing the pH of intracellular vacuoles and interfering with antigen processing and inhibiting T-cell-receptor-induced and B-cell-receptor-induced calcium signaling [178,179]. HCQ also has antithrombotic effects by inhibiting platelet aggregation and arachidonic acid release from stimulated platelets [180]. In the general population, HCQ has been historically used as a prophylactic agent against deep vein thrombosis and pulmonary embolism after hip surgeries [181].

HCQ is now considered an essential therapeutic choice in the management of lupus. HCQ has been shown to decrease the probability of lupus flares, the accrual of damage, and possibly protect SLE patients from vascular and thrombotic events [181-183]. Furthermore, HCQ may facilitate the response to other agents in SLE patients with renal involvement. More recently, chloroquine and HCQ have been shown to improve survival in a cohort of 232 SLE patients after adjusting for patient characteristics and disease activity [184]. It has been recently suggested that HCQ may affect TLR9 activation and IFN-α production and this drug is now considered an essential therapeutic choice in the management of lupus.

In aPL-injected mice, HCQ decreases the thrombus size and the aPL-enhanced thrombus formation in a dose-dependent manner [95]. Furthermore, HCQ inhibits the aPL-induced expression of platelet GPIIb/IIIa receptor (platelet activation) in a dose-dependent fashion [115]. Recently, using 3D atomic microscopy force height images, Rand *et al* showed that HCQ also reverses the binding of aPL-β_2GPI complexes to phospholipids bilayers [185,186]. In SLE patients, those receiving HCQ experienced fewer thrombotic events and in the Baltimore Lupus Cohort, investigators showed a decreased risk of arterial thrombosis [187]. Other investigators demonstrated that HCQ decreases the risk of thrombosis in patients with SLE (OR 0.67). In a Cox multiple failure time analysis, HCQ was shown to protect against thrombosis and increase survival in patients with SLE. In a cross-sectional study in which Erkan *et al* compared 77 APS patients with previous vascular events (65% had no other systemic autoimmune diseases) to 56 asymptomatic (no history of thrombosis or fetal loss) aPL-positive patients (18% had no other systemic autoimmune diseases), logistic regression analysis suggested that HCQ protects against thrombosis in asymptomatic aPL-positive individuals [188]. In summary, although there is experimental and clinical evidence that HCQ might decrease the incidence of thrombosis in patients with SLE, both detailed mechanistic and controlled studies are needed to determine the effectiveness of HCQ for primary and secondary thrombosis prevention in patients with APS. At this time, even though there are insufficient data to recommend HCQ for primary and secondary prevention, it might be reasonable to add HCQ to anticoagulation agents in APS patients who develop recurrent thrombosis despite optimum anticoagulation.

Multiple studies have shown reduction in thrombotic events in SLE patients receiving HCQ [189,182]. However, despite some studies showing a sharp contrast to this demonstrated protective effect, it appears reasonable that HCQ can be used a second line agent, in addition to anti-coagulation, in patients with APS and thrombus. As well, before starting therapy, it is important to screen for macular toxicity with visual field and fundoscopic examination every six to twelve months.

A prospective blind-placebo control clinical trial of persistently aPL-positive individuals will soon be started by an international multicenter collaborative effort under the auspices of APS ACTION (Antiphospholipid Syndrome: Alliance for Clinical Trials and International Networking). The primary objective of this trial is to determine the efficacy of HCQ therapy in primary thrombo-prophylaxis in persistently aPL-positive APS patients with no history of thrombosis or any other systemic autoimmune disease.

c. Rituximab.

Recently, rituximab has been shown to be a good therapeutic agent for life-threatening CAPS in a small number of patients [190-192]. Rituximab has been successfully used in case reports of patients with aPL and auto-immune mediated thrombocytopenia and hemolytic anemia. A systematic review of the off-label use of rituximab in APS revealed the higher rate of therapeutic response in patients with APS (92%) [193] and an increasing number of similar case reports clearly indicates the need for clinical trials to evaluate the effect of rituximab in the treatment of resistant APS. Currently Erkan *et al* are conducting a RITAPS open-label Phase II trial using Rituximab to study patients who are aPL positive and resistant to conventional anticoagulation (Clinical trials.gov Identifier: NCT00537290). In preliminary results reported at a recent annual meeting of the American College of Rheumatology in 2011, the investigators reported that although a net decrease of aPL antibody titers was not seen in patients given rituximab, the drug appeared to have an effect on improving thrombocytopenia, and skin ulcers accompanied by an overall decrease in CD19+ B cells. [194].

11. Concluding remarks

Since the mid-1980s, aPL antibodies and their associated clinical manifestations have attracted great interest among clinicians and investigators. Indeed, the attention directed to aPL often exceeds that for other autoantibodies within the field of autoimmunity; even in systemic lupus erythematosus, which is characterized by a multitude of specificities, the interest in this serological system remains high.

A significant amount of knowledge has been gained in the last 20 years with respect to etio-pathogenesis of this complex disease. In addition, progress has been accomplished on standardization of "criteria" aPL tests as well as new emerging tests and methodologies that may help to improve the diagnosis of APS. Recently, the improved understanding of the intracellular and molecular mechanisms activated during aPL-induced thrombosis has enabled investigators to propose new and possibly more effective - with less harmful side effects - treatments of APS-related clinical manifestations. Clinical trials for these new treatments are urgently needed (some already have been started) to translate bench research into new therapies for affected patients.

12. References

[1] Miyakis S, lockshin MD, Atsumi I et al. International concensus statement on an update of the classification criteria for definite antiphospholipid syndrome (APS). J Thromb Haemost 2006; 4:295-306

[2] McNeil HP, Simpson RJ, Cherterman CN et al. Antiphospholipid antibodies are directed against a complex antigen that includes lipid binding inhibitor of coagulation: β2 glycoprotein I (apolipoprotein H). Proc Natl Acad Sci USA 1990; 87:4120-4

[3] Roubey RA. Antiphospholipid syndrome: antibodies and antigens. Curr Opin Hematol 2000; 7(5):316-320.

[4] Ginsburg KS, Liang MH, Newcomer L et al. Anticardiolipin antibodies and the risk for ischemic stroke and venous thrombosis. Ann Intern Med1992; 117:997-1002
[5] McClain MT, Arbuckle MR, Heinlen LD et al. The prevalence, onset and clinical significance of antiphospholipid antibodies prior to diagnosis of systemic lupus erythematosus. Arthritis Rheum 2004;50:1226-32
[6] Petri M. Update on anti-phospholipid antibodies in SLE: the Hopkins' Lupus Cohort. Lupus 2010; 19:419-23
[7] Asherson RA. Multiorgan failure and antiphospholipid antibodies: the catastrophic antiphospholipid (Asherson's) syndrome. Immunobiology 2005; 210: 727-33
[8] Sailer T, Zaglami C, Kurz C et al. Anti-beta(2)-glycoprotein-I antibodies are associated with pregnancy loss in women with the lupus anticoagulant. Thromb Haemost 2006; 5:796-801.
[9] Moore JE, Mohr CF. Biologically false positive serologic tests for syphilis; type, incidence, and cause. J Am Med Assoc 1952; 150: 467-473
[10] Conley CL, Hartmann RC. A hemorrhagic disorder caused by circulating anticoagulant in patients with disseminated lupus erythematosus. J Clin Invest 1952; 31:621-622
[11] Feinstein DI, Rapaport SI. Acquired inhibitors of blood coagulation. Prog Hemostas Thromb 1972;1:75-95.
[12] Bowie EJ, Thrompson JH Jr, Pascuzzi CA, Owen CA Jr. Thrombosis in Systemic Lupus Erythematosus despite circulating anticoagulants. J Lab Clin Med. 1963; 62:416-30.
[13] Thiagarajan P, Shapiro SS, De Marco L. Monoclonal immunoglobulin M lambda coagulation inhibitor with phospholipid specificity. Mechanism of lupus anticoagulant. J Clin Invest 1980;66:397-405.
[14] Harris EN. Anticardiolipin antibodies: detection by radioimmunoassay and association with thrombosis. Lancet 1983; 2: 1211-1214.
[15] Boey ML, Colaco CB, Gharavi AE, Elkon KB, Loizou S, Hughes GR. Thrombosis in SLE: striking associations with the presence of circulating "lupus anticoagulant" Br Med J. 1983; 287: 1021-3.
[16] Elias M, Eldor A. Thromboembolism in patients with the "lupus" like circulating anticoagulant. Arch Int Med. 1984; 144: 510-515
[17] Harris EN, Pierangeli SS. Primary, secondary, and catastrophic antiphospholipid syndrome: what's in a name? Semin Throm Haemost 2008; 34:219-226
[18] Cervera R, Khamashta MA, Shoenfeld Y, et al. "Morbidity and mortality in the antiphospholipid syndrome during a 5-year period: a multicentre prospective study of 1000 patients." Ann Rheum Dis. 2009; 68: 1428-1432
[19] Cervera R, Tektonidou MG, Espinosa G, et al. "Task Force on Catastrophic Antiphospholipid Syndrome (APS) and Non-Criteria APS Manifestations (I): catastrophic APS, APS nephropathy and heart valve lesions." Lupus. 2011; 20: 165-173.
[20] Bucciarelli S, Espinosa G, Cervera R, et al. "Mortality in the Catastrophic Antiphospholipid Syndrome: Causes of Death and Prognostic Factors in a Series of 250 Patients." Arthritis Rheum. 2006; 54(8): 2568-2576.
[21] Ciubotaru C, Esfahani F, Benedict RHB, Wild LM, Baer AN. "Chorea and Rapidly Progressive Subcortical Dementia in Antiphospholipid Syndrome." J Clin Rheumatol. 2002; 8: 332-339.

[22] Cervera R, Tektonidou MG, Espinosa G, et al. "Task Force on Catastrophic Antiphospholipid Syndrome (APS) and Non-Criteria APS Manifestations (II): thrombocytopenia and skin manifestations." Lupus. 2011; 20: 174-181.
[23] Pierangeli SS, Harris EN. A quarter of a century in anticardiolipin antibody testing and attempted standardization has led us to here, which is?. Semin Thromb Haeemost 2008;334:313-328.
[24] Pierangeli S, Groot P, Dlott J, et al. "Criteria" aPL tests: Report of a task force and preconference workshop at the 13th International Congress on Antiphospholipid Antibodies, Galveston, TX. April 2010.Lupus 2011; 20: 182-190.
[25] Lakos G, Favaloro EJ, Harris EN, Meroni PL, Tincani A, Wong RC et al. International consensus guidelines on anticardiolipin and anti-beta(2) glycoprotein I testing: A report from the APL task force at the 13(th) international congress on antiphospholipid antibodies. Arthritis Rheum 2011 Sep 27. doi: 10.1002/art.33349. [Epub ahead of print]
[26] Pierangeli S, Favaloro EJ, Lakos G, Meroni PL, Tincani A, Wong RC, Harris EN. Standards and reference materials for the anticardiolipin and anti-β(2)glycoprotein I assays: A report of recommendations from the APL Task Force at the 13th International Congress on Antiphospholipid Antibodies. Clin Chim Acta. 2011 Oct 15. [Epub ahead of print]
[27] Bertolaccini ML, Amengual O, Atsumi T,et al. "Non-criteria" aPL tests: report of a task force and preconference workshop at the 13th International Congress on Antiphospholipid Antibodies. Lupus 2011; 20: 191-205.
[28] Permpikul P, Rao LV, Rapaport SI. Functional and binding studies of the roles of prothrombin and beta 2-glycoprotein I in the expression of lupus anticoagulant activity. Blood. 1994 May 15;83(10):2878-92.
[29] de Laat B, Pengo V, Pabinger I, Musial J, Voskuyl AE, Bultink IE et al. The association between circulating antibodies against domain I of beta2-glycoprotein I and thrombosis: an international multicenter study. J Thromb Haemost. 2009 Nov;7(11):1767-73
[30] Martin SJ, Reutelingsperger CP, McGahon AJ, Rader JA, van Schie RC, LaFace DM, Green DR. Early redistribution of plasma membrane phosphatidylserine is a general feature of apoptosis regardless of the initiating stimulus: inhibition by overexpression of Bcl-2 and Abl. J Exp Med. 1995 Nov 1;182(5):1545-56.
[31] Kobayashi K, Kishi M, Atsumi T, Bertolaccini ML, Makino H, Sakairi N et al. Circulating oxidized LDL forms complexes with beta2-glycoprotein I: implication as an atherogenic autoantigen. J Lipid Res. 2003 Apr;44(4):716-26.
[32] Lopez LR, Simpson DF, Hurley BL, Matsuura E. OxLDL/beta2GPI complexes and autoantibodies in patients with systemic lupus erythematosus, systemic sclerosis, and antiphospholipid syndrome: pathogenic implications for vascular involvement. Ann N Y Acad Sci. 2005 Jun;1051:313-22.
[33] Cuadrado MJ, Buendía P, Velasco F et al. Vascular endothelial growth factor expression in monocytes from patients with primary antiphospholipid syndrome. J Thromb Haemost. 2006 Nov;4(11):2461-9

[34] Pierangeli SS, Colden-Stanfield M, Liu X et al. Antiphospholipid antibodies from antiphospholipid syndrome patients activate endothelial cells in vitro and in vivo. Circulation. 1999 Apr 20;99(15):1997-2002
[35] Chamley LW, Duncalf AM, Mitchell MD, Johnson PM. Action of anticardiolipin and antibodies to beta2-glycoprotein-I on trophoblast proliferation as a mechanism for fetal death. Lancet. 1998 Sep 26;352(9133):1037-8
[36] Shi T, Giannakopoulos B, Yan X et al. Anti-beta2-glycoprotein I antibodies in complex with beta2-glycoprotein I can activate platelets in a dysregulated manner via glycoprotein Ib-IX-V. Arthritis Rheum. 2006 Aug;54(8):2558-67
[37] Pierangeli SS, Vega-Ostertag ME, Raschi E et al. Toll-like receptor and antiphospholipid mediated thrombosis: in vivo studies. Ann Rheum Dis. 2007 Oct;66(10):1327-33
[38] Sorice M, Longo A, Capozzi A et al. Anti-beta2-glycoprotein I antibodies induce monocyte release of tumor necrosis factor alpha and tissue factor by signal transduction pathways involving lipid rafts. Arthritis Rheum. 2007 Aug;56(8):2687-97
[39] Romay-Penabad Z, Aguilar-Valenzuela R, Urbanus RT, Derksen H et al. Apolipoprotein E receptor 2′ is involved in the thrombotic complications in a murine model of the antiphospholipid syndrome. Blood. 2011 Jan 27;117(4):1408-14.
[40] Urbanus RT, Pennings MT, Derksen RH, de Groot PG. Platelet activation by dimeric beta2-glycoprotein I requires signaling via both glycoprotein Ibalpha and apolipoprotein E receptor 2'. J Thromb Haemost. 2008 Aug;6(8):1405-12
[41] Sikara MP, Routsias JG, Samiotaki M et al. {beta}2 Glycoprotein I ({beta}2GPI) binds platelet factor 4 (PF4): implications for the pathogenesis of antiphospholipid syndrome. Blood. 2010 Jan 21;115(3):713-23
[42] Chen PP, Giles I. Antibodies to serine proteases in the antiphospholipid syndrome. Curr Rheumatol Rep. 2010 Feb;12(1):45-52.
[43] Rand JH, Wu XX, Guller S et al. Antiphospholipid immunoglobulin G antibodies reduce annexin-V levels on syncytiotrophoblast apical membranes and in culture media of placental villi. Am J Obstet Gynecol. 1997 Oct;177(4):918-23
[44] Nojima J, Kuratsune H, Suehisa E et al. Association between the prevalence of antibodies to beta(2)-glycoprotein I, prothrombin, protein C, protein S, and annexin V in patients with systemic lupus erythematosus and thrombotic and thrombocytopenic complications. Clin Chem. 2001 Jun;47(6):1008-15
[45] Ortona E, Capozzi A, Colasanti T, Conti F, Alessandri C, Longo A et al. Vimentin/cardiolipin complex as a new antigenic target of the antiphospholipid syndrome. Blood. 2010 Oct 21;116(16):2960-7.
[46] Jiang H, Chess L. How the immune system achieves self-nonself discrimination during adaptive immunity. Adv Immunol. 2009;102:95-133.
[47] Gharavi AE, Sammaritano LR, Wen J, Elkon KB. Induction of antiphospholipid autoantibodies by immunization with beta 2 glycoprotein I (apolipoprotein H). J Clin Invest. 1992 Sep;90(3):1105-9
[48] Gharavi AE, Pierangeli SS, Colden-Stanfield M et al. GDKV-induced antiphospholipid antibodies enhance thrombosis and activate endothelial cells in vivo and in vitro. J Immunol. 1999 Sep 1;163(5):2922-7

[49] Gharavi AE, Pierangeli SS, Gharavi EE et al. Thrombogenic properties of antiphospholipid antibodies do not depend on their binding to beta2 glycoprotein 1 (beta2GP1) alone. Lupus. 1998;7(5):341-6.

[50] Gharavi EE, Chaimovich H, Cucurull E et al. Induction of antiphospholipid antibodies by immunization with synthetic viral and bacterial peptides. Lupus. 1999;8(6):449-55

[51] Gharavi AE, Pierangeli SS, Espinola RG et al. Antiphospholipid antibodies induced in mice by immunization with a cytomegalovirus-derived peptide cause thrombosis and activation of endothelial cells in vivo. Arthritis Rheum. 2002 Feb;46(2):545-52

[52] Gharavi AE, Vega-Ostertag M, Espinola RG et al. Intrauterine fetal death in mice caused by cytomegalovirus-derived peptide induced aPL antibodies. Lupus. 2004;13(1):17-23

[53] Blank M, Krause I, Fridkin M et al. Bacterial induction of autoantibodies to beta2-glycoprotein-I accounts for the infectious etiology of antiphospholipid syndrome. J Clin Invest. 2002 Mar;109(6):797-804

[54] Levy Y, Almog O, Gorshtein A, Shoenfeld Y. The environment and antiphospholipid syndrome. Lupus. 2006;15(11):784-90

[55] Uthman IW, Gharavi AE. Viral infections and antiphospholipid antibodies. Semin Arthritis Rheum. 2002 Feb;31(4):256-63.

[56] Sène D, Piette JC, Cacoub P. Antiphospholipid antibodies, antiphospholipid syndrome and viral infections. Rev Med Interne. 2009 Feb;30(2):135-41

[57] VAN Os GM, Meijers JC, Agar C, Seron MV, Marquart JA, Akesson P et al. Induction of anti-β(2) -glycoprotein I autoantibodies in mice by protein H of Streptococcus pyogenes. J Thromb Haemost. 2011 Dec;9(12):2447-56.

[58] Rauch J, Dieudé M, Subang R, Levine JS. The dual role of innate immunity in the antiphospholipid syndrome. Lupus. 2010 Apr;19(4):347-53.

[59] Aguilar-Valenzuela R, Nickerson K, Romay-Penabad Z, Shlomchik MJ, Vargas G, Shilagard T, Pierangeli S. Involvement of TLR7 and TLR9 in the production of antiphospholipid antibodies. Arthritis Rheum 2011; 63(10):s281 (abstract 723)

[60] Hashimoto Y, Kawamura M, Ichikawa K et al. Anticardiolipin antibodies in NZW x BXSB F1 mice. A model of antiphospholipid syndrome. J Immunol. 1992 Aug 1;149(3):1063-8

[61] Kita Y, Sumida T, Iwamoto I, Yoshida S, Koike T. V gene analysis of anti-cardiolipin antibodies from (NZW x BXSB) F1 mice. Immunology. 1994 Jul;82(3):494-501.

[62] Ida A, Hirose S, Hamano Y et al. Multigenic control of lupus-associated antiphospholipid syndrome in a model of (NZW x BXSB) F1 mice. Eur J Immunol. 1998 Sep;28(9):2694-703

[63] Papalardo E, Romay-Penabad Z, Christadoss P, Pierangeli S. Induction of pathogenic antiphospholipid antibodies in vivo are dependent on expression of MHC-II genes. Lupus 2010; 19:496 (abstract)

[64] . Exner T, Barber S, Kronenberg H, Rickard KA. Familial association of the lupus anticoagulant. Br J Haematol. 1980 May;45(1):89-96

[65] Jolidon RM, Knecht H, Humair L, de Torrente A. Different clinical presentations of a lupus anticoagulant in the same family. Klin Wochenschr. 1991 May 24;69(8):340-4

[66] Matthey F, Walshe K, Mackie IJ, Machin SJ. Familial occurrence of the antiphospholipid syndrome. J Clin Pathol. 1989 May;42(5):495-7
[67] Dagenais P, Urowitz MB, Gladman DD, Norman CS. A family study of the antiphospholipid syndrome associated with other autoimmune diseases. J Rheumatol. 1992 Sep;19(9):1393-6
[68] Rouget JP, Goudemand J, Montreuil G et al. Lupus anticoagulant: a familial observation. Lancet. 1982 Jul 10;2(8289):105.
[69] Mackie IJ, Colaco CB, Machin SJ. Familial lupus anticoagulants. Br J Haematol. 1987 Nov;67(3):359-63
[70] May KP, West SG, Moulds J, Kotzin BL. Different manifestations of the antiphospholipid antibody syndrome in a family with systemic lupus erythematosus. Arthritis Rheum. 1993 Apr;36(4):528-33
[71] Arnett FC, Olsen ML, Anderson KL, Reveille JD. Molecular analysis of major histocompatibility complex alleles associated with the lupus anticoagulant. J Clin Invest. 1991 May;87(5):1490-5
[72] Asherson RA, Doherty DG, Vergani D et al. Major histocompatibility complex associations with primary antiphospholipid syndrome. Arthritis Rheum. 1992 Jan;35(1):124-5
[73] Caliz R, Atsumi T, Kondeatis E et al. HLA class II gene polymorphisms in antiphospholipid syndrome: haplotype analysis in 83 Caucasoid patients. Rheumatology (Oxford). 2001 Jan;40(1):31-6
[74] Hashimoto H, Yamanaka K, Tokano Y et al. HLA-DRB1 alleles and beta 2 glycoprotein I-dependent anticardiolipin antibodies in Japanese patients with systemic lupus erythematosus. Clin Exp Rheumatol. 1998 Jul-Aug;16(4):423-7
[75] Wilson WA, Scopelitis E, Michalski JP et al. Familial anticardiolipin antibodies and C4 deficiency genotypes that coexist with MHC DQB1 risk factors. J Rheumatol. 1995 Feb;22(2):227-35
[76] Petri M, Watson R, Winkelstein JA, McLean RH. Clinical expression of systemic lupus erythematosus in patients with C4A deficiency. Medicine (Baltimore). 1993 Jul;72(4):236-44
[77] Bertolaccini ML, Atsumi T, Caliz AR et al. Association of antiphosphatidylserine/ prothrombin autoantibodies with HLA class II genes. Arthritis Rheum. 2000 Mar;43(3):683-8
[78] Vargas-Alarcon G, Granados J, Bekker C et al. Association of HLA-DR5 (possibly DRB1*1201) with the primary antiphospholipid syndrome in Mexican patients. Arthritis Rheum. 1995 Sep;38(9):1340-1
[79] Galeazzi M, Sebastiani GD, Tincani A et al. HLA class II alleles associations of anticardiolipin and anti-beta2GPI antibodies in a large series of European patients with systemic lupus erythematosus. Lupus. 2000;9(1):47-55
[80] Hirose N, Williams R, Alberts AR et al. A role for the polymorphism at position 247 of the beta2-glycoprotein I gene in the generation of anti-beta2-glycoprotein I antibodies in the antiphospholipid syndrome. Arthritis Rheum. 1999 Aug;42(8):1655-61

[81] Chopra N, Koren S, Greer WL et al. Factor V Leiden, prothrombin gene mutation, and thrombosis risk in patients with antiphospholipid antibodies. J Rheumatol. 2002 Aug;29(8):1683-8
[82] Pierangeli SS, Barker JH, Stikovac D, Ackerman D, Anderson G, Barquinero J, Acland R, Harris EN. Effect of human IgG antiphospholipid antibodies on an in vivo thrombosis model in mice.Thromb. Haemostas. 1994; 71(5): 670-4.
[83] Stockmans F, Deckmyn H, Gruwez J, Vermylen J, Acland R. Continuous quantitative monitoring of mural, platelet-dependent, thrombus kinetics in the crushed rat femoral vein. Thromb Haemost. 1991 Apr 8;65(4):425-31.
[84] Barker JH, Gu JM, Anderson GL, O'Shaughenessy M, Pierangeli S, Johnson P, Galletti G, Acland RD. The effects of heparin and dietary fish oil on embolic events and the microcirculation downstream from a small artery repair. Plast. Reconstr. Surg . 1993; 91: 335-342.
[85] Pierangeli SS, Liu X, Barker JH, Anderson G, Harris EN. Induction of thrombosis in a mouse model by IgG, IgM and IgA immunoglobulins from patients with the Antiphospholipid Syndrome. Thrombosis Haemost . 1995; 74(5): 1361-1367.
[86] Olee T, Pierangeli SS, Handley HH, Novotny W, En J, Harris EN, Woods L, Chen PP. Generation and characterization of Monoclonal IgG Anticardiolipin Antibodies from a Patient with the Antiphospholipid Syndrome. Proc Nat Acad Sci. (USA). 1996; 93: 8606-8611.
[87] Pierangeli SS, Liu, XW, Anderson G, Barker JH, Harris EN. Thrombogenic properties of murine anti-cardiolipin antibodies induced by ß$_2$glycoprotein 1 and human IgG antiphospholipid antibodies. Circulation. 1996; 94:1746-1751.
[88] Jankowski M, Vreys I, Wittevrongel C, Boon D, Vermylen J, Hoylaerts MF, Arnout J. Thrombogenicity of beta 2-glycoprotein I-dependent antiphospholipid antibodies in a photochemically induced thrombosis model in the hamster. Blood. 2003 Jan 1;101(1):157-62. Epub 2002 Sep 5.
[89] Fischetti F, Durigutto P, Pellis V, Debeus A, Macor P, Bulla R, Bossi F, Ziller F, Sblattero D, Meroni P, Tedesco F. Thrombus formation induced by antibodies to beta2-glycoprotein I is complement dependent and requires a priming factor. Blood. 2005 Oct 1;106(7):2340-6. Epub 2005 Jun 14.
[90] Arad A, Proulle V, Furie RA, Furie BC, Furie B. β_2-Glycoprotein-1 autoantibodies from patients with antiphospholipid syndrome are sufficient to potentiate arterial thrombus formation in a mouse model. Blood. 2011 Mar 24;117(12):3453-9. Epub 2011 Jan 18.
[91] Pierangeli SS, Espinola RG, Liu X, Harris EN. Thrombogenic effects of antiphospholipid (aPL) antibodies are mediated by intercellular cell adhesion molecule-1(ICAM-1), vascular cell adhesion molecule-1 (VCAM-1) and P-selectin. Circulation Res 2001; 88: 245-250.
[92] Pierangeli SS, Liu Xiaowei, Espinola R, Olee T, Min Zhi, Harris EN and Chen PP. Functional analysis of patient-derived IgG monoclonal anticardiolipin antibodies using in vivo thrombosis and in vivo microcirculation Models. Thrombosis and Haemostasis 2000; 84:388-395.
[93] Pierangeli SS, Espinola RG, Liu X, Harris EN, Salmon J. Identification of an Fc□ receptor independent mechanism by which intravenous immunoglobulin (IVIG

ameliorates antiphospholipid antibody-induced thrombogenic phenotype. Arthritis Rheum 2001;44: 876-883 (2001)

[94] Vega-Ostertag ME, Liu X, Henderson V, Pierangeli SS. A peptide that mimics the Vth Region of □2glycoprotein I reverses antiphospholipid-mediated thrombosis in mice. Lupus. 2006; 15: 358-365.

[95] Edwards M, Pierangeli SS,Liu Xwei, Barker JH, Anderson GH, Harris EN. Hydroxychloroquine Reverses Thrombogenic Properties of Antiphospholipid Antibodies in Mice. Circulation . 1997; 96(12):4380-4384.

[96] Holers VM, Girardi G, Mo L, Guthridge JM, Molina H, Pierangeli SS, Espinola R, Liu X, Mao D, Vialpando CG, Salmon JE. Complement C3 activation is required for antiphospholipid antibody-induced fetal loss. J Exp Med 2002; 195(2): 211-220.

[97] Ferrara DE, Liu X, Espinola RG, Meroni PL, Abujhalaf I, Harris EN, Pierangeli SS. Inhibition of the thrombogenic and inflammatory properties of antiphospholipid antibodies by fluvastatin in an in vivo animal model. Arthritis Rheum. 2003; 48(11): 3272-3279.

[98] Pierangeli SS, Girardi G, Vega-Ostertag ME, Liu X, Espinola RG, Salmon JE. Requirement of activation of complement C3 and C5 for antiphospholipid antibody-mediated thrombophilia. Arthritis Rheum 2005; 52: 2120-2124.

[99] Vega-Ostertag ME, Liu PP, Henderson V, Chen PP, Pierangeli SS. A human monoclonal anti-prothrombin antibody is thrombogenic.in vivo and upregulates expression of tissue factor and E-selectin on endothelial cells. Br. J. Haematology. 2006; 135: 214-219.

[100] Vega-Ostertag ME, Ferrara DE, Romay-Penabad Z, Liu X, Taylor WR, Colden-Stanfield M, Pierangeli SS. Role of p38 mitogen-activated protein kinase in antiphospholipid antibody-mediated thrombosis and endothelial cell activation. J Thromb Haemost 2007; 5: 1828-1834.

[101] Montiel-Manzano G, Romay-Penabad Z, Papalardo de Martinez E, Meillon-Garcia LA, Garcia-Latorre E, Reyes-Maldonado, Pierangeli SS. In vivo effects of an inhibitor of nuclear factor-kappa B on thrombogenic properties of antiphospholipid antibodies. Ann N Y Acad Sci 2007; 1108: 540-553.

[102] Romay-Penabad Z, Liu XX, Montiel-Manzano G, Papalardo de Martinez E, Pierangeli SS. C5a receptor-deficient mice are protected from thrombophilia and endothelial cell activation induced by some antiphospholipid antibodies. Ann N Y Acad Sci 2007; 1108: 554-566.

[103] Ioannou Y, Romay-Penabad Z, Pericleous C, Giles I, Papalardo E, Vargas G, Shilagard T, Latchman DS, Isenberg D, Rahman A, Pierangeli S. A novel concept for the in vivo inhibition of antiphospholipid antibody induced vascular thrombosis through the use of the antigenic target peptide domain I of □2glycoprotein I. J. Thromb Haemost 2009; 7:833-842.

[104] Giles I, Pericleous C, Liu X, Ehsanullaj J, Clarke L, Brogan P, Newton-West M, Swerlick R, Lambrianides N, Chen P, Latchman D, Isenberg D, Pierangeli SS, Rahman A. Thrombin binding predicts the effects of sequence changes in a human monoclonal antiphospholipid antibodies on its in vivo biological actions. J Immunol 2009; 182:4836-4843.

[105] Romay-Penabad Z, Montiel-Manzano G, Shilagard T, Vargas G, Deora A, Wang M, Garcia-Latorre E, Reyes-Maldonado E, Hajjar KA, Pierangeli S. Annexin A2 is involved in antiphospholipid antibody-mediated pathogenic effects in vitro and in vivo. Blood 2009; 114:3074-3083.

[106] Aron AL, Cuellar ML, Brey RL, Mckeown S, Espinoza LR, Shoenfeld Y, Gharavi AE. Early onset of autoimmunity in MRL/++ mice following immunization with beta 2 glycoprotein I. Clin Exp Immunol. 1995 July; 101(1): 78–81

[107] Branch DW, Dudley DJ, Mitchell MD, Creighton KA, Abbott TM, Hammond EH, Daynes RA. Immunoglobulin G fractions from patients with antiphospholipid antibodies cause fetal death in BALB/c mice: a model for autoimmune fetal loss. Am J Obstet. Gynecol. 1990; 163:210-216.

[108] Bakimer R, Fishman P, Blank M et al. Induction of primary antiphospholipid syndrome in mice by immunization with a human monoclonal anticardiolipin antibody (H-3). J Clin Invest 1992; 89: 1558-63.

[109] Gharavi AE, Vega-Ostertag ME, Espinola RG, et al. Intrauterine fetal death in mice caused by cytomegalovirus-derived peptide induced by aPL antibodies. Lupus 2004; 13:17-23.

[110] Fishman P, Falach-Vaknine E, Zigelman, R Bakimer R, Sredni B, Djaldetti M, Shoenfeld Y. Prevention of fetal loss in experimental antiphospholipid syndrome by in vivo administration of recombinant interleukin-3. J Clin Invest. 1993 April; 91(4): 1834–1837.

[111] Girardi G, Berman J, Redecha P et al. Complement C5a receptors and neutrophils mediate fetal injury in the antiphospholipid syndrome. J Clin Invest. 2003 Dec;112(11):1644-54

[112] Girardi G, Redecha P, Salmon JE. Heparin prevents antiphospholipid antibody-induced fetal loss by inhibiting complement activation. Nat Med 2004; 10: 1222–1226.

[113] Khamashta MA, Harris EN, Gharavi AE et al. Immune mediated mechanism for thrombosis: antiphospholipid antibody binding to platelet membranes. Ann Rheum Dis. 1988 Oct;47(10):849-54

[114] Lutters BC, Derksen RH, Tekelenburg WL et al. Dimers of beta 2-glycoprotein I increase platelet deposition to collagen via interaction with phospholipids and the apolipoprotein E receptor 2'. J Biol Chem. 2003 Sep 5;278(36):33831-8

[115] Espinola RG, Pierangeli SS, Gharavi AE, Harris EN. Hydroxychloroquine reverses platelet activation induced by human IgG antiphospholipid antibodies. Thromb Haemost. 2002 Mar;87(3):518-22

[116] Pierangeli SS, Vega-Ostertag M, Harris EN. Intracellular signaling triggered by antiphospholipid antibodies in platelets and endothelial cells: a pathway to targeted therapies. Thromb Res. 2004;114(5-6):467-76

[117] Meroni PL, Raschi E, Camera M et al. Endothelial activation by aPL: a potential pathogenetic mechanism for the clinical manifestations of the syndrome. J Autoimmun. 2000 Sep;15(2):237-40

[118] Simantov R, Lo SK, Gharavi A et al. Antiphospholipid antibodies activate vascular endothelial cells. Lupus. 1996 Oct;5(5):440-1

[119] Amengual O, Atsumi T, Khamashta MA, Hughes GR. The role of the tissue factor pathway in the hypercoagulable state in patients with the antiphospholipid syndrome. Thromb Haemost. 1998 Feb;79(2):276-81
[120] Kornberg A, Blank M, Kaufman S, Shoenfeld Y. Induction of tissue factor-like activity in monocytes by anti-cardiolipin antibodies. J Immunol. 1994 Aug 1;153(3):1328-32
[121] Reverter JC, Tàssies D, Font J et al. Effects of human monoclonal anticardiolipin antibodies on platelet function and on tissue factor expression on monocytes. Arthritis Rheum. 1998 Aug;41(8):1420-7
[122] Alijotas-Reig J, Palacio-Garcia C, Vilardell-Tarres M. Circulating microparticles, lupus anticoagulant and recurrent miscarriages. Eur J Obstet Gynecol Reprod Biol. 2009 Jul;145(1):22-6
[123] López-Pedrera Ch, Buendía P, Cuadrado MJ, et al; Antiphospholipid antibodies from antiphospholipid syndrome patients induce monocyte expression through the simultaneous activation of both NFkB/Rel proteins via p38 MAPK pathway, and the MEK1/ERK pathway. Arthritis Rheum. 2006;54:301–311.
[124] Jajoria P, Murthy V, Papalardo E, Romay-Penabad Z, Gleason C, Pierangeli SS. Statins for the treatment of antiphospholipid syndrome? Ann N Y Acad Sci. 2009 Sep;1173:736-45
[125] Tesser J, et al. Safety and efficacy of the humanized anti-C5a antibody h5G1.1 in patients with rheumatoid arthritis. Arthritis Rheum 2001; 44: s274 (abstract).
[126] Wang Y, Rollins SA, Madri JA, Matis LA. Anti-C5 monoclonal antibody therapy prevents collagen-induced arthritis and ameliorates established disease. Proc Natl Acad Sci USA. 1995; 92: 8955-8959.
[127] Quigg RJ. Use of complement inhibitors in tissue injury. Trends Mol Med 2002; 8:430-436.
[128] Tofukuji M, Stahl GL, Agah A, Metais C, Simons M. Sellke FW. 1998. Anti-C5 monoclonal antibody reduces cardiopulmonary bypass and cardioplegia-induced coronary endothelial dysfunction. J Thorac. Cardiovasc Durg 116:1060-1068.
[129] Arumugam TV, Shiels IA, Strachan AJ, Abbenante G, Fairlie DP, Taylor SM. A small molecule C5a receptor antagonist protects kidneys from ischemia/reperfusion injury in rats. Kidney Int 2003; 63:134-142.
[130] Strachan AJ, Woodruff TM, Haaima G, Fairlie DP, Taylor SM. A new small molecule C5a-receptor antagonist inhibits the reverse-passive Arthus reaction and endotoxic shock in rats. J Immunol 2000; 164: 6560-6565.
[131] Patel KLH, Farrar CA, Hargreaves EG, Sacks SH, Zhou W. Complement activation regulates the capacity of proximal tubular epithelial cell to stimulate alloreactive T cell response. J Am Soc Nephrol 2004; 15:2414-2422.
[132] Finch AM, Wong AK, Paczkowski NJ. Wadi SK, Craik DJ, Fairlie DP, Taylor SM. Low molecular-weight peptidic and cyclic antagonist of the receptor for the complement factor C5a. J Med Chem 1999; 42:1965-1974.
[133] Mastellos D, Papadimitriou JC, Franchini S, Pangiotis AT, Lambris JD. A novel role of complement: mice deficient in the fifth component of complement (C5) exhibit impaired liver regeneration. J Immunol 2001; 166: 2479-2486.

[134] Carrera-Marin AL, Romay-Penabad Z, Machin S, Cohen H, Pierangeli S. C5 inhibitor rEV576 ameliorates in vivo effects of antiphospholipid antibodies. Arthritis Rheum 2011; 63(10):s5 (abstract 12)

[135] Soltys J, Kusner LL, Young A, Richmonds C, Hatala D et al. Novel complement inhibitor limits severity of experimentally myasthenia gravis. Ann Neurol. 2009 Jan;65(1):67-75.

[136] Halstead SK, Humphreys PD, Zitman FM, Hamer J, Plomp JJ, Willison HJ. C5 inhibitor rEV576 protects against neural injury in an in vitro mouse model of Miller Fisher syndrome. J Peripher Nerv Syst. 2008 Sep;13(3):228-35.

[137] De Wolf F, Carreras LO, Moerman P et al. Decidual vasculopathy and extensive placental infarction in a patient with repeated thromboembolic accidents, recurrent fetal loss, and a lupus anticoagulant. Am J Obstet Gynecol. 1982 Apr 1;142(7):829-34

[138] Hanly JG, Gladman DD, Rose TH et al. Lupus pregnancy. A prospective study of placental changes. Arthritis Rheum. 1988 Mar;31(3):358-66

[139] Nayar R, Lage JM. Placental changes in a first trimester missed abortion in maternal systemic lupus erythematosus with antiphospholipid syndrome; a case report and review of the literature. Hum Pathol. 1996 Feb;27(2):201-6

[140] Out HJ, Kooijman CD, Bruinse HW, Derksen RH. Histopathological findings in placentae from patients with intra-uterine fetal death and anti-phospholipid antibodies. Eur J Obstet Gynecol Reprod Biol. 1991 Oct 8;41(3):179-86

[141] Peaceman AM, Rehnberg KA. The effect of immunoglobulin G fractions from patients with lupus anticoagulant on placental prostacyclin and thromboxane production. Am J Obstet Gynecol. 1993 Dec;169(6):1403-6

[142] Rand JH, Wu XX, Guller S et al. Reduction of annexin-V (placental anticoagulant protein-I) on placental villi of women with antiphospholipid antibodies and recurrent spontaneous abortion. Am J Obstet Gynecol. 1994 Dec;171(6):1566-72

[143] Wang X, Campos B, Kaetzel MA, Dedman JR. Annexin V is critical in the maintenance of murine placental integrity. Am J Obstet Gynecol. 1999 Apr;180(4):1008-16

[144] Donohoe S, Kingdom JC, Mackie IJ et al. Ontogeny of beta 2 glycoprotein I and annexin V in villous placenta of normal and antiphospholipid syndrome pregnancies. Thromb Haemost. 2000 Jul;84(1):32-8

[145] McIntyre JA. Immune recognition at the maternal-fetal interface: overview. Am J Reprod Immunol. 1992 Oct-Dec;28(3-4):127-31

[146] Di Simone N, Meroni PL, de Papa N et al. Antiphospholipid antibodies affect trophoblast gonadotropin secretion and invasiveness by binding directly and through adhered beta2-glycoprotein I. Arthritis Rheum. 2000 Jan;43(1):140-50

[147] Katsuragawa H, Kanzaki H, Inoue T et al. Monoclonal antibody against phosphatidylserine inhibits in vitro human trophoblastic hormone production and invasion. Biol Reprod. 1997 Jan;56(1):50-8

[148] Adler RR, Ng AK, Rote NS. Monoclonal antiphosphatidylserine antibody inhibits intercellular fusion of the choriocarcinoma line, JAR. Biol Reprod. 1995 Oct;53(4):905-10

[149] Rote NS, Vogt E, DeVere G et al. The role of placental trophoblast in the pathophysiology of the antiphospholipid antibody syndrome. Am J Reprod Immunol. 1998 Feb;39(2):125-36

[150] Castellucci M, De Matteis R, Meisser A et al. Leptin modulates extracellular matrix molecules and metalloproteinases: possible implications for trophoblast invasion. Mol Hum Reprod. 2000 Oct;6(10):951-8

[151] Di Simone N, Castellani R, Caliandro D, Caruso A. Antiphospholid antibodies regulate the expression of trophoblast cell adhesion molecules. Fertil Steril. 2002 Apr;77(4):805-11

[152] Francis J, Rai R, Sebire NJ et al. Impaired expression of endometrial differentiation markers and complement regulatory proteins in patients with recurrent pregnancy loss associated with antiphospholipid syndrome. Mol Hum Reprod. 2006 Jul;12(7):435-42

[153] Di Simone N, Di Nicuolo F, D'Ippolito S et al. Antiphospholipid antibodies affect human endometrial angiogenesis. Biol Reprod. 2010 Aug 1;83(2):212-9

[154] Borghi MO, Raschi E, Scurati S et al. Effects of a toll-like receptor antagonist and anti-annexin A2 antibodies on binding and activation of decidual cells by anti-β2glycoprotein I antibodies. Clin Exp Rheumatol 2007. 2:35

[155] Quigg RJ, Kozono Y, Berthiaume D et al. Blockade of antibody-induced glomerulonephritis with Crry-Ig, a soluble murine complement inhibitor. J Immunol. 1998 May 1;160(9):4553-60

[156] Redecha P, Tilley R, Tencati M et al. Tissue factor: a link between C5a and neutrophil activation in antiphospholipid antibody induced fetal injury. Blood. 2007 Oct 1;110(7):2423-31

[157] Girardi G, Yarilin D, Thurman JM et al. Complement activation induces dysregulation of angiogenic factors and causes fetal rejection and growth restriction. J Exp Med. 2006 Sep 4;203(9):2165-75

[158] Ruiz-Irastora G, Hunt BJ, Khamashta MA. "A systematic review of secondary thromboprophylaxis in patients with antiphospholipid antibodies." Arthritis Rheum. 2007; 57: 1487-95

[159] Vargas-Hitos JA, Ateka-Barrutia O, Sangle S, Khamashta MA. "Efficacy and safety of long-term low molecular weight heparin in patients with antiphospholipid syndrome." Ann Rheum Dis. 2011; 70: 1652-1654.

[160] Rai R, Cohen H, Dave M, Regan L. "Randomised controlled trial of aspirin and aspirin plus heparin in pregnant women with recurrent miscarriage associated with phospholipid antibodies (or antiphospholipid antibodies)". BMJ. 1997; 314: 253-257.

[161] Alalaf S. "Bemiparin versus low dose aspirin for management of recurrent early pregnancy loss due to antiphospholipid antibody syndrome." Arch Gynecol Obstet. 2011. ePub ahead of print.

[162] Erkan D, Harrison M, Levy R, et al. Aspirin for primary thrombosis prevention in the antiphospholipid syndrome: a randomized, double-blind, placebo-controlled trial in asymptomatic antiphospholipid antibody-positive individuals. Arthritis Rheum 2007; 56: 2382–2391.

[163] Zhou H, Wolberg AS, Roubey AS. Characterization of monocyte tissue factor activity induced by IgG antiphospholipid antibodies and inhibition by dilazep. Blood 2004; 15: 2353-2358

[164] Ostertag MV, Liu X, Henderson V, Pierangeli SS. A peptide that mimics the Vth region of beta-2-glycoprotein I reverses antiphospholipid-mediated thrombosis in mice. Lupus 2006;15:358-65.

[165] Blank M, Shoenfeld Y, Cabilly S, Heldman Y, Fridkin M, Katchalski-Katzir E. of experimental antiphospholipid syndrome and endothelial cell activation by synthetic peptides. Proc Natl Acad Sci U S A 1999;96:5164-8.

[166] Pierangeli SS, Blank M, Liu X, et al. A peptide that shares similarity with bacterial antigens reverses thrombogenic properties of antiphospholipid antibodies in vivo. J Autoimmun 2004;22:217-25.

[167] Carrera-Marin AL, Romay-Penabad Z, Qu HC, et al. A C5a receptor antagonist amerliorates in vivo effects of antiphospholipid antibodies. Arthritis Rheum 2009; 60; s767 (abstract).

[168] Halcox JPJ, Deanfield JE. Beyond the laboratory. Clinical implications for statin pleitropy. Circulation 2004; 109 (suppl II); 42-48

[169] Colli S, Eligini S, Lalli M, et al. Statins inhibit tissue factor in cultured human macrophages. A novel mechanism of protection against atherothrombosis. Arterioscler Thromb Vasc Biol 1997; 17: 265-272.

[170] Aikawa M, Rabkin E, Sugiyama S, et al. An HMG-CoA inhbitor, cerivastatin, suppresses growth of macrophages expressing matrix metalloproteinases and tissue factor in vivo and in vitro, Circulation 2001; 103:276-283.

[171] Baetta R, Camera M, Comparato C, et al. Tremoli E. Fluvastatin reduces tissue factor expression and macrophage accumulation in carotid lesions of cholesterol-fed rabbits in absence of lipid lowering. Arterioscler Thromb Vasc Biol 2002; 22:692-698.

[172] Ridker PM, Danielson E, Fonseca FA, et al: JUPITER Trial Study Group. Reduction in C-reactive protein and LDL cholesterol and cardiovascular event rates after initiation of rosuvastatin: a prospective study of the JUPITER trial. Lancet 2009; 373: 1175-1182.

[173] Meroni PL, Raschi E, Testoni C, et al. Statins prevent endothelial cell activation induced by antiphospholipid (anti-□$_2$glycoprotein I) antibodies: effect on the proadhesive and proinflammatory phenotype. Arthritis Rheum 2001: 44:2870-2878.

[174] Ferrara DE, Swerlick R, Casper K, et al. Fluvastatin inhibits upregulation of tissue factor expression by antiphospholipid antibodies on endothelial cells. J Thromb Haemost 2004; 2: 1558-1563.

[175] Martinez-Martinez LA, Amigo MC, Orozco A, et al. Effect of rosuvastatin on VCAM-1 expression by HIVEC exposed to APS serum in an in vitro model. Clin Exp Rheumatol 2007; 25:18-19.

[176] Murthy V, Erkan D, Jajoria P, Willis R, Vega J, Barilaro B, Basra G, Hsu E, Martinez-Martinez LA, Jatwani S, Papalardo E, Gonzalez EB, Sunkureddi PR, Pierangeli S. Effects of Fluvastatin on Pro-Inflammatory and Pro-Thrombotic Markers in Antiphospholipid Antibody (aPL)-Positive Patients: Preliminary Results from an Open-Label Prospective Pilot Study. Arthritis Rheum 2011; 63(10):s283 (abstract 726)

[177] Cuadrado MJ, Lopez-Pedrera C, Aguirre A, et al. Changes Operated in Protein Pattern of Monocytes from Patients with Antiphospholipid Syndrome Treated with Statins. Arthritis Rheum 2007; 56: S782 (abstract)

[178] Lombard-Platlet S, Bertolino P, Deng H, Gerlier D, Rabourdin-Combe C. Inhibition by chloroquine of the class II major histocompatibility complex-restricted presentation of endogenous antigens varies according to the cellular origin of the antigen-presenting cells, the nature of the T-cell epitope, and the responding T cell. Immunology 1993; 80: 566–573.

[179] Goldman FD, Gilman AL, Hollenback C, et al. Hydroxychloroquine inhibits calcium signals in T cells: a new mechanism to explain its immunomodulatory properties. Blood 2000; 95: 3460–3466.

[180] Jancinova V, Nosal R, Petrikova M. On the inhibitory effect of chloroquine on blood platelet aggregation. Thromb Res 1994; 74: 495–504.

[181] Johnson R, Charnley J. Hydroxychloroquine in prophylaxis of pulmonary embolism following hip arthroplasty. Clin Orthop Relat Res 1979; 144: 174–177.

[182] Erkan D, Yazici Y, Peterson MG et al. A cross-sectional study of clinical thrombotic risk factors and preventive treatments in antiphospholipid syndrome. Rheumatology (Oxford) 2002; 41:9249-929.

[183] Ho KT, Ahn CW, Alarcon GS, et al. Systemic lupus erythematosus in a multiethnic cohort (LUMINA): XXVIII. Factors predictive of thrombotic events. Rheumatology (Oxford) 2005; 44:1303-1307.

[184] Tektonidou MG, Laskari K, Panagiotakis DB, Moutsopoulos HM. Risk factors for thrombosis and primary thrombosis prevention in patients with systemic lupus erythematosus with or without antiphospholipid antibodies. Arthritis Rheum 2009; 61:29-35.

[185] Rand JH. Wu XX, Quinn AS, et al. Hydroxychloroquine directly reduces the binding of antiphospholipid antibody-beta2-glycoprotein I complexes to phospholipid bilayers. Blood 2008; 112: 1687–1695.

[186] Rand JH. Wu XX, Quinn AS, et al. Hydroxychloroquine protects the annexin A5 anticoagulant shield from disruption by antiphospholipid antibodies: evidence for a novel effect for an old antimalarial drug. Blood. 2009 Nov 30. [Epub ahead of print]

[187] Petri M. Lupus in Baltimore: evidence-based 'clinical pearls' from the Hopkins Lupus Cohort Lupus 2005; 14: 970-973.

[188] Kaiser R, Cleveland CM, Criswell LA. Risk and protective factors for thrombosis in systemic lupus erythematosus: results from a large, multi-ethnic cohort. Ann Rheum Dis Ann Rheum Dis 2009; 68: 238-241.

[189] Ruiz-Irastorza G. Egurbide MV, Pijoan JL, et al. Effect of antimalarials on thrombosis and survival in patients with systemic lupus erythematosus. Lupus 2006; 15: 577–583.

[190] Rubenstein E, Arkfeld DG, Metyas S, et al. Rituximab treatment for resistant antiphospholipid syndrome. J Rheumatol 2006; 33: 355–357.

[191] Tenedious F, Erkan D, Lockshin MD. Rituximab in the primary antiphospholipid antibody syndrome. Arthritis Rheum 2005; 52: 4078 (abstract).

[192] Erdozain JG, Ruiz-Irastorza G, Egurbide MV, et al. Sustained response to rituximab of autoimmune hemolytic anemia associated with antiphospholipid syndrome. Haematologica 2004;89:ECR34 [abstract].

[193] Erre GL, Pardini S, Faedda R, et al. Effect of rituximab on clinical and laboratory features of antiphospholipid syndrome: a case report and a review of literature. Lupus 2008; 17: 50–55.

[194] Erkan D, Vega J, Ramon G, Kozora E, Lockshin MD. Rituximab in Antiphospholipid Syndrome (RITAPS)—A Pilot Open-Label Phase II Prospective Trial for Non-Criteria Manifestations of Antiphospholipid Antibodies (aPL). Arthritis Rheum 2011; 63(10):s283 (abstract 727)